THE BOOK OF LIFE – NATURAL HEALING

D - N

VOL 2

By

Niddia Alexander

This book is a work of non-fiction. The information contained herein is intended for educational purposes only and is not a substitute for professional medical advice, diagnosis, or treatment. Always consult with a qualified healthcare provider before making any changes to your diet, health routines, or lifestyle.

ISBN (Paperback): 979-8-9997306-7-1

Published by: ***Book of Life – Natural Healing***

Library of Congress Control Number: 20252921175

Cover Design: Niddia Alexander

Interior Layout and Design: Niddia Alexander

Printed in the United States of America

First Edition VOL 2

For more information or to contact the author, please visit: https://authorniddiaalexander.com/

"So do not fear, for I am with you; do not be dismayed, for I am your God. I will strengthen you and help you; I will uphold you with my righteous right hand."

Isaiah 41:10

This verse is often cited as a source of comfort and encouragement, reminding believers that God is present with them, offering strength, help, and support, especially during times of fear or distress. It emphasizes the idea of trust and reliance on God's protection and guidance.

DEDICATION

This book is dedicated to two extraordinary forces in my life, whose unwavering support and guidance have been instrumental in bringing this work to fruition.

To God, the source of all wisdom and inspiration, I offer my deepest gratitude for choosing me for this sacred assignment. Your divine guidance has illuminated my path and filled my heart with purpose and conviction. May this book serve as a testament to Your grace and infinite wisdom, and may it be a source of hope, healing, and transformation for all who encounter its pages.

To my dear mother, whose love, encouragement, and unwavering support have been my constant source of strength throughout this journey. Your belief in me has been a beacon of light, guiding me through the challenges and triumphs of writing this book. Your dedication and sacrifice inspire me every day, and I am eternally grateful for your presence in my life.

With love and gratitude,

Niddia Alexander

ACKNOWLEDGMENT

I would like to take this opportunity to express my heartfelt gratitude to the Almighty God for His divine guidance and inspiration throughout the journey of writing this book, “The Book of Life – Natural Healing” or "Natural Ways to a Healthy Life." It is with humility and reverence that I acknowledge His profound wisdom and grace, which have illuminated my path and empowered me to undertake this endeavor.

God's assignment and vision for this book have been a beacon of light, guiding my thoughts, words, and actions as I sought to impart knowledge and insights into the pursuit of a healthy and fulfilling life. His unwavering presence has provided me with strength, courage, and clarity, enabling me to navigate the complexities of health and wellness with diligence and compassion.

I am deeply grateful for the opportunity to serve as a vessel for His message of hope, healing, and transformation. May His divine blessings continue to flow abundantly, touching the hearts and minds of all who engage with this work, and may it inspire positive change and empower individuals to embrace a lifestyle that nurtures both body and soul.

In closing, I offer my sincerest thanks to God for entrusting me with this sacred task and for blessing me with the resources, opportunities, and support needed to bring this vision to fruition. May His infinite love and grace guide us all on the path to wholeness and vitality.

With profound gratitude and humility,

Niddia Alexander

TABLE OF CONTENTS

DEDICATION i
ACKNOWLEDGMENT ii
AUTHOR'S NOTE 2
INTRODUCTION 4
Dandelion 5
Dates 11
Dill 17
Dulse 24
Echinacea 30
Eggplant 37
Endive 45
Fennel 52
Figs 60
Flax Seed 68
Fonio 74
Galangal 80
Garlic 85
Ginger 92
Ginkgo 100
Ginseng 105
Grapefruit 111
Grapes 117
Green Beans 124
Green Peas 132
Guava 139
Hazelnuts 145
Hemp Seed 152
Hijiki 158
Honey 165
Honeydew 171

Horseradish ... 177
Hyssop ... 183
Irish Moss / Sea Moss ... 189
Kale ... 196
Kelp (Kombu) ... 203
Kidney Beans ... 213
Kiwi ... 219
Lavender ... 224
Leaf of Life ... 229
Leeks ... 237
Lemon ... 243
Lemongrass / Fever Grass ... 249
Lentils ... 255
Lettuce ... 261
Licorice ... 266
Lima Beans / Butter Beans ... 274
Lime ... 281
L-Theanine ... 286
Mango ... 289
Millet ... 295
Mulberries ... 302
Mullein ... 307
Mushrooms ... 312
Mustard Greens ... 321
Naseberry ... 330
Nettle ... 336
Nori ... 344
Nutmeg ... 351
Essential Nutrients for Optimal Health ... 356
- What is Carbohydrate? ... 358
- What is Protein? ... 361
- Fats (Healthy Fats) ... 364

What is Vitamin A? 367
Vitamin B1 (Thiamine) 370
Vitamin B2 (Riboflavin) 373
Vitamin B3 (Niacin) 376
Vitamin B5 (Pantothenic Acid): 379
Vitamin B6 (Pyridoxine): 382
Vitamin B7 *(Biotin)* 385
Vitamin B9 (Folate or Folic Acid): 387
Vitamin B12 (Cobalamin) 389
Other Foods High in Vitamin B12 (Cobalamin) 391
Vitamin C (Ascorbic Acid) 393
Vitamin D 397
Natural Foods High in Vitamin D 398
Vitamin E (Tocopherol) 400
Vitamin K 403
Essential Minerals 406
Calcium 409
Magnesium 412
Phosphorus 415
Sodium 418
Potassium 421
Chloride 424
Iron 426
Zinc 429
Copper 433
Selenium 436
Iodine 439
Manganese 441
Fluoride 444
Chromium 447
Molybdenum 450
Choline 453

Water 456
Fiber 458
Phytonutrients........ 460
Omega-3 Fatty Acids 462
Antioxidant -Essential Compounds........ 464
Free Radicals 466
Plant-Based Foods Beneficial for Diabetes........ 467
Oxidative Stress........ 469
Cardiovascular Disease (CVD)........ 470
Unhealthy Diet 478
Plant-Based Foods Beneficial for Cancer Prevention and Support 480
Plant-Based Foods Beneficial for Chronic Obstructive Pulmonary Disease (COPD) 482
Plant-Based Foods Beneficial for Cold and Flu 484
Plant-Based Foods Beneficial for Diabetes 486
Plant-Based Foods Beneficial for Heart Disease 488
Plant-Based Foods Beneficial for Hypertension (High Blood Pressure)........ 490
Plant-Based Foods Beneficial for Kidney Disease 492
Plant-Based Foods Beneficial for Mental Health 494
Plant-Based Foods Beneficial for Osteoarthritis........ 496
Plant-Based Foods Beneficial for Osteoporosis 498
Plant-Based Foods Beneficial for Respiratory Infectious Disease 500
Nutrients Daily Recommendations 502
Nutrient-Rich Foods that Grows in less than 100 Days........ 504
Conclusion 520

"Jesus looked at them and said, 'With man this is impossible, but with God all things are possible.'"

Matthew 19:26

This verse comes from a passage in which Jesus is speaking to his disciples about the difficulty of the rich entering the kingdom of heaven. It emphasizes the power and sovereignty of God, highlighting that what may seem impossible to humans is achievable through God's intervention and grace. It serves as a reminder of the limitless possibilities and the importance of faith in God's ability to accomplish what seems impossible from a human perspective.

AUTHOR'S NOTE

My name is Niddia Alexander, and I am honored to welcome you to the pages of this book. Before delving into the heart of its content, I feel compelled to introduce myself and shed light on the inspiration behind this transformative work on plant-based foods for natural healing.

As a mother of four beautiful children, I cherish every moment spent nurturing and motivating them to embrace the best versions of themselves. Alongside my role as a parent, I find solace in the simple joys of life – whether it's immersing myself in the wisdom of motivational speakers, indulging in the beauty of nature, or seeking refuge in the tranquil embrace of the beach.

While my passions may span from trading in the forex market to envisioning investment properties, one consistent thread defines my journey – a steadfast belief in the natural way of life. Whenever faced with ailments or discomforts, I instinctively turn to wholesome foods to restore balance and vitality to my body. For me, nourishing foods brimming with nutritional benefits have always been a cornerstone of well-being.

It was amidst this backdrop of reverence for nature and holistic living that I experienced a profound series of dreams and visions. Guided by the whispers of the Holy Spirit, I was entrusted with a divine assignment – to pen a book that would illuminate the path to health and wellness through plant-based nutrition. With unwavering faith and obedience, I embarked on this daunting task, surrendering myself to the guidance of a higher power.

Though initially daunted by the magnitude of the task before me, I found solace in the assurance that if God had called me to this mission, He would undoubtedly see me through it. Each morning, I approached my assignment with reverence, seeking divine guidance through prayer and worship. Along the way, I gleaned invaluable lessons and experienced the profound joy of being a conduit for a greater purpose.

As the words flowed onto the page, I realized that I was merely a vessel, channeling the wisdom and grace bestowed upon me by my Heavenly Father. All praise and gratitude belong to Him, for without His guidance, this book would not have come to fruition. It is my sincere prayer that the insights shared within these pages will empower you on your journey towards optimal health and wellness.

"Be strong and courageous. Do not be afraid or terrified because of them, for the Lord your God goes with you; he will never leave you nor forsake you."

Deuteronomy 31:6

This verse is part of Moses' final words to the Israelites before they enter the Promised Land. It serves as a source of encouragement and reassurance, reminding the Israelites to trust in God's presence and protection as they face challenges and uncertainties. It emphasizes the importance of courage and faith, knowing that God will always be with them, never abandoning them, no matter what difficulties they encounter.

INTRODUCTION

In an era marked by the hustle and bustle of modern life, the pursuit of a healthy lifestyle has become an increasingly paramount endeavor for individuals seeking vitality, longevity, and overall well-being. Amidst the myriad of trends, diets, and fads, one timeless truth stands unwavering: the profound impact of nature's bounty on our health and vitality.

In this book, titled "The Book of Life: Natural Healing," we embark on a journey to explore the transformative power of plant-based foods in nurturing a life of vitality and wellness. Rooted in ancient wisdom and modern science, this comprehensive guide offers a holistic approach to achieving optimal health through the consumption of nutrient-rich, plant-derived foods.

Drawing upon the latest research and centuries-old practices, "The Book of Life – Natural Healing" delves into the myriad benefits of embracing a plant-based lifestyle, from enhanced physical health to heightened mental clarity and spiritual well-being. Through a wealth of information, delicious recipes, and evidence-based insights, readers will discover the abundant riches that nature provides for nourishing body, mind, and soul.

This book is not just a guide to healthy eating; it is a celebration of the inherent connection between humanity and our God given natural world. It invites readers to rekindle their relationship with the earth, embracing the abundance of fruits, vegetables, grains, nuts, seeds, and legumes that sustain and nourish us at the deepest levels.

As we journey together through the pages of "The Book of Life – Natural Healing," let us awaken to the profound wisdom that lies within the embrace of plant-based wellness. May this book serve as a beacon of inspiration and empowerment, guiding us towards a life of radiant health, vitality, and harmony with the natural world.

Welcome to the transformative journey of "The Book of Life – Natural Healing: Embracing Plant-Based Wellness."

Warm regards,

Niddia Alexander

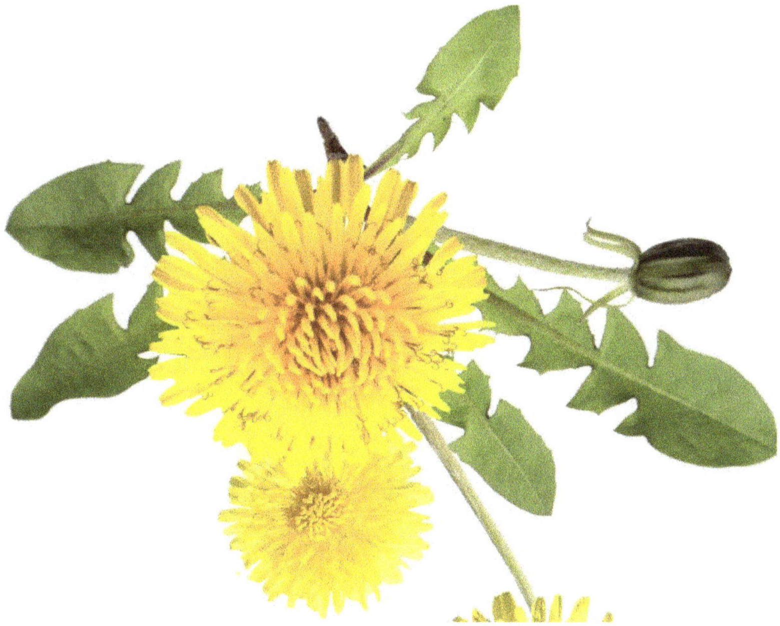

Dandelion

Health Wonders of Dandelion: Benefits and Versatile Uses of Dandelion Leaves

Dandelion, often dismissed as a pesky weed, is a treasure trove of health benefits, with its vibrant yellow blooms and luscious green leaves holding remarkable medicinal properties. Beyond its reputation as a lawn intruder, dandelion leaves are gaining recognition for their potential to promote well-being. Let's delve into the diverse benefits and versatile uses of dandelion leaves, unlocking the secrets of this humble herb.

Nutritional Powerhouse:

Dandelion leaves are a nutritional powerhouse, packed with essential vitamins and minerals. Rich in vitamin A, C, and K, dandelion leaves contribute to immune support, skin health, and blood clotting. They are also a good source of calcium, iron, and potassium, vital for bone health, oxygen transport, and electrolyte balance.

Vitamins:

Vitamin A: Important for vision health, immune function, and skin health. It supports the growth and repair of tissues and helps maintain healthy skin and mucous membranes.

Vitamin C: Acts as an antioxidant to protect cells from damage, boosts the immune system, and promotes collagen synthesis for healthy skin and connective tissues.

Vitamin K: Essential for blood clotting and bone health. It helps regulate calcium levels in the blood and supports bone mineralization.

Vitamin E: Provides antioxidant properties that protect cells from oxidative stress and supports immune function. It also promotes skin health and may reduce the risk of chronic diseases.

Minerals:

Calcium: Important for bone health, muscle function, and nerve transmission. It also plays a role in blood clotting and hormone secretion.

Potassium: Helps regulate blood pressure, fluid balance, and muscle contractions. It supports heart health and may reduce the risk of stroke and kidney stones.

Iron: Necessary for the formation of hemoglobin, which carries oxygen in the blood. It helps prevent iron deficiency anemia and supports energy metabolism.

Magnesium: Supports muscle and nerve function, regulates blood sugar levels, and contributes to bone health. It also plays a role in energy metabolism and protein synthesis.

Antioxidants:

Flavonoids: Have antioxidant properties that protect cells from oxidative damage and inflammation. They may reduce the risk of chronic diseases such as heart disease and cancer.

Beta-carotene: Converts to vitamin A in the body and acts as an antioxidant. It supports eye health, immune function, and skin health.

Lutein and zeaxanthin: Carotenoids that accumulate in the retina and may reduce the risk of age-related macular degeneration. They support eye health and vision.

Chlorogenic acid: Has antioxidant and anti-inflammatory properties. It may help lower blood pressure, reduce blood sugar levels, and protect against chronic diseases.

Liver Detoxification:

One of the standout benefits of dandelion leaves is their ability to support liver health. Traditionally used in herbal medicine, dandelion is believed to stimulate liver function and promote the detoxification of harmful substances. The diuretic properties of dandelion leaves may aid in flushing out toxins, contributing to overall liver well-being.

Anti-Inflammatory and Antioxidant Properties:

Dandelion leaves boast anti-inflammatory and antioxidant properties attributed to compounds like beta-carotene and polyphenols. These properties make dandelion a potential ally in reducing inflammation in the body and protecting cells from oxidative stress. As a result, incorporating dandelion leaves into your diet may contribute to managing chronic inflammatory conditions.

Digestive Aid and Weight Management:

The mild diuretic nature of dandelion leaves, coupled with their fiber content, can support healthy digestion. Dandelion has been traditionally used to alleviate digestive issues, such as bloating and constipation. The fiber promotes a feeling of fullness, making it a valuable addition to a weight management plan by reducing overall calorie intake.

Medicinal Herb in Traditional Medicine:

- **Historical Use:** Dandelion leaves have a rich history as a medicinal herb in traditional medicine systems, particularly in Europe and Asia. Ancient cultures utilized dandelion leaves for their diuretic properties, employing them to promote kidney health and urinary tract function. The leaves were also recognized for their potential to alleviate digestive issues, such as indigestion and bloating.

Liver Tonic:

- **Historical Use:** In traditional herbal medicine, dandelion leaves were commonly used as a liver tonic. The belief in their ability to stimulate liver function and promote detoxification led to their inclusion in remedies for liver ailments. The diuretic nature of dandelion leaves was thought to assist in flushing out toxins from the liver, contributing to overall liver health.

Culinary Ingredient in Ancient Greece and Rome:

- **Historical Use:** Dandelion leaves were a prized culinary ingredient in ancient Greek and Roman cultures. They were consumed in salads for their unique flavor and believed digestive benefits. The bitter and peppery taste of dandelion leaves added depth to various dishes, and they were appreciated not only for their culinary appeal but also for their potential health-promoting properties.

Native American Medicinal Uses:

- **Historical Use:** Native American tribes utilized dandelion leaves for various medicinal purposes. The leaves were often brewed into teas or infusions to address issues such as water retention, digestive discomfort, and as a general tonic. Dandelion leaves were valued for their versatility and considered a part of the herbal pharmacopoeia for promoting overall well-being.

These historical uses of dandelion leaves highlight their longstanding reputation as a valuable herb with diverse benefits. From traditional medicine to culinary applications, dandelion leaves have played a significant role in various cultures throughout history, earning recognition for their potential contributions to health and wellness.

Nutritional Content

The nutritional content of 1 cup (about 55 grams) of raw dandelion greens is approximately as follows:

- **Carbohydrates:** 5.1 grams
- **Fiber:** 1.9 grams
- **Protein:** 1.5 grams
- **Fat:** 0.4 grams

Please note that these values are approximate and can vary slightly based on factors such as the specific variety of dandelion greens and how they are prepared. Dandelion greens are low in calories and carbohydrates but are a good source of fiber, vitamins, and minerals, making them a nutritious addition to your diet.

Versatile Culinary Uses:

Dandelion leaves are not just limited to medicinal use; they can also be a flavorful addition to your culinary repertoire. Here are some creative culinary uses:

Salads: Add fresh dandelion leaves to salads for a peppery and slightly bitter flavor, enhancing the nutritional profile of your meal.

Smoothies: Blend dandelion leaves into smoothies for a nutrient-packed, green boost that adds a unique twist to your beverage.

Tea: Brew dandelion leaf tea for a caffeine-free alternative with potential digestive benefits and a mild, earthy taste.

Sauteed Greens: Sauté dandelion leaves with garlic and olive oil for a delicious side dish that complements various main courses.

Here are two recipes featuring dandelion:

Dandelion Salad with Honey Mustard Dressing:

Ingredients:

- 4 cups fresh dandelion greens, washed and chopped
- 1/2 cup cherry tomatoes, halved

- 1/4 cup sliced red onion
- 1/4 cup crumbled feta cheese (optional)
- 1/4 cup chopped walnuts or almonds
- Salt and pepper to taste

Honey Mustard Dressing:

- 2 tablespoons olive oil
- 1 tablespoon apple cider vinegar
- 1 tablespoon honey
- 1 teaspoon Dijon mustard
- Salt and pepper to taste

Instructions:

1. In a large bowl, combine the dandelion greens, cherry tomatoes, red onion, feta cheese (if using), and chopped nuts.
2. In a separate small bowl, whisk together the olive oil, apple cider vinegar, honey, Dijon mustard, salt, and pepper to make the dressing.
3. Pour the dressing over the salad and toss until well coated.
4. Serve immediately as a refreshing and nutritious salad.

Dandelion Flower Fritters:

Ingredients:

1. 1 cup dandelion flowers, washed and dried
2. 1/2 cup all-purpose flour
3. 1/2 cup cornmeal
4. 1 teaspoon baking powder
5. 1/2 teaspoon salt
6. 1/2 cup milk (or plant-based milk)
7. 1 egg

8. Vegetable oil for frying

Instructions:

1. In a medium bowl, whisk together the flour, cornmeal, baking powder, and salt.
2. In another bowl, whisk together the milk and egg until well combined.
3. Gradually add the wet ingredients to the dry ingredients, stirring until a smooth batter forms.
4. Heat vegetable oil in a skillet over medium heat.
5. Dip each dandelion flower into the batter, coating it evenly.
6. Carefully place the battered flowers into the hot oil and fry until golden brown and crispy, about 2-3 minutes per side.
7. Use a slotted spoon to remove the fritters from the oil and place them on a paper towel-lined plate to drain excess oil.
8. Serve the dandelion flower fritters warm as a tasty appetizer or snack. Optional: Serve with a dipping sauce of your choice, such as ranch dressing or marinara sauce.

These recipes showcase the versatility of dandelion and how it can be incorporated into delicious dishes. Enjoy experimenting with these nutritious and flavorful recipes!

Conclusion:

Dandelion leaves, once dismissed as a garden nuisance, emerge as a potent source of health benefits and culinary inspiration. From liver support to anti-inflammatory properties, this versatile herb has much to offer. Whether consumed in salads, smoothies, or as a soothing tea, dandelion leaves present a delicious and nutritious addition to your wellness journey. Embrace the beauty and benefits of dandelion and discover the myriad ways it can contribute to a healthier and more vibrant life.

If you have specific health concerns, allergies, or conditions, it's advisable to consult with a healthcare professional or a registered dietitian before making significant changes to your diet.

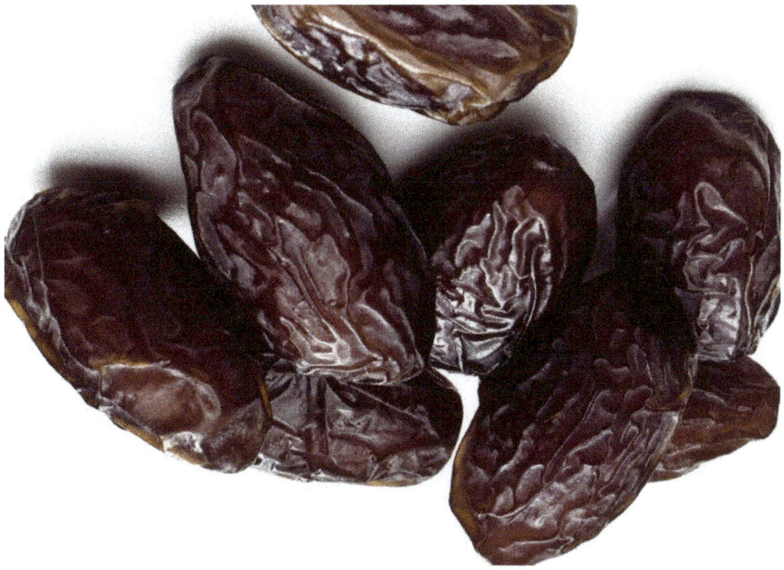

Dates

Exploring the Benefits and Uses of Dates

Dates, the succulent fruit derived from the date palm tree, have been a staple in human diets for thousands of years. Packed with natural sweetness and a plethora of health benefits, dates have earned their place not only as a delicious snack but also as a versatile ingredient in various culinary traditions around the world.

Nutritional Powerhouse:

One of the key reasons dates have maintained their popularity is their impressive nutritional profile. Rich in essential vitamins and minerals, dates provide a quick and convenient energy boost. They are an excellent source of natural sugars, including glucose, fructose, and sucrose, making them an ideal choice for a quick pick-me-up during a busy day.

Vitamins and Minerals:

Vitamin B6 (Pyridoxine):

- **Benefits:** Important for brain development and function, helps the body convert food into energy, supports the nervous and immune systems.

Folate (Vitamin B9):

- **Benefits:** Essential for DNA synthesis and repair, aids in red blood cell formation, supports fetal development during pregnancy.

Vitamin K:

- **Benefits:** Vital for blood clotting and bone health, helps regulate calcium in the blood.

Vitamin A:

- **Benefits:** Supports vision health, immune function, and skin health, acts as an antioxidant.

Vitamin C:

- **Benefits:** Boosts the immune system, aids in collagen production for skin health, acts as an antioxidant.

Vitamin E:

- **Benefits:** Acts as an antioxidant, supports skin health, protects cells from damage.

Niacin (Vitamin B3):

- **Benefits:** Essential for energy production, supports the nervous system, contributes to skin health.

Riboflavin (Vitamin B2):

- **Benefits:** Important for energy production, supports normal vision and skin health.

Thiamine (Vitamin B1):

- **Benefits:** Essential for energy metabolism, supports nerve function.

Pantothenic Acid (Vitamin B5):

- **Benefits:** Important for energy production, helps synthesize fatty acids and hormones.

Calcium:

- **Benefits:** Essential for bone and teeth health, supports muscle function, plays a role in blood clotting.

Iron:

- **Benefits:** Critical for the formation of hemoglobin and oxygen transport in the blood, supports energy metabolism.

Magnesium:

- **Benefits:** Important for muscle and nerve function, supports bone health, regulates blood sugar levels.

Phosphorus:

- **Benefits:** Essential for bone and teeth health, involved in energy metabolism.

Potassium:

- **Benefits:** Helps regulate blood pressure, supports heart and muscle function, aids in fluid balance.

Zinc:

- **Benefits:** Supports immune function, plays a role in wound healing, involved in DNA synthesis.

Copper:

- **Benefits:** Important for iron absorption, supports the formation of red blood cells.

Manganese:

- **Benefits:** Contributes to bone formation, supports metabolism, acts as an antioxidant.

Fiber Content:

Dates are also a significant source of dietary fiber, which plays a crucial role in promoting digestive health. Fiber aids in preventing constipation and promoting regular bowel movements. Additionally, the fiber content helps to maintain a feeling of fullness, making dates a satisfying and healthy snack option.

Rich in Antioxidants:

Dates are abundant in antioxidants, including flavonoids, carotenoids, and phenolic acid. These compounds help neutralize harmful free radicals in the body, protecting cells from oxidative stress. Regular consumption of dates may contribute to reducing the risk of chronic diseases and supporting overall well-being.

Energy Boost:

The natural sugars present in dates, primarily glucose, fructose, and sucrose, provide a quick and sustained energy boost. This makes dates an excellent choice for athletes and those looking for a natural source of energy before or after physical activities. The combination of carbohydrates and essential nutrients makes dates an efficient and healthy energy snack.

Heart Health:

Dates have been associated with heart health benefits. Studies suggest that regular consumption of dates may contribute to lowering levels of LDL (bad) cholesterol while increasing HDL (good) cholesterol. Additionally, the potassium content in dates supports heart health by helping regulate blood pressure.

Nutritional Content
The nutritional content of 1 cup of dates (approximately 147 grams) typically includes:

- Calories: Approximately 415 kcal
- Carbohydrates: Around 110 grams
- Protein: Roughly 3 grams
- Fiber: About 12 grams
- Fat: Less than 1 gram
- Sugar: Around 93 grams

Please note that these values are approximate and can vary slightly depending on factors such as variety and ripeness of the dates.

Versatile Culinary Uses:

Dates are not only a nutritious snack but also a versatile ingredient in cooking and baking. They can be used in both sweet and savory dishes, adding a natural sweetness and chewy texture. Dates can be blended into smoothies, chopped and added to salads, or used to sweeten desserts and snacks. They are also a popular ingredient in energy bars and balls, providing a natural alternative to processed sugars.

Here are two delicious recipes that feature dates as a key ingredient:

Date and Nut Energy Balls:

Ingredients:

- 1 cup pitted dates
- 1 cup mixed nuts (almonds, walnuts, cashews)
- 1/2 cup rolled oats
- 2 tablespoons chia seeds
- 1/4 cup honey or maple syrup
- 1 teaspoon vanilla extract
- A pinch of salt
- Desiccated coconut for rolling (optional)

Instructions:

1. In a food processor, combine pitted dates, mixed nuts, rolled oats, chia seeds, honey or maple syrup, vanilla extract, and a pinch of salt.
2. Pulse the ingredients until a sticky dough forms.

3. Scoop out small portions and roll them into bite-sized balls.
4. Optional: Roll the energy balls in desiccated coconut for an extra layer of flavor.
5. Refrigerate the energy balls for at least 30 minutes to firm up.
6. Enjoy these nutritious and energy-boosting date and nut energy balls as a snack or a quick on-the-go treat!

Stuffed Medjool Dates with Goat Cheese and Pistachios:

Ingredients:

- Medjool dates, pitted
- Goat cheese
- Pistachios, shelled and chopped
- Honey, for drizzling (optional)

Instructions:

1. Preheat the oven to 350°F (180°C).
2. Carefully slit the dates lengthwise and remove the pits.
3. Fill each date with a small amount of goat cheese and top with chopped pistachios.
4. Place the stuffed dates on a baking sheet and bake for 5-7 minutes or until the cheese is slightly melted and the dates are warmed.
5. Remove from the oven and let them cool for a few minutes.
6. Optional: Drizzle honey over the stuffed dates for added sweetness.
7. Serve these stuffed Medjool dates as a delightful appetizer or a unique dessert at your next gathering.

These recipes showcase the versatility of dates, whether used in wholesome energy balls or paired with savory goat cheese and pistachios for a delightful appetizer. Enjoy experimenting with these delicious date-based creations!

Natural Sweetener:

The high natural sugar content in dates makes them an excellent alternative to refined sugars in cooking and baking. Date paste or pureed dates can be used as a sweetener in various recipes, offering a healthier option without sacrificing flavor.

Conclusion:

Dates stand out not only for their delicious taste but also for their numerous health benefits. Packed with essential nutrients, fiber, and antioxidants, dates support digestive health, provide a natural energy boost, and contribute to overall well-being. If you have specific health concerns, allergies, or conditions, it's advisable to consult with a healthcare professional or a registered dietitian before making significant changes to your diet.

Whether enjoyed as a snack on their own, blended into smoothies, or incorporated into a variety of recipes, dates are a versatile and nutritious addition to a balanced diet. Embracing the benefits of dates can be a flavorful and health-conscious choice for individuals seeking a naturally sweet and nutrient-dense food option.

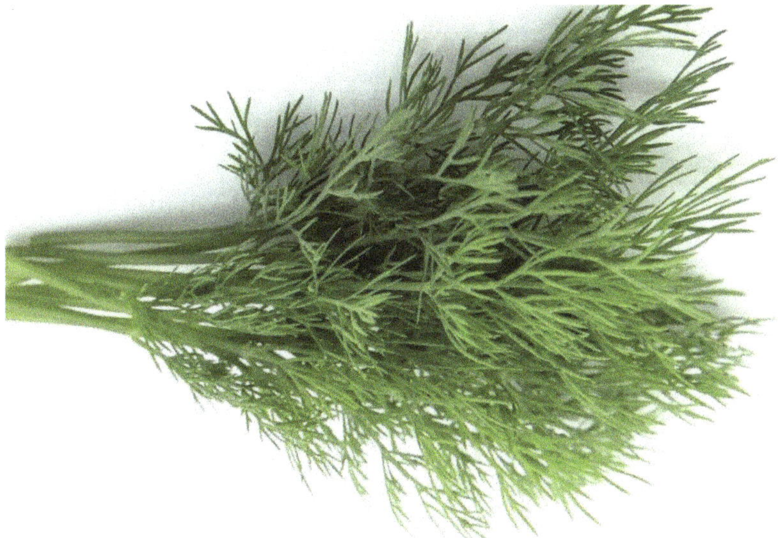

Dill

A Versatile Herb with Remarkable Benefits and Uses

Dill, scientifically known as Anethum graveolens, is an aromatic herb that has been cherished for its culinary and medicinal properties for centuries. Belonging to the same family as parsley, celery, and carrots, dill is native to the Mediterranean region but is now cultivated worldwide. With its delicate feathery leaves and distinctive flavor profile, dill adds a unique touch to various dishes, while also offering a range of health benefits.

Dill is a nutrient-rich herb that contains a variety of vitamins, minerals, and antioxidants, each offering unique health benefits. Here's a list of the key nutrients found in dill and their potential health benefits:

Vitamins:

Vitamin A: Important for vision health, immune function, and skin health. It also plays a role in cell growth and differentiation.

Vitamin C: A powerful antioxidant that boosts the immune system, promotes healthy skin, and aids in wound healing. It also helps the body absorb iron from plant-based foods.

Vitamin K: Essential for blood clotting and bone health. Vitamin K also supports heart health and may help reduce the risk of osteoporosis.

Folate (Vitamin B9): Vital for cell division and DNA synthesis. Folate is especially important during pregnancy for fetal development and helps prevent neural tube defects.

Niacin (Vitamin B3): Supports energy metabolism and helps maintain healthy skin, nerves, and digestion.

Riboflavin (Vitamin B2): Necessary for energy production, metabolism of fats, proteins, and carbohydrates, and maintaining healthy skin and eyes.

Pyridoxine (Vitamin B6): Involved in more than 100 enzyme reactions in the body, including protein metabolism, neurotransmitter synthesis, and immune function.

Minerals:

Calcium: Essential for bone health, muscle function, and nerve transmission. Calcium also plays a role in blood clotting and hormone secretion.

Iron: Important for transporting oxygen in the blood and maintaining energy levels. Iron deficiency can lead to anemia.

Magnesium: Supports muscle and nerve function, regulates blood sugar levels, and is involved in over 300 biochemical reactions in the body.

Potassium: Helps regulate blood pressure, muscle contractions, and fluid balance. Potassium also supports heart health and kidney function.

Manganese: Necessary for bone formation, collagen production, and antioxidant defense. Manganese also plays a role in metabolism and wound healing.

Phosphorus: Vital for bone and teeth health, energy metabolism, and DNA synthesis. Phosphorus also helps maintain acid-base balance in the body.

Zinc: Essential for immune function, wound healing, and DNA synthesis. Zinc also supports growth and development during childhood, adolescence, and pregnancy.

Antioxidants:

Flavonoids: Antioxidant compounds found in dill that help neutralize free radicals and reduce oxidative stress. Flavonoids have anti-inflammatory and anti-cancer properties.

Monoterpenes: Phytochemicals with antioxidant and anti-inflammatory effects. Monoterpenes found in dill may help protect against chronic diseases and support overall health.

Incorporating dill into your diet can help boost your intake of these essential nutrients, supporting overall health and well-being. Whether added to salads, soups, sauces, or seafood dishes, dill adds both flavor and nutrition to your meals.

Health Benefits of Dill

In addition to its culinary uses, dill offers a plethora of health benefits, thanks to its rich nutrient profile and unique phytochemicals:

Digestive Aid: Dill has long been used as a digestive aid, helping to alleviate symptoms such as bloating, gas, and indigestion. Its essential oils and compounds stimulate digestive juices and promote healthy gut function.

Antioxidant Properties: Dill contains potent antioxidants, including flavonoids, polyphenols, and vitamin C, which help neutralize harmful free radicals in the body, reducing the risk of chronic diseases such as heart disease, cancer, and diabetes.

Anti-inflammatory Effects: Compounds found in dill, such as monoterpenes and flavonoids, possess anti-inflammatory properties that may help reduce inflammation and alleviate symptoms of inflammatory conditions like arthritis and asthma.

Antimicrobial Activity: Dill exhibits antimicrobial properties, thanks to its essential oils, which have been shown to inhibit the growth of bacteria, fungi, and other harmful microorganisms, thereby supporting immune health and reducing the risk of infections.

Menstrual Relief: Dill has been traditionally used to alleviate menstrual cramps and discomfort. Its antispasmodic properties may help relax uterine muscles and reduce pain associated with menstruation.

Incorporating Dill into Your Diet

Adding dill to your culinary repertoire is a simple and delicious way to enjoy its flavor and reap its health benefits. Here are some tips for incorporating dill into your diet:

Fresh Dill: Use fresh dill leaves as a garnish for salads, soups, sandwiches, and seafood dishes. Chop dill finely and sprinkle it over cooked vegetables or roasted potatoes for added flavor.

Dill Seeds: Crush dill seeds and sprinkle them over grilled meats, fish, or roasted vegetables. Add them to homemade pickles, marinades, or spice blends for a burst of flavor.

Dill Sauce: Make a creamy dill sauce by combining chopped dill with yogurt, sour cream, mayonnaise, lemon juice, and garlic. Use it as a dip for vegetables, a sauce for grilled meats or fish, or a dressing for salads.

Dill Infusions: Brew dill tea by steeping fresh or dried dill leaves in hot water for a soothing and aromatic herbal infusion. Add honey or lemon for sweetness and enjoy as a calming beverage.

Culinary Uses of Dill

Dill is perhaps most renowned for its culinary uses, where its fresh leaves and seeds are prized for their flavor and aroma. Here are some common culinary applications of dill:

Seasoning: Dill's bright, tangy flavor pairs well with a variety of dishes, including seafood, poultry, salads, and vegetables. It adds depth and complexity to soups, stews, sauces, and marinades.

Pickling: Dill is a key ingredient in pickling brines, where its seeds infuse vegetables such as cucumbers, carrots, and green beans with a distinctive dill flavor. Dill pickles are a beloved condiment enjoyed worldwide.

Baking: Dill can be incorporated into bread, scones, crackers, and savory pastries to add a subtle herbal note and aroma.

Garnish: Fresh dill leaves make an attractive garnish for a wide range of dishes, adding a pop of color and freshness to salads, sandwiches, dips, and appetizers.

Here are two delicious recipes that feature dill as a key ingredient:

Creamy Dill Salmon:

- Ingredients:
    - 4 salmon fillets
    - Salt and pepper to taste
    - 2 tablespoons olive oil
    - 2 cloves garlic, minced
    - 1 cup heavy cream
    - 2 tablespoons Dijon mustard
    - 2 tablespoons chopped fresh dill
    - 1 tablespoon lemon juice
- Instructions:
    1. Season the salmon fillets with salt and pepper.
    2. In a large skillet, heat the olive oil over medium heat. Add the salmon fillets and cook for 4-5 minutes on each side, or until cooked through. Remove the salmon from the skillet and set aside.
    3. In the same skillet, add the minced garlic and sauté for 1-2 minutes, until fragrant.
    4. Stir in the heavy cream, Dijon mustard, chopped dill, and lemon juice. Cook for 2-3 minutes, stirring occasionally, until the sauce thickens slightly.
    5. Return the salmon fillets to the skillet, spooning the sauce over them. Cook for an additional 1-2 minutes to heat through.
    6. Serve the creamy dill salmon hot, garnished with extra dill leaves if desired. Enjoy with steamed vegetables or rice.

Cucumber Dill Salad:

- Ingredients:
    0. 2 large cucumbers, thinly sliced
    1. 1/2 red onion, thinly sliced
    2. 1/4 cup chopped fresh dill
    3. 1/4 cup Greek yogurt
    4. 1 tablespoon olive oil
    5. 1 tablespoon lemon juice
    6. Salt and pepper to taste
- Instructions:
    1. In a large mixing bowl, combine the sliced cucumbers, sliced red onion, and chopped dill.
    2. In a small bowl, whisk together the Greek yogurt, olive oil, lemon juice, salt, and pepper to make the dressing.
    3. Pour the dressing over the cucumber mixture and toss gently to coat.
    4. Cover the salad and refrigerate for at least 30 minutes to allow the flavors to meld.
    5. Serve the cucumber dill salad chilled, as a refreshing side dish or accompaniment to grilled meats or seafood.

These recipes showcase the vibrant flavor of dill and its versatility in both savory and creamy dishes. Enjoy experimenting with dill in your culinary creations!

Historical Uses:

Dill (Anethum graveolens) has a long history of use, dating back thousands of years. Here are two historical uses of dill:

Ancient Egypt and Greece:

- Dill has been documented as a culinary and medicinal herb in ancient civilizations such as Egypt and Greece.
- In Ancient Egypt, dill was used both as a flavoring agent in food and beverages and for its purported medicinal properties. It was often incorporated into herbal remedies and ointments.
- In Ancient Greece, dill was considered a symbol of vitality and used for its aromatic qualities in cooking. Greek physicians, including Hippocrates, recognized dill for

its digestive benefits and prescribed it to aid digestion and alleviate gastrointestinal discomfort.

Medieval Europe:

- Dill continued to be valued during the medieval period in Europe, where it was cultivated in monastery gardens and used in culinary and medicinal preparations.
- In medieval European cuisine, dill was commonly used to flavor meats, fish, soups, and sauces. It was also used in pickling brines to preserve vegetables and meats.
- Dill was believed to have various medicinal properties during this time, including its use as a digestive aid and as a remedy for flatulence and colic.

These historical uses of dill highlight its significance as both a culinary herb and a medicinal plant throughout the ages. Today, dill remains popular in kitchens around the world for its distinctive flavor and aroma, as well as its potential health benefits.

Tips on Growing Dill

Dill (Anethum graveolens) is a relatively fast-growing herb that can be cultivated from seed to harvest in a relatively short period. Here's a detailed overview of the growth stages and timeline for dill:

1. **Germination (7-14 days)**:
    - Dill seeds typically germinate within 7 to 14 days when planted in moist, well-draining soil with temperatures ranging between 60°F to 70°F (15°C to 21°C). Providing consistent moisture during this stage is crucial for successful germination.
2. **Seedling Stage (2-4 weeks)**:
    - After germination, dill seedlings emerge from the soil. During this stage, they develop their first true leaves and establish their root system. Dill seedlings are delicate and may require protection from harsh weather conditions, pests, and diseases.
3. **Vegetative Growth (4-6 weeks)**:
    - As the dill seedlings mature, they enter a phase of vegetative growth, focusing on developing foliage and stems. With adequate sunlight, water, and nutrients, dill plants grow rapidly during this stage, reaching heights of 18 to 24 inches (45 to 60 centimeters).
4. **Flowering (6-8 weeks)**:
    - Dill plants typically begin to flower about 6 to 8 weeks after planting. The flowers are small, yellow, and arranged in umbrella-like clusters called umbels. Flowering

signals that the dill plant is nearing maturity and transitioning from vegetative growth to seed production.

5. **Seed Formation (2-3 weeks)**:

    - After flowering, dill plants focus on producing seeds. The seeds develop within the umbels and gradually change from green to brown as they mature. It's essential to allow some of the seeds to fully mature on the plant if you want to collect them for future planting.

6. **Harvesting (8-10 weeks)**:

    - Dill leaves can be harvested as soon as the plants reach a suitable size, typically about 8 to 10 weeks after planting. Snip off individual leaves as needed or cut the entire plant down to about 2 inches (5 centimeters) above the soil level to encourage regrowth.
    - If you're harvesting dill seeds, wait until the seeds are fully mature and turning brown on the plant. Cut the seed heads from the plant and hang them upside down in a well-ventilated area to dry. Once dry, shake the seed heads to release the seeds, and store them in an airtight container for future use.

By following this timeline and providing proper care and maintenance, you can enjoy a bountiful harvest of fresh dill leaves or seeds within a relatively short timeframe.

Conclusion:

Dill is much more than just a flavorful herb – it's a powerhouse of nutrition and wellness. Whether you're enhancing the flavor of your favorite dishes or harnessing its health-promoting properties, dill deserves a place in your kitchen and your holistic health routine. So, next time you're at the market, pick up a bunch of fresh dill and let its aromatic charm and beneficial qualities enrich your culinary creations and nourish your body and soul.

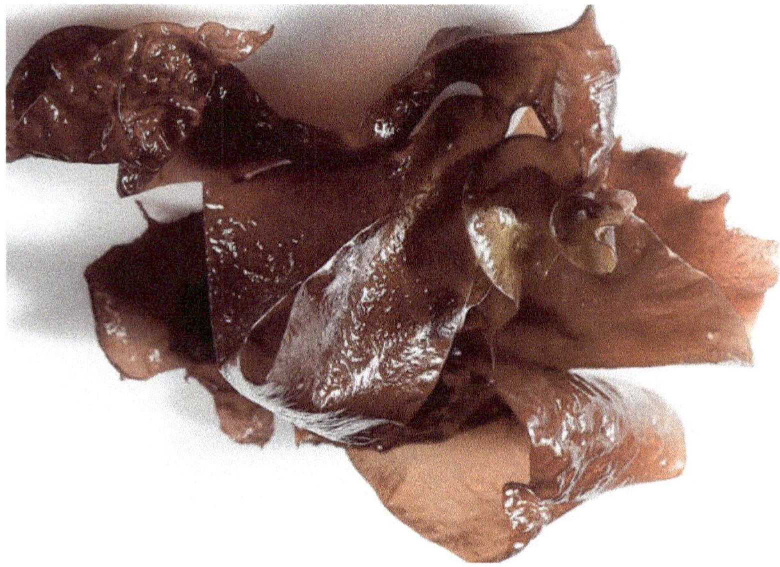

Dulse

The Nutrient-Rich Seaweed with Health Benefits and Culinary Versatility

Dulse, a red algae that thrives along the Northern Atlantic and Pacific coastlines, has long been celebrated for its unique flavor, vibrant color, and impressive nutritional profile. This seaweed variety, scientifically known as Palmaria palmata, offers a plethora of health benefits and a versatility that extends from traditional medicine to culinary creations. Let's explore the wonders of dulse, delving into its benefits and diverse uses.

Nutritional Powerhouse:

Dulse stands out as a nutrient-dense food, packed with essential vitamins, minerals, and other beneficial compounds. Here are some key nutritional components found in dulse:

Protein:

- Dulse is surprisingly rich in protein, making it a valuable addition to plant-based diets.

Iron:

- An essential mineral, iron is crucial for oxygen transport in the blood and overall energy metabolism. Dulse provides a plant-based source of iron.

Vitamins:

Dulse contains various vitamins, including vitamin C, vitamin A, and the B-vitamin complex. These vitamins play roles in immune function, vision, and energy metabolism.

Dulse, a red seaweed, is a nutrient-dense food that provides a range of essential vitamins and minerals. While the exact nutrient composition can vary depending on factors like harvesting location and processing methods, here is a general list of key vitamins and minerals found in dulse:

Vitamins:

Vitamin C: A powerful antioxidant that supports the immune system and skin health.

Vitamin A: Essential for vision, immune function, and skin health.

Vitamin B12: Though the amount is relatively small compared to animal sources, dulse contains some B12, making it valuable for plant-based diets.

Vitamin E: An antioxidant that helps protect cells from oxidative damage.

Vitamin K: Important for blood clotting and bone health.

Minerals:

Iodine: Dulse is known for its relatively high iodine content, which is crucial for thyroid health and hormone production.

Iron: Essential for oxygen transport in the blood and energy metabolism.

Potassium: Important for maintaining fluid balance, supporting muscle and nerve function, and promoting heart health.

Magnesium: Involved in muscle and nerve function, blood glucose control, and bone health.

Calcium: Crucial for bone and teeth health, as well as various cellular processes.

Phosphorus: Important for bone and teeth formation, energy metabolism, and acid-base balance.

Sodium: Present in dulse, sodium is an electrolyte essential for maintaining fluid balance and supporting nerve function.

Dietary Fiber:

- With a notable fiber content, dulse contributes to digestive health, supporting regular bowel movements and aiding in satiety.

Omega-3 Fatty Acids:

- Dulse is a source of omega-3 fatty acids, particularly alpha-linolenic acid (ALA), which is known for its anti-inflammatory properties and potential cardiovascular benefits.

Health Benefits:

Thyroid Support:

- Dulse is considered a good source of iodine, a crucial mineral for thyroid health. Adequate iodine intake is essential for the production of thyroid hormones, which regulate metabolism.

Heart Health:

- The omega-3 fatty acids in dulse may contribute to cardiovascular health by reducing inflammation and supporting optimal cholesterol levels.

Antioxidant Properties:

Dulse contains various antioxidants, including polyphenols and flavonoids, which help combat oxidative stress and protect cells from damage.

Polyphenols:

- Dulse contains various polyphenolic compounds, including flavonoids and phenolic acids. These compounds have antioxidant properties and contribute to the overall health-promoting effects of dulse.

Flavonoids:

- Flavonoids are a diverse group of antioxidants found in plants. They have been associated with anti-inflammatory and anti-cancer properties. Dulse may contain flavonoids that contribute to its antioxidant activity.

Beta-carotene:

- Dulse contains beta-carotene, a precursor to vitamin A. Beta-carotene is a powerful antioxidant that helps protect cells from damage caused by free radicals.

Ascorbic Acid (Vitamin C):

- Vitamin C is a well-known antioxidant present in dulse. It plays a crucial role in neutralizing free radicals, supporting the immune system, and promoting skin health.

Tocopherols (Vitamin E):

- Dulse contains vitamin E, including tocopherols, which are fat-soluble antioxidants known for their ability to protect cell membranes from oxidative damage.

Carotenoids:

- Apart from beta-carotene, dulse may contain other carotenoids with antioxidant properties. Carotenoids contribute to the seaweed's color and offer potential health benefits.

Phycobilins:

- Phycobilins are water-soluble pigments found in red algae, including dulse. These pigments have antioxidant and anti-inflammatory properties and contribute to the vibrant red color of the seaweed.

Antioxidants play a crucial role in neutralizing free radicals, which are reactive molecules that can damage cells and contribute to aging and various diseases. Including antioxidant-rich foods like dulse in your diet may contribute to overall well-being and support a healthy lifestyle. However, it's essential to consume a variety of nutrient-rich foods to ensure a balanced intake of antioxidants and other essential nutrients.

Culinary Uses:

Dulse's culinary versatility extends from traditional seaweed dishes to innovative creations in modern cuisine. Here are some popular uses:

Salads and Soups:

- Dulse can be added to salads, providing a unique umami flavor and a nutritional boost. It can also be used to enhance the depth of flavor in soups and stews.

Snacks:

- Roasted or dried dulse makes for a nutritious and savory snack, offering a crunchy texture and a sea-inspired taste.

Smoothies:

- Incorporate dried or powdered dulse into smoothies for an extra nutrient kick without overpowering the flavor.

Wraps and Rolls:

- Use dulse sheets as a wrap for sushi rolls or sandwich fillings, adding a seafood-like essence to your dishes.

Condiments:

- Dulse flakes or powder can be used as a seasoning or condiment, sprinkled over dishes for a burst of flavor and nutrition.

Dulse, with its unique flavor and nutritional benefits, can be incorporated into various recipes.

Here are two delicious recipes featuring dulse:

Dulse and Avocado Nori Rolls:

Ingredients:

- Nori sheets
- 1 cup cooked quinoa or sushi rice
- 1 avocado, sliced
- Dulse flakes or whole dulse leaves
- 1 cucumber, julienned
- Carrots, julienned
- Soy sauce or tamari for dipping
- Pickled ginger and wasabi (optional)

Instructions:

1. Lay a sheet of nori on a bamboo sushi rolling mat.
2. Spread a thin layer of cooked quinoa or sushi rice evenly over the nori sheet, leaving about an inch of space at the top.
3. Place avocado slices, julienned cucumber, julienned carrots, and dulse flakes along the center of the rice.
4. Carefully roll the nori sheet from the bottom using the bamboo mat, applying gentle pressure to create a tight roll.
5. Wet the top edge of the nori sheet with water to seal the roll.
6. Slice the roll into bite-sized pieces using a sharp knife.
7. Serve the dulse and avocado nori rolls with soy sauce or tamari for dipping. Add pickled ginger and wasabi on the side if desired.

Dulse and Chickpea Salad:

Ingredients:

- 1 can (15 oz) chickpeas, drained and rinsed
- 1/2 cup diced red onion
- 1/2 cup diced cucumber
- 1/2 cup cherry tomatoes, halved
- 1/4 cup chopped fresh parsley

- Dulse flakes or whole dulse leaves
- 2 tablespoons olive oil
- 1 tablespoon lemon juice
- Salt and pepper to taste

Instructions:

1. In a large bowl, combine chickpeas, diced red onion, diced cucumber, cherry tomatoes, and chopped parsley.
2. Add dulse flakes or torn dulse leaves to the salad, adjusting the amount to your liking.
3. In a small bowl, whisk together olive oil and lemon juice. Season with salt and pepper.
4. Pour the dressing over the salad and toss gently to combine.
5. Allow the salad to marinate for a few minutes to let the flavors meld.
6. Serve the dulse and chickpea salad as a side dish or a light main course. It can also be served over a bed of greens or with crusty bread.

These recipes showcase the versatility of dulse, adding a flavorful and nutritious element to sushi rolls and a hearty chickpea salad. Enjoy the unique taste and health benefits that dulse brings to these dishes!

Conclusion:

Dulse, with its rich nutritional content and versatile culinary applications, is a true gem from the sea. Whether enjoyed for its health benefits or used to elevate the taste of various dishes, this red seaweed continues to captivate the palates of those seeking both nourishment and gastronomic delight. If you have specific health concerns, allergies, or conditions, it's advisable to consult with a healthcare professional or a registered dietitian before making significant changes to your diet.

Embrace the potential of dulse in your kitchen and explore the myriad ways it can contribute to your well-being and culinary adventures.

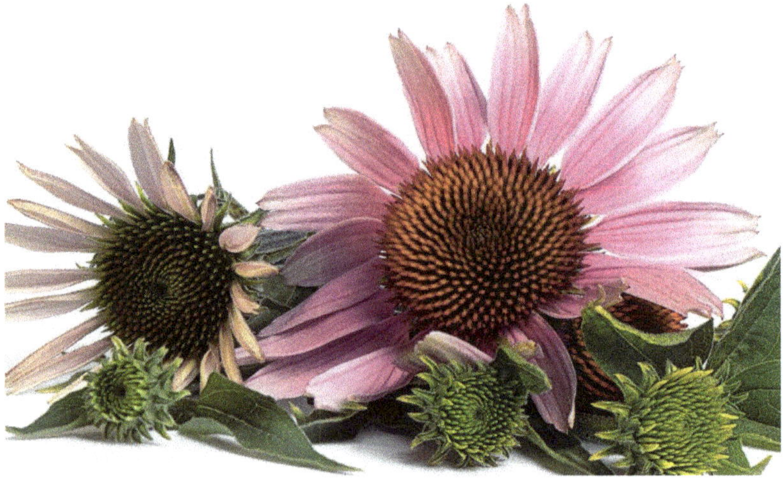

Echinacea

Unveiling the Benefits and Diverse Uses of This Herbal Wonder

Echinacea, a vibrant and resilient herb, has long been celebrated for its numerous health benefits and versatile applications. Commonly known as the purple coneflower, Echinacea has earned a reputation as a potent herbal remedy with immune-boosting properties. In this article, we will explore the various benefits and wide-ranging uses of Echinacea.

Immune System Support:

Echinacea is renowned for its ability to bolster the immune system. Rich in active compounds such as flavonoids, polysaccharides, and alkamides, Echinacea stimulates the production and activity of immune cells. Regular consumption or use of Echinacea supplements may help reduce the risk of infections and shorten the duration of colds and flu. It acts as a natural shield, empowering the body's defenses against pathogens.

Respiratory Health:

Echinacea's anti-inflammatory and antimicrobial properties make it a valuable ally in promoting respiratory health. It is often used to alleviate symptoms of respiratory infections, such as the common cold and bronchitis. Echinacea's ability to reduce inflammation in the respiratory tract can ease congestion and support overall respiratory well-being.

Wound Healing and Skincare:

Echinacea's natural antibacterial and anti-inflammatory qualities extend to skincare. The herb can be applied topically to wounds, cuts, and skin irritations to promote healing. Echinacea creams and ointments are known for their soothing effects on the skin, making them useful for conditions like eczema and psoriasis. The herb's regenerative properties contribute to the overall health and vitality of the skin.

Anti-inflammatory Benefits:

Echinacea contains compounds that exhibit anti-inflammatory effects, making it beneficial for conditions characterized by inflammation, such as arthritis. Regular use of Echinacea supplements or extracts may help reduce joint pain and inflammation, providing relief for individuals with inflammatory conditions.

Antioxidant Powerhouse:

Loaded with antioxidants, Echinacea helps combat oxidative stress in the body. Antioxidants play a crucial role in neutralizing free radicals, which can contribute to aging and various chronic diseases. By incorporating Echinacea into your routine, you support your body's defense against oxidative damage.

Bioactive Compounds and Benefits:

Echinacea is a herbal remedy rather than a traditional dietary source of nutrients. However, it contains various bioactive compounds that contribute to its health benefits. Here are some key constituents found in Echinacea and their associated benefits:

Alkamides:

- **Benefit:** Alkamides are bioactive compounds found in Echinacea that contribute to its immune-boosting properties. These compounds are believed to enhance the activity of immune cells, supporting the body's defense against infections. Alkamides may play a role in reducing the severity and duration of colds and flu.

Polysaccharides:

- **Benefit:** Echinacea contains polysaccharides, which are complex carbohydrates with immune-modulating properties. Polysaccharides stimulate the activity of white blood cells and enhance the overall immune response. This contributes to Echinacea's effectiveness in supporting the immune system and combating various infections.

Flavonoids:

- **Benefit:** Flavonoids are antioxidants found in Echinacea that help neutralize free radicals in the body. These compounds contribute to Echinacea's overall antioxidant activity, providing protection against oxidative stress. Antioxidants play a crucial role in preventing cellular damage and reducing the risk of chronic diseases.

Essential Oils:

- **Benefit:** Echinacea contains essential oils, including volatile compounds like caryophyllene and germacrene D. These oils contribute to the herb's anti-inflammatory and antimicrobial properties. Essential oils in Echinacea may help alleviate respiratory symptoms, reduce inflammation, and contribute to its overall therapeutic effects.

Holistic Wellness:

Beyond its targeted benefits, Echinacea contributes to holistic wellness. Its adaptogenic properties help the body adapt to stress, promoting a balanced and resilient system. Echinacea teas, tinctures, or capsules can be incorporated into a wellness routine to support overall health and vitality.

Echinacea is primarily known for its medicinal uses, and it is not a traditional culinary herb. However, some creative chefs and herbal enthusiasts have explored unconventional culinary applications for Echinacea. Here are three culinary uses:

Echinacea Infused Honey:

- Create a unique and flavorful honey infusion by combining dried Echinacea flowers with honey. This can be done by placing Echinacea petals in a jar and covering them with honey. Allow the mixture to sit for several weeks to allow the honey to absorb the herbal essence. The resulting Echinacea-infused honey can be drizzled over desserts, added to tea, or used as a sweetener in various recipes. It provides a subtle floral and earthy flavor to dishes.

Echinacea Tea Blends:

- Incorporate Echinacea into homemade tea blends for a delightful and potentially immune-boosting beverage. Combine dried Echinacea flowers with other herbal ingredients like chamomile, mint, or lemon balm to create a soothing herbal tea. The addition of Echinacea adds a mild earthy note to the tea, and when combined with complementary herbs, it can result in a well-balanced and flavorful infusion.

Echinacea-Infused Vinegar:

- Make a unique herbal vinegar by infusing Echinacea with apple cider vinegar or white wine vinegar. Place dried Echinacea petals in a clean, sterilized jar and cover them with vinegar. Let the mixture steep for a few weeks, ensuring the petals are fully submerged. The resulting Echinacea-infused vinegar can be used as a flavorful addition to salad dressings, marinades, or even as a tangy drizzle over roasted vegetables.

Echinacea, a popular herb known for its potential immune-boosting properties, can be incorporated into various recipes.

Here are two recipes that use echinacea:

Echinacea Tea:

Ingredients:

- 1 tablespoon dried echinacea root or 2-3 echinacea tea bags

- 2 cups water
- Honey (optional, for sweetness)
- Lemon slices (optional, for flavor)

Instructions:

1. Bring 2 cups of water to a boil in a saucepan.
2. Add the dried echinacea root or echinacea tea bags to the boiling water.
3. Reduce heat and let the echinacea steep in the water for about 10-15 minutes.
4. Remove the saucepan from heat and strain the echinacea tea into a cup.
5. Add honey and lemon slices if desired for flavor.
6. Stir well and enjoy your soothing echinacea tea, especially during cold and flu season to support immune health.

Echinacea Immune-Boosting Smoothie:

Ingredients:

1. 1 ripe banana
2. 1 cup mixed berries (such as strawberries, blueberries, raspberries)
3. 1/2 cup spinach leaves
4. 1/2 cup plain Greek yogurt or dairy-free yogurt alternative
5. 1/2 cup orange juice or apple juice
6. 1 teaspoon echinacea powder or echinacea extract
7. 1 tablespoon honey or maple syrup (optional, for sweetness)
8. Ice cubes (optional, for a colder smoothie)

Instructions:

1. In a blender, combine the ripe banana, mixed berries, spinach leaves, Greek yogurt or dairy-free yogurt, orange juice or apple juice, echinacea powder or extract, and honey or maple syrup (if using).
2. Add ice cubes if you prefer a colder smoothie.
3. Blend all the ingredients until smooth and creamy.
4. Taste the smoothie and adjust sweetness or thickness by adding more honey, maple syrup, or liquid as desired.

5. Pour the immune-boosting echinacea smoothie into glasses and serve immediately.
6. Enjoy this nutritious and delicious smoothie as part of your daily routine to support your immune system and overall well-being.

These recipes offer tasty ways to incorporate echinacea into your diet to potentially support immune health and overall wellness.

It's important to note that while these culinary uses of Echinacea may add interesting flavors to dishes, the primary reputation of Echinacea lies in its medicinal properties. When using Echinacea for culinary purposes, be mindful of the quantity to avoid potential overconsumption. Additionally, individuals with allergies to plants in the Asteraceae family (such as ragweed) should exercise caution when using Echinacea in any form.

Echinacea is not a conventional source of vitamins and minerals, its bioactive compounds offer a range of health benefits, primarily in supporting the immune system and promoting overall well-being. It's important to note that Echinacea is often consumed as a supplement, tea, or tincture rather than as a food source.

Historical Uses:

Echinacea, also known as purple coneflower, has a rich history of traditional use by various indigenous peoples in North America. Here are two historical uses of echinacea:

Native American Medicinal Herb: Native American tribes, particularly the Plains Indians, used echinacea for various medicinal purposes. It was commonly used as a remedy for ailments such as infections, wounds, toothaches, sore throats, and snakebites. The indigenous peoples prepared echinacea as infusions or poultices made from the roots, leaves, or flowers of the plant. Echinacea was highly valued for its purported immune-stimulating properties and was considered a versatile herbal medicine for promoting overall health and well-being.

Early American Settlers' Medicinal Plant: European settlers in North America learned about the medicinal uses of echinacea from Native American tribes and began incorporating it into their own traditional medicine practices. Echinacea gained popularity among early American settlers as a valuable medicinal herb for treating various infections and illnesses. It was often used as a remedy for colds, flu, respiratory infections, and other common ailments. Echinacea preparations, such as teas, tinctures, and poultices, were commonly used by early American settlers to support immune health and alleviate symptoms of illness.

These historical uses of echinacea highlight its long-standing reputation as a medicinal plant with potential health benefits, particularly for immune support and treating various infections and illnesses. While modern scientific research continues to explore the efficacy of echinacea, its historical significance as a traditional herbal remedy remains an important aspect of its cultural heritage.

Tips on Growing Echinacea

Echinacea, also known as coneflower, is a beautiful and beneficial perennial herb that is commonly grown for its medicinal properties and ornamental value. Here's a detailed breakdown of the time it takes for Echinacea to grow:

1. **Germination**: Echinacea seeds typically germinate within 10 to 20 days after planting, depending on factors such as soil temperature, moisture levels, and seed quality. Germination can be faster with warmer soil temperatures, ideally around 70 to 75°F (21 to 24°C).
2. **Seedling Stage**: After germination, Echinacea seedlings will emerge from the soil. During this stage, the seedlings will develop their first true leaves. This process usually takes another 2 to 3 weeks after germination.
3. **Early Growth Phase**: Once the seedlings have established themselves, they will begin to grow more rapidly. Echinacea plants typically form a rosette of leaves during the first growing season. This phase can last for several weeks to a couple of months, depending on environmental conditions and the variety of Echinacea.
4. **Overwintering (for Perennial Varieties)**: If you're growing perennial varieties of Echinacea, they will go through a period of dormancy during the winter months. In regions with cold winters, the plants may die back to the ground, but their roots will remain alive underground. Echinacea typically emerges from dormancy and starts growing again in the spring.
5. **Vegetative Growth and Flowering**: As the weather warms up in the spring, Echinacea plants will resume vegetative growth and may start forming flower buds. Depending on the variety and growing conditions, Echinacea plants usually begin flowering in their second or third year of growth. The flowering period can last several weeks to a couple of months, depending on the specific variety and environmental conditions.
6. **Seed Production**: After flowering, Echinacea plants produce seed heads containing seeds. The seeds mature over several weeks, eventually becoming ready for harvest. If you're growing Echinacea for its ornamental value, you may choose to deadhead spent flowers to encourage continuous blooming and prevent self-seeding.

Overall, from planting Echinacea seeds to seeing mature flowering plants, the process can take approximately 1 to 2 years, depending on the variety and growing conditions. However, Echinacea plants will continue to grow and thrive for many years once established, providing you with beautiful blooms and potential medicinal benefits for years to come.

Conclusion:

Echinacea stands as a botanical marvel, offering a spectrum of benefits that extend from immune system support to skincare and beyond. Whether consumed as a supplement, brewed into a tea, or applied topically, Echinacea has proven its worth in promoting well-being and resilience. Embrace the power of this herbal wonder and integrate Echinacea into your lifestyle for a holistic approach to health and vitality. As with any herbal remedy, it's advisable to consult with a healthcare professional before incorporating Echinacea into your routine, especially if you have underlying health conditions or are taking medications.

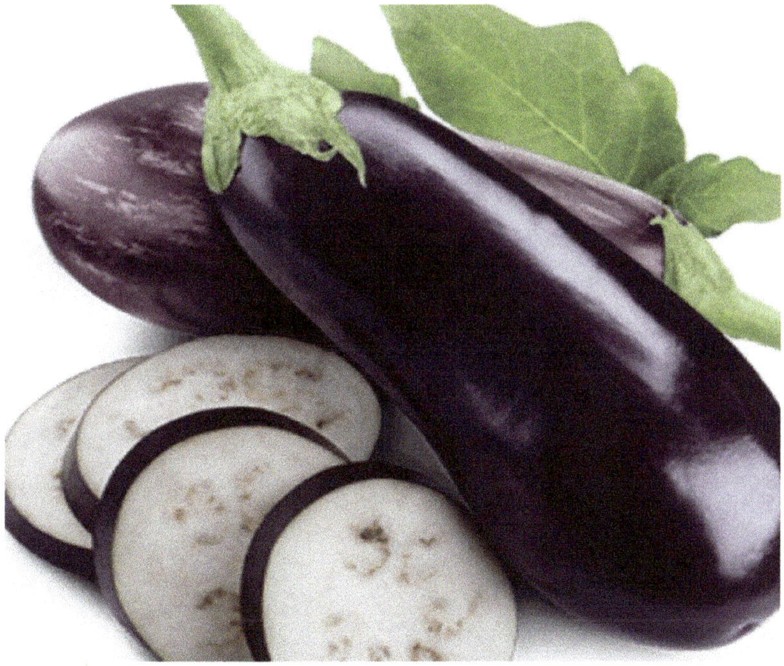

Eggplant

Exploring Its Benefits and Versatile Uses

Eggplant, scientifically known as Solanum melongena, is a popular vegetable with a unique taste and texture that has been enjoyed in cuisines around the world for centuries. Believed to have originated in India, eggplant is now cultivated globally and prized for its culinary versatility, as well as its potential health benefits. Let's delve deeper into the benefits and uses of this fascinating vegetable.

Nutritional Profile of Eggplant

Eggplant is a low-calorie, nutrient-dense vegetable that offers an array of vitamins, minerals, and phytonutrients. Here's a glimpse into its nutritional profile:

Vitamins:

Eggplant is a good source of vitamins such as vitamin C, vitamin K, vitamin B6, and folate, which play essential roles in supporting overall health and wellbeing.

Vitamin C:

- Benefits: Vitamin C is a powerful antioxidant that supports the immune system, promotes collagen production for healthy skin, and aids in the absorption of iron from plant-based foods.

Vitamin K:

- Benefits: Vitamin K plays a crucial role in blood clotting and bone health. It helps regulate calcium in the body and contributes to bone mineralization, reducing the risk of osteoporosis.

Vitamin B6 (Pyridoxine):

- Benefits: Vitamin B6 is involved in over 100 enzyme reactions in the body, including protein metabolism, neurotransmitter synthesis, and immune function. It also helps regulate blood sugar levels and supports cognitive health.

Folate (Vitamin B9):

- Benefits: Folate is essential for DNA synthesis and cell division, making it crucial for fetal development during pregnancy. It also supports red blood cell formation and helps prevent neural tube defects in infants.

Vitamin A:

- Benefits: Vitamin A is important for vision health, immune function, and skin health. It acts as an antioxidant, protecting cells from damage caused by free radicals, and is necessary for the proper functioning of the retina.

Vitamin E:

- Benefits: Vitamin E is a fat-soluble antioxidant that helps protect cell membranes from oxidative damage. It supports immune function, skin health, and may have anti-inflammatory properties.

Vitamin B3 (Niacin):

- Benefits: Vitamin B3 is involved in energy metabolism, DNA repair, and cell signaling. It helps convert food into energy and supports nervous system function.

Vitamin B1 (Thiamine):

- Benefits: Vitamin B1 is essential for energy metabolism and nerve function. It helps convert carbohydrates into energy and plays a role in the synthesis of neurotransmitters.

Vitamin B2 (Riboflavin):

- Benefits: Vitamin B2 is involved in energy production, antioxidant defense, and red blood cell formation. It helps convert food into energy and supports healthy skin, eyes, and mucous membranes.

Vitamin B5 (Pantothenic Acid):

- Benefits: Vitamin B5 is essential for synthesizing coenzyme A, which plays a central role in energy metabolism and fatty acid synthesis. It also supports hormone production and helps maintain healthy skin and hair.

Including eggplant in your diet can provide a variety of vitamins that support overall health and wellbeing.

Minerals

Eggplant contains minerals like potassium, magnesium, and manganese, which are important for maintaining electrolyte balance, bone health, and metabolic functions.

Potassium:

- Benefits: Potassium is an essential mineral that plays a vital role in regulating blood pressure, maintaining fluid balance, and supporting proper muscle and nerve function. It helps counteract the effects of sodium, promoting heart health and reducing the risk of stroke.

Manganese:

- Benefits: Manganese is involved in various metabolic processes, including carbohydrate metabolism, bone formation, and antioxidant defense. It supports collagen production, helps regulate blood sugar levels, and may have anti-inflammatory properties.

Magnesium:

- Benefits: Magnesium is essential for over 300 biochemical reactions in the body, including energy production, muscle and nerve function, and protein synthesis. It supports bone health, heart health, and may help alleviate muscle cramps and promote relaxation.

Copper:

- Benefits: Copper is necessary for the formation of red blood cells, connective tissues, and neurotransmitters. It plays a role in energy metabolism, iron absorption, and antioxidant defense. Copper also supports immune function and may help reduce the risk of osteoporosis.

Iron:

- Benefits: Iron is a crucial component of hemoglobin, the protein in red blood cells that carries oxygen from the lungs to tissues throughout the body. It's essential for oxygen transport, energy production, and immune function. Iron deficiency can lead to anemia and fatigue.

Phosphorus:

- Benefits: Phosphorus is involved in bone mineralization, energy metabolism, and cell membrane structure. It plays a role in DNA and RNA synthesis, as well as in the regulation of acid-base balance in the body.

Calcium:

- Benefits: Calcium is well-known for its role in bone health, but it's also involved in muscle contraction, nerve signaling, blood clotting, and enzyme regulation. It's essential for maintaining strong bones and teeth, as well as for proper heart and muscle function.

Zinc:

- Benefits: Zinc is important for immune function, wound healing, and DNA synthesis. It supports growth and development, reproductive health, and may have antioxidant properties. Zinc also plays a role in taste perception and hormone regulation.

Selenium:

- Benefits: Selenium is a powerful antioxidant that helps protect cells from oxidative damage and supports immune function. It's involved in thyroid hormone metabolism, DNA synthesis, and reproductive health. Selenium may also help reduce inflammation and lower the risk of certain chronic diseases.

Phytonutrients:

- Benefits: While not minerals in the traditional sense, phytonutrients found in eggplant, such as chlorogenic acid and nasunin, also offer health benefits. They have antioxidant and anti-inflammatory properties and may help protect against chronic diseases like heart disease and cancer.

Including eggplant in your diet can provide a variety of minerals that support overall health and wellbeing.

Dietary Fiber:

Eggplant is rich in dietary fiber, particularly insoluble fiber, which supports digestive health, regulates bowel movements, and may help lower cholesterol levels.

Antioxidants:

Eggplant contains potent antioxidants, including phenolic compounds like chlorogenic acid and anthocyanins, which help neutralize harmful free radicals and reduce oxidative stress in the body.

Anthocyanins:

- Benefits: Anthocyanins are water-soluble pigments responsible for the deep purple color of eggplant skin. They have potent antioxidant properties that help neutralize free radicals, reduce inflammation, and protect against chronic diseases such as heart disease, cancer, and neurodegenerative disorders. Anthocyanins may also support cognitive function and vascular health.

Chlorogenic Acid:

- Benefits: Chlorogenic acid is a polyphenol antioxidant found in high concentrations in eggplant. It has been associated with various health benefits, including reducing oxidative stress, lowering blood pressure, improving insulin sensitivity, and protecting against liver damage. Chlorogenic acid may also have anti-inflammatory and antimicrobial properties.

Nasunin:

- Benefits: Nasunin is a unique antioxidant found in the skin of eggplant, particularly in the purple varieties. It has been shown to have potent free radical scavenging activity and may help protect cell membranes from oxidative damage. Nasunin may also support brain health by inhibiting the production of reactive oxygen species (ROS) and reducing oxidative stress in neural tissues.

Flavonoids:

- Benefits: Flavonoids are a diverse group of polyphenolic compounds found in eggplant that have antioxidant, anti-inflammatory, and anti-cancer properties. They help protect cells from oxidative damage, reduce inflammation, and support cardiovascular health. Flavonoids may also promote skin health, improve cognitive function, and enhance immune function.

Vitamin C:

- Benefits: Vitamin C is a potent water-soluble antioxidant found in eggplant that helps protect cells from oxidative damage and supports immune function. It scavenges free radicals, regenerates other antioxidants like vitamin E, and enhances iron absorption. Vitamin C may also promote collagen synthesis, improve skin health, and reduce the risk of chronic diseases.

Vitamin E:

- Benefits: Vitamin E is a fat-soluble antioxidant found in eggplant that helps protect cell membranes from oxidative damage. It scavenges free radicals, reduces inflammation, and supports immune function. Vitamin E may also promote heart health, improve skin health, and protect against age-related cognitive decline.

Carotenoids (such as lutein and zeaxanthin):

- Benefits: Carotenoids are pigments found in eggplant that have antioxidant properties and help protect the eyes from oxidative damage caused by ultraviolet (UV) radiation and blue light. They support eye health, reduce the risk of age-related macular degeneration (AMD), and may improve visual acuity and contrast sensitivity.

Incorporating eggplant into your diet can provide a variety of antioxidants that help protect against oxidative stress and promote overall health and wellbeing.

Health Benefits of Eggplant:

Incorporating eggplant into your diet can offer a range of health benefits, thanks to its nutrient-rich composition:

Heart Health: The fiber, potassium, and antioxidants in eggplant may help promote heart health by lowering blood pressure, reducing cholesterol levels, and protecting against oxidative damage to blood vessels.

Weight Management: With its low calorie and high fiber content, eggplant can be a satisfying addition to a weight loss or weight management diet. Its fiber content helps keep you feeling full and satisfied, reducing the likelihood of overeating.

Blood Sugar Control: Some research suggests that compounds found in eggplant may help improve insulin sensitivity and regulate blood sugar levels, making it a potentially beneficial food for individuals with diabetes or prediabetes.

Cancer Prevention: The antioxidants in eggplant, particularly chlorogenic acid and anthocyanins, have been studied for their potential anti-cancer effects. They may help inhibit the growth of cancer cells and protect against certain types of cancer, although more research is needed in this area.

Nutritional Content

One cup (about 82 grams) of raw eggplant contains approximately:

- Calories: 20
- Carbohydrates: 4.8 grams
- Protein: 0.8 grams
- Fiber: 2.5 grams
- Fat: 0.2 grams
- Sugar: 2.4 grams

These values are approximate and can vary slightly depending on factors such as the size and variety of the eggplant. Eggplant is low in calories and fat, and it's a good source of dietary fiber, making it a healthy addition to a balanced diet.

Versatile Uses of Eggplant in Cooking

Eggplant's mild flavor and meaty texture make it a versatile ingredient in a wide range of culinary preparations. Here are some popular ways to enjoy eggplant:

Roasted Eggplant: Roasting eggplant enhances its natural sweetness and imparts a smoky flavor. Simply slice or cube the eggplant, toss with olive oil, salt, and pepper, and roast in the oven until tender and caramelized. Enjoy as a side dish, salad topping, or sandwich filling.

Eggplant Parmesan: A classic Italian dish, eggplant Parmesan features breaded and fried eggplant slices layered with marinara sauce and melted cheese. It's a hearty and satisfying vegetarian main course that's sure to please.

Baba Ganoush: A Middle Eastern dip made from roasted eggplant, tahini, garlic, lemon juice, and olive oil, baba ganoush is creamy, flavorful, and perfect for dipping pita bread or fresh vegetables.

Ratatouille: Ratatouille is a French vegetable stew made with eggplant, tomatoes, zucchini, bell peppers, onions, and garlic, simmered in olive oil and herbs until tender and fragrant. It's a rustic and comforting dish that celebrates the flavors of summer.

Tips on Growing Eggplant

The time it takes for eggplants to grow from planting to harvest varies depending on several factors, including the variety of eggplant, growing conditions, and climate. However, on average, it takes about 70 to 85 days for most eggplant varieties to reach maturity and become ready for harvest. Here's a detailed overview of the stages involved in the growth of eggplants:

1. **Seed Germination (7-10 days)**:
    - The first stage in the growth of eggplants is seed germination. Eggplant seeds typically germinate within 7 to 10 days when planted in warm and moist soil conditions. During this stage, the seeds absorb water and begin to sprout, sending out roots and shoots.
2. **Seedling Stage (2-4 weeks)**:
    - After germination, the eggplant seeds develop into seedlings. During this stage, the seedlings require adequate sunlight, water, and nutrients to grow strong and healthy. They develop their first true leaves and start to establish their root system.
3. **Transplanting (6-8 weeks)**:
    - Once the seedlings have grown to a suitable size and have developed a few sets of true leaves, they are ready to be transplanted into the garden or larger containers. This typically occurs 6 to 8 weeks after germination, once the danger of frost has passed and the weather has warmed up.

4. **Vegetative Growth (4-6 weeks)**:

    - After transplanting, the eggplant plants enter a period of vegetative growth, where they focus on developing foliage and establishing a strong root system. During this stage, the plants require regular watering, fertilization, and protection from pests and diseases.

5. **Flowering (6-8 weeks)**:

    - Eggplant plants typically begin to flower about 6 to 8 weeks after transplanting. The flowers are usually small and star-shaped, and they may be purple, white, or lavender in color. Each flower has the potential to develop into a fruit (eggplant) if pollinated.

6. **Fruit Development (4-6 weeks)**:

    - After pollination, the flowers develop into small, green fruits, which gradually grow larger and mature over the next 4 to 6 weeks. During this stage, it's essential to provide the plants with adequate water and nutrients to support fruit development.

7. **Harvesting (70-85 days)**:

    - Eggplants are typically ready for harvest about 70 to 85 days after transplanting, depending on the variety. The fruits should be firm, glossy, and fully colored, with a slight give when pressed gently. Use a sharp knife or pruning shears to cut the eggplants from the plant, leaving a short stem attached.

By following proper growing practices and providing optimal growing conditions, you can help ensure a successful eggplant harvest within the expected timeframe.

Conclusion:

Eggplant is a versatile and nutritious vegetable that offers a myriad of culinary possibilities and potential health benefits. Whether roasted, grilled, fried, or stewed, eggplant adds depth and richness to dishes while providing essential vitamins, minerals, and antioxidants. So, the next time you're at the market, pick up a few eggplants and explore the endless culinary delights they have to offer. Your taste buds and your body will thank you! If you have specific health concerns, allergies, or conditions, it's advisable to consult with a healthcare professional or a registered dietitian before making significant changes to your diet.

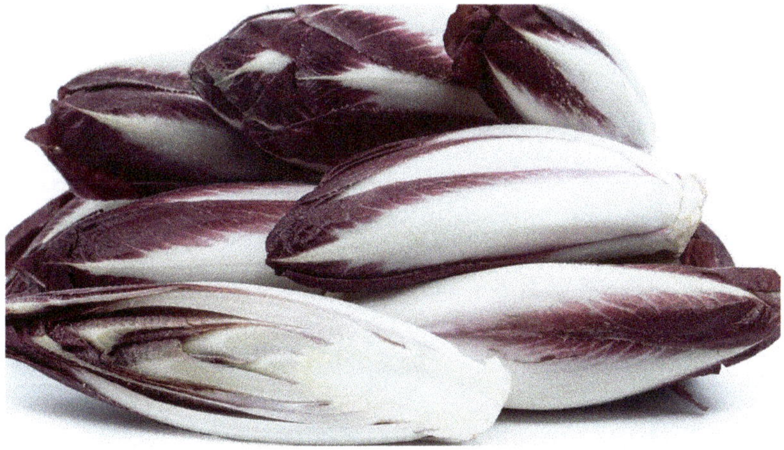

Endive

The Nutritional Treasure Trove

In the realm of leafy greens, endive often finds itself overshadowed by its more popular counterparts like kale, spinach, and romaine lettuce. However, despite its less prominent status, endive boasts a myriad of health benefits and culinary uses that make it a valuable addition to any diet. From its impressive nutritional profile to its versatility in the kitchen, endive is a true gem waiting to be discovered. Let's delve into the world of endive to uncover its hidden treasures.

Nutritional Powerhouse

Endive may be small in size, but it packs a nutritional punch that rivals many other vegetables. Low in calories and carbohydrates while high in fiber, endive is an excellent choice for those seeking to maintain a healthy weight and support digestive health. It's also a rich source of vitamins and minerals, including vitamin K, vitamin A, folate, potassium, and calcium. Vitamin K, in particular, plays a crucial role in bone health and blood clotting, making endive a valuable addition to a balanced diet.

Here's a list of vitamins and minerals found in endive along with their benefits:

Vitamins:

Vitamin K: Essential for blood clotting and bone health. It helps maintain bone density and may reduce the risk of fractures.

Vitamin A: Important for vision, immune function, and skin health. It acts as an antioxidant, helping to protect cells from damage.

Vitamin C: A powerful antioxidant that supports the immune system, aids in collagen production for healthy skin, and enhances iron absorption.

Vitamin E: Another antioxidant that helps protect cells from damage caused by free radicals. It may also play a role in immune function.

Vitamin B9 (Folate): Necessary for DNA synthesis and cell growth. Adequate folate intake is especially important during pregnancy to prevent neural tube defects in the developing fetus.

Minerals:

Potassium: Helps regulate blood pressure by counteracting the effects of sodium. It also plays a role in muscle function and fluid balance.

Calcium: Essential for bone and teeth health. It also plays a role in muscle function, nerve transmission, and hormone secretion.

Phosphorus: Important for bone and teeth health, as well as energy metabolism. It also plays a role in cell membrane structure and function.

Magnesium: Required for over 300 biochemical reactions in the body, including energy production, muscle function, and protein synthesis. It also contributes to bone health and may help regulate blood sugar levels.

Iron: Necessary for the production of hemoglobin, which carries oxygen in the blood. Iron is also involved in energy metabolism and immune function.

Zinc: Essential for immune function, wound healing, and DNA synthesis. It also plays a role in taste perception and may have antioxidant properties.

Copper: Important for the formation of red blood cells and connective tissues. It also acts as an antioxidant and contributes to energy production.

Manganese: Required for bone formation, blood clotting, and energy metabolism. It also serves as a cofactor for several enzymes involved in antioxidant defense.

Incorporating endive into your diet can provide you with a diverse array of vitamins and minerals that support various aspects of health, including bone strength, immune function, and antioxidant protection.

Antioxidant-Rich

One of the standout features of endive is its impressive antioxidant content. Antioxidants help combat oxidative stress in the body, which can contribute to chronic diseases and premature aging. Endive contains compounds such as kaempferol and quercetin, which have been linked to various health benefits, including reduced inflammation and improved heart health. Incorporating endive into your diet can thus help bolster your body's defenses against oxidative damage and support overall well-being.

Here's a list of antioxidants found in endive and their benefits:

Kaempferol: This flavonoid antioxidant has anti-inflammatory properties and may help protect against chronic diseases such as heart disease and cancer. Kaempferol also exhibits neuroprotective effects and may support brain health.

Quercetin: Quercetin is a potent antioxidant with anti-inflammatory and antiviral properties. It may help reduce inflammation, lower blood pressure, and improve heart health. Quercetin also shows promise in supporting immune function and combating allergies.

Vitamin C: Ascorbic acid, or vitamin C, is a well-known antioxidant that plays a crucial role in immune function and collagen production. It helps protect cells from damage, supports wound healing, and enhances the absorption of iron from plant-based foods.

Vitamin E: Tocopherols, a group of compounds that include vitamin E, act as antioxidants, protecting cell membranes from oxidative damage. Vitamin E may help reduce the risk of chronic diseases such as heart disease and certain cancers. It also supports skin health and may have anti-aging effects.

Beta-carotene: Beta-carotene is a precursor to vitamin A and serves as a powerful antioxidant in its own right. It helps protect cells from damage caused by free radicals, supports immune function, and promotes healthy vision. Beta-carotene also contributes to skin health and may have anti-cancer properties.

Lutein and zeaxanthin: These carotenoid antioxidants are particularly beneficial for eye health. They help protect the eyes from age-related macular degeneration and cataracts by filtering harmful blue light and reducing oxidative damage to the retina.

Chlorogenic acid: Found in various fruits and vegetables, including endive, chlorogenic acid exhibits antioxidant and anti-inflammatory properties. It may help regulate blood sugar levels, support cardiovascular health, and protect against neurodegenerative diseases.

Incorporating endive into your diet can provide you with a diverse array of antioxidants that work synergistically to promote overall health and well-being. By reducing oxidative stress and inflammation, these antioxidants help protect against chronic diseases and support various bodily functions, from immune function to skin health and beyond.

Heart-Healthy

Endive's nutrient profile makes it a heart-healthy choice that can contribute to cardiovascular wellness. Its high potassium content helps regulate blood pressure by counteracting the effects of sodium, while its fiber content supports healthy cholesterol levels. Additionally, the presence of folate in endive is essential for metabolizing homocysteine, an amino acid that, when elevated, is associated with an increased risk of heart disease. By including endive in your meals, you can nourish your heart and promote cardiovascular health.

Nutritional Content

The nutritional content of 1 cup (approximately 50 grams) of endive typically includes:

- Carbohydrates: Less than 1 gram
- Protein: Less than 1 gram
- Fiber: Approximately 1.6 grams

- Fat: Less than 0.2 grams

Endive is a low-calorie, low-carbohydrate vegetable that is primarily composed of water and fiber. It contains minimal amounts of protein and fat. This nutritional profile makes endive an excellent choice for those following low-carb diets or looking to increase their fiber intake. Additionally, endive's high water content contributes to its hydrating properties and makes it a refreshing addition to salads and other dishes.

Culinary Versatility

Beyond its nutritional benefits, endive shines in the kitchen thanks to its versatility. Its crisp texture and slightly bitter flavor make it a refreshing addition to salads, providing a delightful contrast to sweeter ingredients like fruits or honey. Endive leaves also serve as excellent vessels for dips, fillings, and appetizers, offering a convenient and elegant way to present bite-sized snacks at gatherings and parties.

Additionally, endive can be cooked in various ways to bring out its unique flavor profile. Whether grilled, roasted, sautéed, or braised, endive develops a caramelized sweetness that complements savory dishes beautifully. It can be paired with ingredients like cheese, nuts, herbs, and citrus fruits to create complex and satisfying flavor combinations that tantalize the taste buds.

Here are two delicious recipes that incorporate endive:

Endive and Apple Salad with Walnuts and Blue Cheese:

Ingredients:

- 2 heads of endive, trimmed and thinly sliced
- 1 apple, thinly sliced
- 1/4 cup walnuts, chopped
- 2-3 tablespoons crumbled blue cheese
- 2 tablespoons extra-virgin olive oil
- 1 tablespoon apple cider vinegar
- 1 teaspoon honey
- Salt and pepper to taste

Instructions:

1. In a large bowl, combine the sliced endive, apple slices, chopped walnuts, and crumbled blue cheese.
2. In a small bowl, whisk together the extra-virgin olive oil, apple cider vinegar, honey, salt, and pepper to make the dressing.
3. Drizzle the dressing over the salad and toss gently to coat all the ingredients evenly.

4. Serve immediately as a refreshing and flavorful appetizer or side dish.

Grilled Endive with Balsamic Glaze:

Ingredients:

- 2 heads of endive, halved lengthwise
- 2 tablespoons extra-virgin olive oil
- Salt and pepper to taste
- Balsamic glaze for drizzling (store-bought or homemade)

Instructions:

1. Preheat your grill to medium-high heat.
2. Brush the cut sides of the endive halves with olive oil and season with salt and pepper.
3. Place the endive halves on the grill, cut side down, and cook for 3-4 minutes, or until lightly charred.
4. Carefully flip the endive halves and continue to grill for another 3-4 minutes, or until tender.
5. Transfer the grilled endive to a serving platter and drizzle with balsamic glaze.
6. Serve hot as a flavorful and elegant side dish or appetizer.

These recipes showcase the versatility of endive and its ability to add both flavor and nutrition to your meals. Whether enjoyed raw in a refreshing salad or grilled to perfection, endive is sure to delight your taste buds and impress your guests.

Tips on Growing Endive

The time it takes for endive to grow depends on several factors, including the variety of endive, growing conditions, and desired harvest size. Here's a detailed timeline of the typical growth stages of endive:

1. Seed Germination (7-14 days):

- Endive is typically grown from seeds, which are sown directly into the soil or started indoors and transplanted later.
- Germination usually occurs within 7 to 14 days under optimal conditions, including adequate moisture, warmth, and light.

2. Seedling Stage (2-4 weeks):

- After germination, endive seedlings emerge from the soil and begin to develop their first true leaves.

- During this stage, seedlings require consistent moisture and moderate temperatures to establish healthy root systems and foliage.

3. Vegetative Growth (4-6 weeks):

- As the seedlings mature, they enter a phase of vegetative growth, during which they develop additional leaves and establish a strong root system.
- Endive plants require regular watering and sufficient sunlight or artificial light to support healthy growth.

4. Head Formation (6-8 weeks):

- Endive leaves continue to grow and form a compact head or rosette at the center of the plant.
- The duration of this stage can vary depending on the specific variety of endive and growing conditions.

5. Harvesting (8-12 weeks):

- Endive can be harvested at various stages of maturity, depending on the desired size and flavor preferences.
- Baby endive leaves can be harvested as soon as they reach a usable size, typically within 8 to 10 weeks after planting.
- Full-sized endive heads are usually ready for harvest within 10 to 12 weeks after planting, once they have reached their mature size and developed a crisp texture.

Factors Affecting Growth Time:

- Temperature: Endive grows best in cool temperatures between 60°F and 70°F (15°C to 21°C). Warmer temperatures may accelerate growth, while extreme heat can cause bolting (premature flowering).
- Soil Conditions: Endive prefers well-draining, fertile soil with a pH between 6.0 and 7.0. Amending the soil with compost or organic matter can promote healthy growth.
- Watering: Consistent moisture is essential for endive growth, but overwatering can lead to root rot. Water the plants deeply and evenly, allowing the soil to dry slightly between waterings.
- Light: Endive requires ample sunlight or artificial light to photosynthesize and produce healthy foliage. Providing 6 to 8 hours of sunlight per day is ideal for optimal growth.

By following these guidelines and providing proper care, you can expect to harvest flavorful and nutritious endive within 8 to 12 weeks of planting, depending on the specific growing conditions and variety chosen.

Conclusion:

Endive may be an underappreciated vegetable, but its benefits and uses make it a valuable addition to any diet. From its nutritional richness to its culinary versatility, endive offers a plethora of reasons to incorporate it into your meals. Whether enjoyed raw in salads, cooked in savory dishes, or used as a creative garnish, endive has the potential to elevate your culinary creations while supporting your health and well-being. So why not give endive a try and unlock its full potential in your kitchen today?

If you have specific health concerns, allergies, or conditions, it's advisable to consult with a healthcare professional or a registered dietitian before making significant changes to your diet.

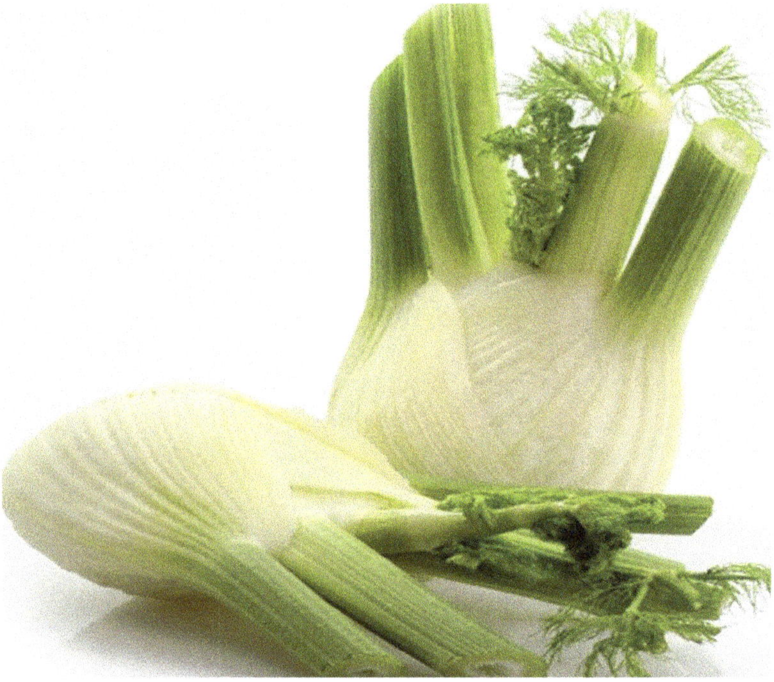

Fennel

The Wonders of Fennel

Fennel, an aromatic and flavorful herb native to the Mediterranean region, has been cherished for its culinary and medicinal properties for centuries. With its delicate fronds and crunchy bulb, fennel not only adds a unique flavor to dishes but also boasts a plethora of health benefits. Let's delve into the fascinating world of fennel, exploring its many virtues and versatile uses.

Nutritional Powerhouse

Fennel is a nutritional powerhouse packed with essential vitamins, minerals, and antioxidants. It is particularly rich in vitamin C, potassium, folate, and fiber, making it a valuable addition to a healthy diet. Its low calorie and high fiber content also make it a great choice for those looking to manage their weight and support digestive health.

Vitamin C:

- Benefits: Acts as a powerful antioxidant, supporting the immune system, promoting collagen production for healthy skin, and aiding in wound healing.

Potassium:

- Benefits: Essential for maintaining fluid balance, regulating blood pressure, supporting muscle function, and promoting heart health.

Folate (Vitamin B9):

- Benefits: Vital for DNA synthesis, cell division, and red blood cell formation, especially important during pregnancy for fetal development and preventing neural tube defects.

Calcium:

- Benefits: Essential for bone health, teeth strength, muscle function, nerve transmission, and blood clotting.

Magnesium:

- Benefits: Supports nerve function, muscle relaxation, bone health, regulates blood sugar levels, aids in energy metabolism, and contributes to cardiovascular health.

Manganese:

- Benefits: Acts as a cofactor for several enzymes involved in metabolism, bone formation, and antioxidant defense.

Iron:

- Benefits: Necessary for oxygen transport in the blood, energy production, immune function, and cognitive development.

Copper:

- Benefits: Plays a role in iron metabolism, collagen synthesis, nerve function, and antioxidant defense.

Zinc:

- Benefits: Essential for immune function, wound healing, DNA synthesis, cell division, and proper sense of taste and smell.

Phosphorus:

- Benefits: Important for bone and teeth health, energy metabolism, cell signaling, and maintaining pH balance in the body.

Vitamin A:

- Benefits: Essential for vision, immune function, skin health, reproduction, and cell communication.

Vitamin K:

- Benefits: Required for blood clotting, bone metabolism, and may have a role in heart health and regulating blood sugar levels.

Vitamin E:

- Benefits: Acts as an antioxidant, protecting cell membranes from damage, supporting immune function, and promoting skin health.

Riboflavin (Vitamin B2):

- Benefits: Important for energy metabolism, growth, red blood cell production, and maintaining healthy skin and vision.

Niacin (Vitamin B3):

- Benefits: Essential for energy metabolism, nervous system function, digestive health, and skin maintenance.

These vitamins and minerals found in fennel contribute to its overall health-promoting properties, making it a valuable addition to a balanced diet.

Digestive Aid:

One of fennel's most celebrated benefits is its ability to aid digestion. The natural compounds found in fennel, such as anethole, help relax the muscles of the digestive tract, reducing bloating, gas, and indigestion. Consuming fennel seeds or tea after meals is a time-honored tradition in many cultures to promote digestion and alleviate gastrointestinal discomfort.

Anti-inflammatory Properties:

Fennel contains potent anti-inflammatory compounds that can help reduce inflammation throughout the body. This makes it beneficial for conditions such as arthritis, asthma, and inflammatory bowel diseases. Regular consumption of fennel may contribute to overall wellness by combating chronic inflammation.

Rich in Antioxidants:

Antioxidants play a crucial role in protecting the body against oxidative stress and cellular damage caused by free radicals. Fennel is abundant in antioxidants like flavonoids, phenolic compounds, and vitamin C, which help neutralize free radicals and support cellular health. Incorporating fennel into your diet can thus contribute to a stronger immune system and reduced risk of chronic diseases.

Flavonoids:

- Benefits: Flavonoids are powerful antioxidants with anti-inflammatory properties. They may help reduce the risk of chronic diseases such as heart disease, cancer, and neurodegenerative disorders.

Phenolic Compounds:

- Benefits: Phenolic compounds exhibit antioxidant and anti-inflammatory effects, contributing to cardiovascular health, improved digestion, and reduced risk of chronic diseases.

Vitamin C:

- Benefits: Ascorbic acid (vitamin C) is a potent antioxidant that supports immune function, collagen synthesis, wound healing, and protects cells from oxidative damage.

Vitamin E:

- Benefits: Tocopherols and tocotrienols (forms of vitamin E) act as antioxidants, protecting cell membranes from oxidative damage, supporting immune function, and promoting skin health.

Beta-carotene:

- Benefits: Beta-carotene is a precursor to vitamin A and acts as a powerful antioxidant. It supports vision health, immune function, and may reduce the risk of certain cancers and cardiovascular diseases.

Lutein:

- Benefits: Lutein is a carotenoid antioxidant that plays a crucial role in eye health, protecting against age-related macular degeneration and cataracts.

Quercetin:

- Benefits: Quercetin is a flavonoid antioxidant with anti-inflammatory properties. It may help reduce allergy symptoms, lower blood pressure, and protect against heart disease and cancer.

Kaempferol:

- Benefits: Kaempferol is a flavonoid antioxidant known for its anti-inflammatory and cardioprotective effects. It may also have anticancer properties and support brain health.

Apigenin:

- Benefits: Apigenin is a flavonoid antioxidant with anti-inflammatory and anticancer properties. It may also have neuroprotective effects and support mental health.

Caffeic Acid:

- Benefits: Caffeic acid is a phenolic antioxidant that exhibits anti-inflammatory and antimicrobial properties. It may help protect against oxidative stress and reduce the risk of chronic diseases.

These antioxidants found in fennel contribute to its overall health-promoting properties, helping to protect cells from damage, reduce inflammation, and support various aspects of health and well-being. Incorporating fennel into your diet can be an excellent way to harness the benefits of these valuable antioxidants.

Culinary Delight:

Fennel's delightful flavor profile adds depth and complexity to a wide range of culinary creations. The bulb, stalks, fronds, and seeds are all edible and can be used in various dishes. The bulb can be sliced thinly and enjoyed raw in salads or roasted with other vegetables for a caramelized sweetness. The aromatic seeds can be toasted and ground to add a warm, anise-like flavor to soups, stews, bread, and desserts.

Here are two delicious recipes that feature fennel as a key ingredient:

Roasted Fennel and Parmesan Salad:

- **Ingredients:**
  - 2 fennel bulbs, trimmed and thinly sliced
  - 2 tablespoons olive oil
  - Salt and pepper to taste
  - 1/4 cup grated Parmesan cheese
  - 2 tablespoons lemon juice
  - 2 cups mixed greens (arugula, spinach, or your choice)
  - 1/4 cup toasted pine nuts
- **Instructions:**
  1. Preheat your oven to 400°F (200°C).
  2. In a large bowl, toss the sliced fennel with olive oil, salt, and pepper until evenly coated.
  3. Spread the fennel slices in a single layer on a baking sheet lined with parchment paper.
  4. Roast in the preheated oven for 20-25 minutes, or until the fennel is tender and lightly caramelized.

5. Remove from the oven and let cool slightly.
6. In a serving bowl, combine the roasted fennel with mixed greens.
7. Drizzle lemon juice over the salad and toss gently to combine.
8. Sprinkle grated Parmesan cheese and toasted pine nuts on top.
9. Serve immediately as a flavorful side dish or light lunch.

Sautéed Shrimp with Fennel and Garlic:

- **Ingredients:**
    0. 1 lb large shrimp, peeled and deveined
    1. 2 fennel bulbs, trimmed and thinly sliced
    2. 4 cloves garlic, minced
    3. 2 tablespoons olive oil
    4. Salt and pepper to taste
    5. 1/4 cup white wine (optional)
    6. Fresh parsley for garnish
- **Instructions:**
    1. Heat olive oil in a large skillet over medium heat.
    2. Add minced garlic and sliced fennel to the skillet, and sauté for 5-7 minutes, or until the fennel is softened and lightly browned.
    3. Season the shrimp with salt and pepper, then add them to the skillet with the fennel and garlic.
    4. Cook the shrimp for 2-3 minutes on each side, or until they turn pink and opaque.
    5. If using, pour white wine into the skillet and let it simmer for 1-2 minutes to deglaze the pan and reduce slightly.
    6. Remove from heat and garnish with fresh parsley.
    7. Serve the sautéed shrimp and fennel hot, accompanied by crusty bread or over cooked pasta, if desired.

These recipes showcase the versatility of fennel and highlight its unique flavor in both salads and main dishes. Enjoy experimenting with fennel in your cooking!

Versatile Uses: Beyond its culinary applications, fennel finds its way into herbal remedies and alternative therapies. Fennel tea, made by steeping crushed fennel seeds in hot water, is a popular remedy for digestive issues, menstrual cramps, and respiratory congestion. The essential oil extracted from fennel is used in aromatherapy for its calming and digestive properties.

Fennel

The time it takes for fennel to grow from seed to harvest can vary depending on various factors such as climate, soil conditions, and the specific variety of fennel being grown. However, on average, fennel takes approximately 80 to 100 days to reach maturity. Here's a detailed breakdown of the growth stages of fennel:

1. **Seed Germination (7-14 days):**
    - Fennel seeds typically germinate within 7 to 14 days under optimal conditions. During this stage, the seeds absorb water and sprout, forming seedlings.
2. **Seedling Stage (2-4 weeks):**
    - After germination, fennel enters the seedling stage, where the young plants develop their first true leaves and establish a root system. During this period, it's essential to ensure adequate moisture and sunlight for healthy growth.
3. **Vegetative Growth (4-6 weeks):**
    - As the seedlings mature, they continue to grow and develop more leaves, stems, and roots. Fennel plants require consistent watering and well-drained soil to thrive during this stage.
4. **Bulb Formation (6-10 weeks):**
    - Depending on the variety, some types of fennel produce a bulbous, edible base. Bulb formation typically occurs around 6 to 10 weeks after planting. During this period, the plants may require additional nutrients, such as nitrogen, to support bulb development.
5. **Maturation (10-14 weeks):**
    - Fennel reaches maturity approximately 10 to 14 weeks after planting. At this stage, the bulbs are fully developed and ready for harvest. The foliage may also become dense and lush.
6. **Harvesting:**
    - Fennel can be harvested once the bulbs have reached the desired size, typically about 3 to 4 inches in diameter for most varieties. Harvesting can be done by cutting the bulbs at ground level using a sharp knife or shears. It's essential to harvest fennel promptly to ensure optimal flavor and texture.

7. **Post-Harvest Care:**

    - After harvesting, remove any remaining foliage and roots from the plants. Fennel bulbs can be stored in the refrigerator for several weeks or used fresh in various culinary dishes. The seeds of fennel can also be harvested once the plant has matured and dried, typically around 100 to 120 days after planting.

By following these general timelines and care practices, you can successfully grow fennel and enjoy its flavorful bulbs, fronds, and seeds in your garden or culinary creations.

Conclusion:

Fennel's myriad benefits and versatile uses make it a cherished herb with a rich history and a promising future. Whether enjoyed in culinary creations, sipped as a soothing tea, or used medicinally, fennel continues to captivate hearts and palates around the world. Embrace the wonders of fennel and let its aromatic essence elevate your health and well-being.

If you have specific health concerns, allergies, or conditions, it's advisable to consult with a healthcare professional or a registered dietitian before making significant changes to your diet.

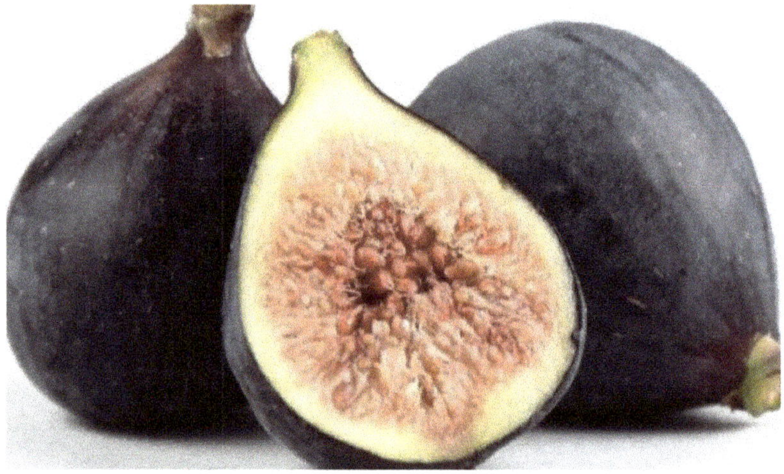

Figs
The Sweet Bounty of Nature

Exploring the Benefits and Uses of Figs

Figs, with their succulent sweetness and distinctive taste, have graced tables and delighted palates for centuries. Originating from the Middle East, these luscious fruits have not only been prized for their flavor but also for their numerous health benefits. In this article, we will delve into the rich tapestry of benefits that figs offer and explore the diverse ways in which they can be enjoyed.

Nutrient-Rich Goodness:

Figs are a nutrient-dense fruit, packed with a variety of essential vitamins and minerals that contribute to overall well-being. Here's a glimpse of the nutritional profile of figs:

Dietary Fiber: Figs are an excellent source of dietary fiber, promoting digestive health, aiding in weight management, and contributing to a feeling of fullness.

Vitamins:

Figs contain vitamins such as vitamin A, vitamin B6, niacin, riboflavin, and vitamin K, providing a spectrum of health benefits, including immune support, energy metabolism, and blood clotting.

Vitamin A: Essential for vision, immune function, and skin health. Figs contain beta-carotene, a precursor to vitamin A.

Vitamin B6 (Pyridoxine): Crucial for brain development, the production of neurotransmitters, and the metabolism of amino acids.

Niacin (Vitamin B3): Essential for DNA repair, energy metabolism, and the proper functioning of the nervous system.

Riboflavin (Vitamin B2): Plays a key role in energy production, cell growth, and the maintenance of healthy skin.

Folate (Vitamin B9): Important for DNA synthesis and cell division. Adequate folate intake is particularly important during pregnancy for fetal development.

Vitamin K: Crucial for blood clotting and bone health.

Vitamin C: An antioxidant that supports immune function, helps the body absorb iron, and promotes healthy skin.

Vitamin E: An antioxidant that helps protect cells from damage caused by free radicals.

Pantothenic Acid (Vitamin B5): Involved in the synthesis of fatty acids, amino acids, and other important molecules.

Choline: While not a vitamin, choline is an essential nutrient found in figs that plays a role in various bodily functions, including brain health and metabolism.

Figs' diverse vitamin profile makes them a valuable addition to a balanced and nutrient-rich diet. Including figs in your meals or snacks can contribute to meeting your daily vitamin requirements and promoting overall health.

Minerals:

Rich in essential minerals like potassium, magnesium, calcium, iron, and copper, figs contribute to bone health, blood pressure regulation, and oxygen transport in the body.

Potassium: Important for maintaining proper heart and muscle function, regulating fluid balance, and supporting overall cardiovascular health.

Calcium: Essential for bone and teeth health, blood clotting, and muscle function.

Magnesium: Crucial for muscle and nerve function, energy metabolism, and bone health.

Phosphorus: Vital for bone and teeth health, energy production, and acid-base balance.

Iron: Important for the formation of hemoglobin, which carries oxygen in the blood.

Copper: Involved in the formation of red blood cells, maintenance of bones and nerves, and the immune system.

Manganese: Plays a role in bone formation, blood clotting, and reducing inflammation.

Zinc: Essential for immune function, wound healing, and DNA synthesis.

Sodium: While sodium is typically present in smaller amounts, it is important for maintaining fluid balance and nerve function.

Selenium: An antioxidant that supports thyroid function and immune system health.

Phytosterols: While not a mineral, phytosterols are plant compounds found in figs that may contribute to heart health by lowering cholesterol levels.

Figs' diverse mineral content makes them a valuable addition to a balanced and nutrient-rich diet. Including figs in your meals or snacks can contribute to meeting your daily mineral requirements and promoting overall health.

Antioxidants:

Figs are loaded with antioxidants, including phenols and flavonoids, which help neutralize free radicals, protect cells from oxidative stress, and reduce inflammation.

Phenols: Figs contain various phenolic compounds, including chlorogenic acid, coumarins, and flavonoids, which contribute to their antioxidant properties.

Flavonoids: Figs are a source of flavonoids, such as quercetin, rutin, and catechins. These compounds have been associated with anti-inflammatory and antioxidant effects.

Carotenoids: Figs contain carotenoids, including beta-carotene, which is a precursor to vitamin A and has antioxidant properties.

Lutein and Zeaxanthin: These carotenoids found in figs contribute to eye health and have antioxidant functions.

Cryptoxanthin: Another carotenoid present in figs, cryptoxanthin, has antioxidant properties.

Vitamin C: Figs contain vitamin C, an antioxidant that supports immune function and helps protect cells from oxidative stress.

Vitamin E: Figs contain vitamin E, a fat-soluble antioxidant that helps protect cell membranes from oxidative damage.

Polyphenols: Figs are rich in polyphenols, which encompass a broad category of compounds with antioxidant and anti-inflammatory properties.

Chlorophyll: Chlorophyll, the green pigment in figs, has antioxidant properties and may contribute to overall health.

Quercetin: Found in figs, quercetin is a flavonoid with antioxidant and anti-inflammatory effects.

Epicatechin: An antioxidant flavonoid found in figs that contributes to their overall antioxidant capacity.

It's important to note that the antioxidant content of figs can vary depending on factors such as the variety of fig, ripeness, and growing conditions. Including a variety of antioxidant-rich foods, such as figs, in your diet can help support overall health and well-being.

Health Benefits:

Heart Health: The high potassium content in figs supports heart health by helping to regulate blood pressure and reduce the risk of cardiovascular diseases.

Digestive Health: The fiber in figs aids in digestion, prevents constipation, and supports a healthy gastrointestinal tract.

Weight Management: Figs, being a low-calorie and high-fiber fruit, can contribute to weight management by promoting satiety and reducing overall calorie intake.

Blood Sugar Control: The soluble fiber in figs helps regulate blood sugar levels, making them a suitable option for individuals managing diabetes.

Nutritional Content

Here's the approximate nutritional content in 1 cup (about 151 grams) of fresh figs:

- **Carbohydrates:** Around 39 grams
- **Protein:** Approximately 2 grams
- **Fiber:** Roughly 5.5 grams
- **Fat:** Less than 1 gram
- **Sugar:** About 29 grams

Please note that these values can vary slightly depending on factors such as the specific variety of figs and their ripeness. Figs are a nutritious fruit rich in fiber, vitamins, and minerals, making them a healthy addition to your diet.

Culinary Uses:

Figs' natural sweetness and versatility make them a delightful addition to a range of culinary creations. Here are some popular ways to enjoy figs:

Fresh and Raw: Enjoy figs in their purest form by eating them fresh and raw. Their natural sweetness is a treat on its own.

Salads: Slice figs and add them to salads for a burst of sweetness, complementing the savory elements. They pair well with greens, nuts, and cheese.

Preserves and Jams: Create delicious fig preserves or jams to spread on toast, pancakes, or as an accompaniment to cheeses.

Baking: Incorporate figs into baking recipes for muffins, cakes, and tarts. Their sweet and chewy texture adds depth to baked goods.

Dried Figs: Drying figs concentrates their sweetness, resulting in a chewy and flavorful snack. Dried figs can be enjoyed on their own or added to trail mixes.

Stuffed Figs: Stuff figs with ingredients like goat cheese, nuts, or honey for an elegant and tasty appetizer or dessert.

Figs' sweet and luscious flavor makes them a versatile ingredient in both savory and sweet dishes. ***Here are two delicious recipes featuring figs:***

Fig and Goat Cheese Salad with Balsamic Glaze:

Ingredients:

- 1 cup fresh figs, halved
- 4 cups mixed salad greens (arugula, spinach, or mixed greens)
- 1/2 cup crumbled goat cheese
- 1/3 cup chopped walnuts or pecans
- 2 tablespoons balsamic glaze
- 2 tablespoons extra-virgin olive oil
- Salt and pepper to taste

Instructions:

1. **Prepare the Salad:**
    - In a large salad bowl, combine the mixed greens, halved figs, crumbled goat cheese, and chopped nuts.
2. **Make the Dressing:**
    - In a small bowl, whisk together the balsamic glaze and extra-virgin olive oil. Season with salt and pepper to taste.
3. **Assemble the Salad:**
    - Drizzle the dressing over the salad and gently toss to coat the ingredients evenly.
4. **Serve:**
    - Divide the salad among individual plates.
    - Optionally, garnish with additional goat cheese and nuts.
5. **Enjoy a refreshing and flavorful Fig and Goat Cheese Salad as a light and satisfying appetizer or side dish.**

Honey-Roasted Figs with Vanilla Greek Yogurt:

Ingredients:

- 8-10 fresh figs, halved
- 2 tablespoons honey
- 1 teaspoon vanilla extract
- 1 cup Greek yogurt
- Fresh mint leaves for garnish

Instructions:

1. **Prepare the Figs:**
    - Preheat the oven to 375°F (190°C).
    - Place the halved figs on a baking sheet.
2. **Drizzle with Honey:**
    - Drizzle the figs with honey and sprinkle with vanilla extract.
3. **Roast the Figs:**
    - Roast the figs in the preheated oven for about 12-15 minutes or until they are soft and caramelized.
4. **Serve with Greek Yogurt:**
    - Spoon Greek yogurt onto serving plates.
    - Arrange the honey-roasted figs on top of the yogurt.
5. **Garnish and Serve:**
    - Garnish with fresh mint leaves for a burst of freshness.
6. Enjoy a delightful and simple dessert of Honey-Roasted Figs with Vanilla Greek Yogurt. The warm, caramelized figs paired with creamy yogurt create a perfect balance of flavors.

These recipes showcase the versatility of figs, whether used in a refreshing salad or a simple and elegant dessert. Feel free to customize these recipes based on your preferences and enjoy the unique and delightful taste of fresh figs.

Historical uses:

Figs have a rich history and have been cultivated and consumed by various civilizations for thousands of years. Here are two historical uses of figs:

Ancient Mediterranean and Middle Eastern Cultures:

Figs hold significant historical importance in the Mediterranean and Middle Eastern cultures, dating back to ancient times. In ancient Greece and Rome, figs were considered a staple food and were often used as a symbol of abundance and fertility. The cultivation of figs spread throughout the region, becoming an integral part of the Mediterranean diet.

Culinary Use:

- Figs were commonly used in both savory and sweet dishes. They were enjoyed fresh, dried, or preserved in honey.
- Figs were often incorporated into traditional Mediterranean desserts, and their sweet flavor made them a natural choice for enhancing the taste of various dishes.

Symbolism:

- In ancient Greek mythology, the fig tree was associated with Dionysus, the god of wine and revelry. Figs were considered a sacred fruit and were featured in religious rituals.
- Figs were also used symbolically in ancient Middle Eastern cultures, representing fertility and prosperity.

Traditional Medicine in Ancient Egypt:

Figs were valued not only for their culinary uses but also for their perceived medicinal properties in ancient civilizations. In ancient Egypt, figs were utilized in traditional medicine, and they held a place in the daily life of the people.

Medicinal Use:

- Figs were believed to have digestive benefits, and they were often recommended to treat digestive issues such as constipation.
- The latex from the fig tree, known as "milky juice," was used topically for various skin conditions and to promote wound healing.
- Ancient Egyptian healers recognized the potential health benefits of figs and incorporated them into their herbal remedies.

Religious Significance:

- Figs had religious significance in ancient Egyptian culture. The fig tree was associated with fertility, and the fruit was considered a symbol of life and abundance.
- Figs were often depicted in ancient Egyptian art and were featured in burial rituals, where they were placed in tombs as offerings for the deceased.

These historical uses of figs highlight their versatility in both culinary and medicinal contexts, as well as their cultural and symbolic significance in various ancient civilizations. Figs continue to be appreciated today for their rich flavor, nutritional benefits, and cultural importance.

Conclusion:

Figs, with their delectable taste and myriad health benefits, exemplify the bountiful offerings of nature. Whether enjoyed fresh, dried, or incorporated into various dishes, figs add a touch of sweetness and nutritional richness to our culinary experiences. If you have specific health concerns, allergies, or conditions, it's advisable to consult with a healthcare professional or a registered dietitian before making significant changes to your diet.

Embrace the versatility of figs and savor the wholesome goodness they bring to both the kitchen and the table. From enhancing heart health to tantalizing taste buds, figs stand as a testament to the delightful fusion of flavor and wellness in the world of fruits.

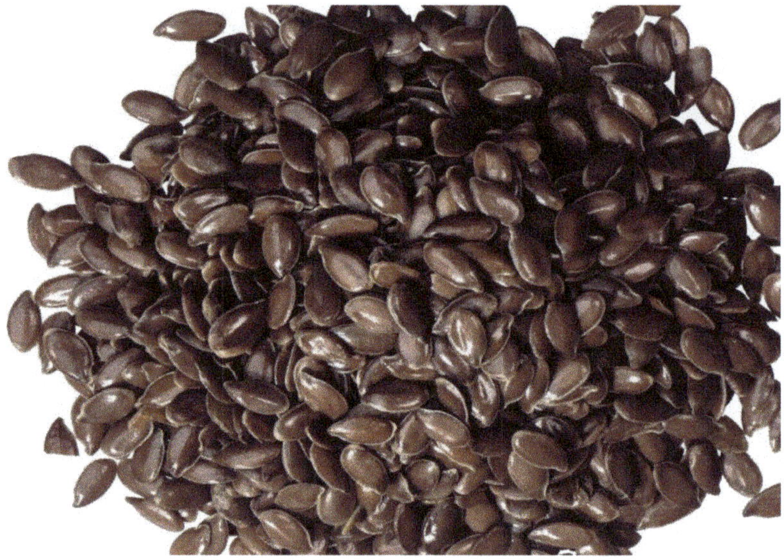

Flax Seed

The Power of Nature: Unveiling the Benefits and Versatile Uses of Flaxseed

Flaxseed, also known as linseed, has emerged as a nutritional powerhouse and versatile ingredient, celebrated for its numerous health benefits and culinary applications. Derived from the flax plant (Linum usitatissimum), flaxseed has been cultivated for centuries and cherished for its rich nutritional profile. In this article, we will explore the myriad benefits of flaxseed and discover the creative ways it can be incorporated into a balanced and wholesome diet.

Nutritional Content:

Flaxseed is a nutritional powerhouse, packed with essential nutrients that contribute to overall well-being. Here are some key components found in flaxseed:

Omega-3 Fatty Acids:

- **Benefits:**
    - Supports heart health by reducing inflammation and promoting healthy cholesterol levels.
    - Essential for brain function and may contribute to cognitive well-being.

Dietary Fiber:

- **Benefits:**
    - Aids in digestion and promotes regular bowel movements.
    - Contributes to a feeling of fullness, supporting weight management.

Lignans:

- **Benefits:**
    - Flaxseed is rich in lignans, which have antioxidant properties.
    - May have potential anti-cancer properties and hormonal balance benefits.

Protein:

- **Benefits:**
    - Provides a plant-based source of protein essential for muscle repair and overall body function.

Vitamins in Flaxseed:

Vitamin E:

- **Benefits:**
    - Acts as a powerful antioxidant, protecting cells from damage caused by free radicals.
    - Supports skin health and may contribute to a healthy immune system.

Vitamin B1 (Thiamine):

- **Benefits:**
    - Plays a crucial role in energy metabolism, helping convert food into energy.
    - Supports proper nerve function and overall nervous system health.

Vitamin B6 (Pyridoxine):

- **Benefits:**
    - Essential for brain development and function.
    - Aids in the synthesis of neurotransmitters, such as serotonin and dopamine.

Minerals in Flaxseed:

Manganese:

- **Benefits:**
    - Supports bone health and the formation of connective tissues.
    - Acts as a cofactor for various enzymes involved in energy metabolism.

Magnesium:

- **Benefits:**
    - Essential for muscle and nerve function.
    - Contributes to bone health and supports the body's energy production.

Phosphorus:

- **Benefits:**
    - Crucial for the formation and maintenance of strong bones and teeth.
    - Plays a role in energy metabolism and the synthesis of DNA and RNA.

Incorporating flaxseed into your diet provides these essential vitamins and minerals, contributing to overall health and supporting various physiological functions in the body. The nutrient-rich profile of flaxseed makes it a valuable addition to a balanced and wholesome diet.

Health Benefits:

Heart Health:

- The omega-3 fatty acids in flaxseed contribute to cardiovascular health by reducing inflammation and improving lipid profiles, thereby reducing the risk of heart disease.

Digestive Health:

- The high fiber content aids in digestive regularity, preventing constipation and promoting a healthy gut.

Weight Management:

- The combination of fiber and healthy fats in flaxseed contributes to a feeling of fullness, supporting weight management and reducing overeating.

Hormonal Balance:

- Lignans in flaxseed have been studied for their potential to balance hormones, particularly in women, and may offer benefits for conditions like menopausal symptoms.

Culinary Uses:

Ground Flaxseed in Smoothies:

- Add a tablespoon of ground flaxseed to your morning smoothies for an extra boost of fiber, omega-3s, and a nutty flavor.

Flaxseed Oil in Salad Dressings:

- Incorporate flaxseed oil into homemade salad dressings for a light, nutty taste and a dose of heart-healthy omega-3s.

Flaxseed in Baking:

- Use ground flaxseed as an egg substitute in baking recipes for a vegan-friendly option that adds moisture and nutritional value.

Flaxseed in Yogurt or Oatmeal:

- Sprinkle ground flaxseed over yogurt or oatmeal to enhance the texture and provide a nutrient boost.

Here are 2 recipe using flaxseed:

Flaxseed and Banana Smoothie:

- **Ingredients:**
    - 1 ripe banana
    - 1 cup almond milk (or any milk of your choice)
    - 1 tablespoon ground flaxseed
    - 1 tablespoon almond butter
    - 1/2 teaspoon cinnamon
    - Ice cubes (optional)
- **Instructions:**

1. In a blender, combine the ripe banana, almond milk, ground flaxseed, almond butter, and cinnamon.
2. Blend until smooth and creamy.
3. If desired, add ice cubes and blend again for a refreshing chill.
4. Pour into a glass and sprinkle a little extra ground flaxseed on top for added texture.
5. Enjoy this nutrient-packed flaxseed and banana smoothie as a delicious and satisfying breakfast or snack.

Flaxseed-Coated Baked Chicken Tenders:

- **Ingredients:**
    - 1 pound chicken tenders
    - 2 tablespoons ground flaxseed

  - 1/4 cup whole wheat flour
  - 1 teaspoon paprika
  - 1/2 teaspoon garlic powder
  - Salt and pepper to taste
  - 2 eggs, beaten
  - Cooking spray

- **Instructions:**

1. Preheat the oven to 400°F (200°C) and line a baking sheet with parchment paper.
2. In a shallow bowl, combine ground flaxseed, whole wheat flour, paprika, garlic powder, salt, and pepper.
3. Dip each chicken tender into the beaten eggs, then coat evenly with the flaxseed mixture, pressing gently to adhere.
4. Place the coated chicken tenders on the prepared baking sheet.
5. Lightly spray the tops of the tenders with cooking spray to promote browning.
6. Bake in the preheated oven for 15-20 minutes or until the chicken is cooked through and the coating is crispy.
7. Serve the flaxseed-coated baked chicken tenders with your favorite dipping sauce for a nutritious twist on a classic dish.

These recipes showcase the versatility of flaxseed, whether incorporated into a nutrient-packed smoothie or used as a coating for baked chicken tenders. Enjoy the benefits of flaxseed in delicious and creative ways as part of a healthy and balanced diet.

Historical Uses:

Flaxseed has a long history of traditional use for various purposes. Here are two historical uses of flaxseed:

Ancient Medicinal and Culinary Uses:

Flaxseed has been cultivated for thousands of years, dating back to ancient civilizations such as those in Mesopotamia and Egypt. In ancient times, flaxseed was valued for both its medicinal properties and its culinary uses. Ancient Egyptians used flaxseed as a dietary staple and also applied it topically for its soothing properties on the skin. Additionally, historical records indicate that flaxseed was used as a remedy for digestive issues, such as constipation, and as a poultice for external wounds and inflammation.

Traditional Fiber Production:

Historically, flaxseed was primarily cultivated for the production of fiber, specifically linen. Flax fibers extracted from the stem of the flax plant were spun and woven into linen textiles, which were highly prized for their strength, durability, and versatility. Linen fabric was used for clothing, bedding, household textiles, and even as a form of currency in some ancient societies. Flaxseed cultivation played a crucial role in the economy and trade of many civilizations throughout history, particularly in regions with suitable climate conditions for flax cultivation.

These historical uses of flaxseed highlight its significance as a versatile and valuable plant with applications in medicine, nutrition, and textile production throughout human history.

Conclusion:

Flaxseed stands as a testament to the nutritional benefits that nature offers. From promoting heart health to supporting digestive well-being and hormonal balance, flaxseed has rightfully earned its place as a superfood in the realm of healthy living. It's crucial to emphasize that most people can safely enjoy flaxseed as part of a balanced diet. If you have specific health concerns or are taking medications, it's advisable to consult with a healthcare professional before making significant changes to your diet. Embrace the versatility of flaxseed by incorporating it into your daily meals and unlock the myriad benefits that this small seed has to offer. Whether ground, in oil form, or as a baking ingredient, flaxseed invites you to harness the power of nature for a nourished and vibrant life.

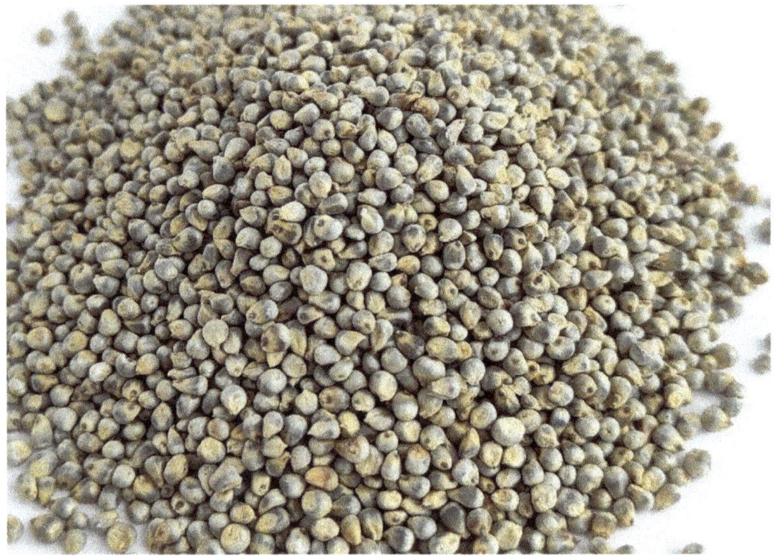

Fonio

The Ancient Grain with Modern Appeal

In recent years, there has been a growing interest in ancient grains and traditional foods that offer both nutritional benefits and culinary versatility. Among these ancient grains, fonio stands out as a nutrient-rich, gluten-free grain with a long history of cultivation in West Africa. While fonio may be lesser-known in many parts of the world, its impressive nutritional profile and culinary potential are gaining attention globally. Let's delve into the benefits and uses of this remarkable grain.

Nutritional Benefits

Fonio, scientifically known as Digitaria exilis and Digitaria iburua, is a species of millet that has been cultivated for thousands of years in West Africa, particularly in countries like Senegal, Mali, Nigeria, and Guinea. Despite its small size, fonio packs a nutritional punch:

Rich in Protein: Fonio is a complete protein, containing all nine essential amino acids that the body needs for muscle growth, repair, and overall health. This makes it an excellent source of plant-based protein, particularly for individuals following vegetarian or vegan diets.

High in Fiber: Fonio is rich in dietary fiber, which promotes digestive health, aids in weight management, and helps regulate blood sugar levels. Fiber also contributes to feelings of fullness and satiety, making fonio a satisfying and nutritious food choice.

Gluten-Free: Fonio is naturally gluten-free, making it suitable for individuals with celiac disease, gluten sensitivity, or those who choose to follow a gluten-free diet. It provides a safe and nutritious alternative to wheat and other gluten-containing grains.

Packed with Nutrients

Fonio is a good source of essential vitamins and minerals, including iron, zinc, magnesium, phosphorus, and B vitamins. These nutrients play key roles in various bodily functions, such as energy metabolism, immune function, and bone health.

Vitamins:

Vitamin B1 (Thiamine): Essential for energy metabolism, nerve function, and carbohydrate metabolism.

Vitamin B2 (Riboflavin): Important for energy production, red blood cell formation, and antioxidant activity.

Vitamin B3 (Niacin): Supports energy metabolism, DNA repair, and skin health.

Vitamin B6 (Pyridoxine): Necessary for amino acid metabolism, neurotransmitter synthesis, and immune function.

Vitamin B9 (Folate): Vital for DNA synthesis, cell division, and fetal development during pregnancy.

Vitamin E: Provides antioxidant properties that protect cells from oxidative damage and support immune function.

Minerals:

Iron: Essential for oxygen transport in the blood and energy production.

Zinc: Supports immune function, wound healing, and DNA synthesis.

Magnesium: Important for muscle and nerve function, bone health, and blood sugar regulation.

Phosphorus: Necessary for bone and teeth formation, energy metabolism, and cell membrane structure.

Potassium: Helps regulate blood pressure, fluid balance, and muscle contractions.

Calcium: Crucial for bone and teeth health, muscle function, and nerve transmission.

Antioxidants:

Phenolic Compounds: Have antioxidant properties that help neutralize free radicals and reduce oxidative stress, potentially lowering the risk of chronic diseases such as heart disease and cancer.

Flavonoids: Provide anti-inflammatory and antioxidant effects, supporting heart health, brain function, and immune function.

Carotenoids: Act as antioxidants, protecting cells from damage caused by harmful free radicals.

Amino Acids:

Essential Amino Acids: Fonio contains all nine essential amino acids, including:

- **Lysine:** Important for protein synthesis, collagen production, and calcium absorption.
- **Methionine:** Provides sulfur for various biochemical processes, including protein synthesis and metabolism.
- **Threonine:** Supports immune function, collagen production, and fat metabolism.
- **Tryptophan:** Precursor to serotonin, a neurotransmitter that regulates mood and sleep.
- **Valine, Leucine, Isoleucine (Branched-Chain Amino Acids):** Essential for muscle growth, repair, and energy production.
- **Histidine:** Important for growth and development in infants and for maintaining healthy tissues in adults.

Low Glycemic Index:

Fonio has a low glycemic index, meaning it causes a gradual rise in blood sugar levels compared to high-glycemic foods. This makes it an ideal choice for individuals managing diabetes or those looking to maintain stable blood sugar levels.

Nutritional Content

The exact nutritional content can vary slightly depending on factors such as processing methods and brand, but here's an approximate breakdown of the nutritional content in 1 cup (about 170 grams) of cooked fonio:

- Carbohydrates: Approximately 41-43 grams
- Protein: Approximately 2-3 grams
- Fiber: Approximately 1-2 grams
- Fat: Approximately 0.5-1 gram
- Calories: Approximately 170-200 calories

Please note that these values are approximate and can vary. Additionally, if you are using raw fonio, the values may differ as well.

Culinary Uses:

Fonio has been a staple food in West African cuisine for centuries, prized for its nutritional value, quick cooking time, and versatility in recipes. Here are some popular culinary uses of fonio:

Fonio Porridge: Fonio can be cooked into a creamy porridge by simmering it with water or milk and sweetening it with honey, sugar, or fruit. Fonio porridge is a comforting and nourishing breakfast dish enjoyed in many West African countries.

Fonio Pilaf: Fonio can be cooked pilaf-style by sautéing it with onions, garlic, and spices before adding broth and simmering until tender. Fonio pilaf makes a flavorful and satisfying side dish or base for hearty main courses.

Fonio Salad: Cooked fonio can be cooled and tossed with a variety of fresh vegetables, herbs, nuts, and dressing to create a refreshing and nutritious salad. Fonio salad is perfect for light lunches or as a side dish for summer gatherings.

Fonio Flour: Fonio can be ground into flour and used in baking recipes to make bread, pancakes, muffins, and other baked goods. Fonio flour adds a nutty flavor and delicate texture to baked treats while boosting their nutritional value.

Fonio Soup: Fonio grains can be added to soups, stews, and broths to add texture, thickness, and nutritional content. Fonio soup is a hearty and comforting dish enjoyed across West Africa, often featuring a variety of vegetables, meats, and spices.

Here are two recipes that use fonio:

Fonio Salad with Vegetables:

Ingredients:

- 1 cup fonio
- 2 cups water or vegetable broth
- 1 cucumber, diced
- 1 tomato, diced
- 1 bell pepper, diced
- 1/4 cup red onion, finely chopped
- 1/4 cup fresh parsley, chopped
- Juice of 1 lemon
- 2 tablespoons olive oil
- Salt and pepper to taste

Instructions:

1. Rinse the fonio under cold water to remove any debris. Drain well.
2. In a saucepan, bring the water or vegetable broth to a boil. Add the rinsed fonio, reduce heat to low, cover, and simmer for about 5 minutes or until the fonio is cooked and water is absorbed. Fluff the fonio with a fork and let it cool slightly.
3. In a large mixing bowl, combine the cooked fonio, diced cucumber, tomato, bell pepper, red onion, and chopped parsley.
4. In a small bowl, whisk together the lemon juice, olive oil, salt, and pepper to make the dressing.
5. Pour the dressing over the salad ingredients and toss gently to coat everything evenly.
6. Taste and adjust seasoning if needed. Serve the fonio salad immediately or chill it in the refrigerator for a couple of hours before serving.

Fonio Porridge with Coconut Milk:

Ingredients:

- 1 cup fonio
- 2 cups coconut milk
- 1/4 teaspoon ground cinnamon
- 1 tablespoon honey or maple syrup (optional)
- Fresh fruit for topping (such as sliced bananas, berries, or mango)

Instructions:

1. Rinse the fonio under cold water and drain well.
2. In a saucepan, combine the coconut milk and fonio. Bring to a simmer over medium heat.
3. Reduce the heat to low, cover, and let the fonio cook for about 5-7 minutes, stirring occasionally, until it absorbs the coconut milk and reaches a creamy consistency.
4. Stir in the ground cinnamon and sweeten with honey or maple syrup if desired.
5. Serve the fonio porridge hot, topped with your choice of fresh fruit.

Enjoy these delicious fonio recipes!

Historical Uses

Fonio has a rich history of traditional uses, especially in West Africa, where it's been cultivated for centuries. Here are two historical uses of fonio:

Culinary Staple: Fonio has been a staple food in West African cuisines for thousands of years. It's often used to make various dishes such as porridges, couscous-like side dishes, flatbreads, and even fermented beverages. Its versatility and nutritional value have made it a crucial part of the diet in regions where it's grown. Fonio grains were traditionally hand-pounded to remove the husks before being ground into flour or cooked whole.

Cultural and Ceremonial Significance: Fonio holds cultural significance in many West African societies. It's not just a food source but also plays a role in traditional ceremonies, rituals, and social gatherings. For example, in some cultures, fonio may be used in religious ceremonies or offered as a symbol of hospitality and goodwill during communal feasts and celebrations. Its presence in various cultural practices underscores its importance beyond mere sustenance and highlights its deep-rooted connection to the cultural fabric of the region.

Conclusion:

Fonio is a versatile and nutritious grain with a rich history and a promising future. Whether enjoyed as breakfast porridge, a savory pilaf, or a gluten-free flour in baking, fonio offers endless culinary possibilities. As global interest in diverse and sustainable foods continues to grow, fonio's role in promoting health and culinary innovation is sure to expand, making it a grain worth exploring and incorporating into a balanced diet.

If you have specific health concerns, allergies, or conditions, it's advisable to consult with a healthcare professional or a registered dietitian before making significant changes to your diet.

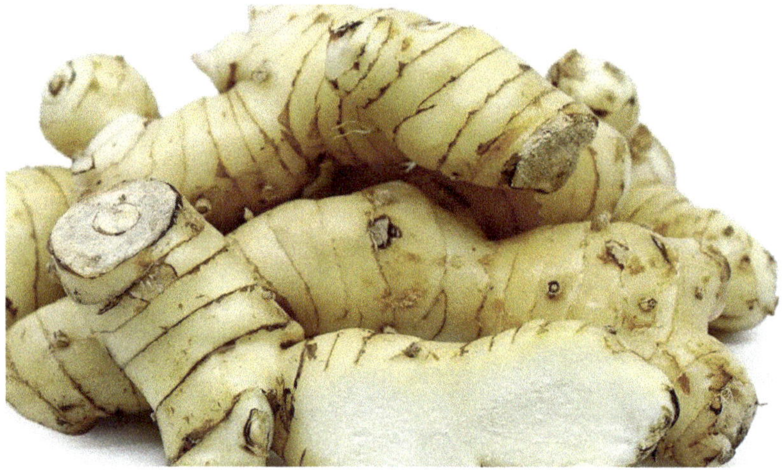

Galangal

Galangal: Exploring Its Wonders in Health and Cuisine

Galangal, with its aromatic fragrance and unique flavor, has been cherished for centuries in various cultures for its culinary and medicinal properties. This rhizomatous herb, belonging to the ginger family, is native to Southeast Asia and is widely used in traditional Asian cuisines as well as herbal medicine. Let's delve into the world of galangal and uncover its myriad benefits and uses.

A Closer Look at Galangal

Galangal (Alpinia galanga) is a perennial plant characterized by its knobby rhizomes, which resemble ginger root but have a distinct spicy, citrusy flavor. There are two main varieties of galangal: greater galangal (Alpinia galanga) and lesser galangal (Alpinia officinarum). While greater galangal is more commonly used in cooking, both varieties offer similar health benefits.

Nutritional Profile and Health Benefits

Galangal is not only prized for its culinary appeal but also for its potential health-promoting properties. Here are some of the key benefits of galangal:

Digestive Health: Galangal has long been used in traditional medicine to support digestive health. It contains compounds that stimulate digestive enzymes, promote bile production, and alleviate symptoms of indigestion, bloating, and nausea.

Anti-inflammatory and Antioxidant Properties: Galangal contains bioactive compounds such as flavonoids and phenolic acids, which possess anti-inflammatory and antioxidant properties. These compounds help reduce inflammation, neutralize free radicals, and protect against oxidative stress, thus supporting overall health and longevity.

Immune Support: Galangal is rich in immune-boosting nutrients such as vitamins C and A, as well as minerals like iron and zinc. These nutrients help strengthen the immune system, enhance immune response to infections, and protect against colds, flu, and other illnesses.

Antimicrobial Activity: Galangal exhibits antimicrobial activity against various pathogens, including bacteria, viruses, and fungi. It contains compounds such as galangin and alpinin, which have been shown to inhibit the growth of harmful microorganisms and support immune function.

Anti-Cancer Potential: Preliminary research suggests that galangal may have anti-cancer properties, thanks to its ability to inhibit the growth and spread of cancer cells. Certain compounds found in galangal, such as galangin and 1'-acetoxychavicol acetate (ACA), have shown promising results in laboratory studies for their potential anti-cancer effects.

Culinary Uses

In addition to its medicinal properties, galangal is prized for its culinary versatility and unique flavor profile. Here are some popular culinary uses of galangal:

Soups and Curries: Galangal is a key ingredient in many Southeast Asian soups, stews, and curries, imparting a warm, spicy flavor and aromatic fragrance to dishes such as Tom Yum soup and Thai green curry.

Stir-fries and Stir-fry Pastes: Galangal is often used in stir-fries and stir-fry pastes, adding depth of flavor and complexity to dishes such as Indonesian sambal and Malaysian rendang.

Marinades and Sauces: Galangal can be finely grated or pounded into marinades and sauces, infusing meats, seafood, and vegetables with its distinctive taste and aroma.

Herbal Teas and Infusions: Galangal tea is a popular herbal remedy for digestive complaints, colds, and flu. Simply steep sliced galangal rhizome in hot water for a soothing and aromatic beverage.

Here are two delicious recipes featuring galangal:

Thai Coconut Soup with Galangal (Tom Kha Gai):

- **Ingredients:**
  - 2 cups chicken broth or vegetable broth
  - 1 can (13.5 oz) coconut milk
  - 1 stalk lemongrass, bruised and chopped into 2-inch pieces
  - 3-4 slices galangal (about 1-inch each)
  - 2-3 kaffir lime leaves, torn into pieces
  - 2 boneless, skinless chicken breasts, thinly sliced

- 1 cup sliced mushrooms (such as straw mushrooms or cremini mushrooms)
- 1 tablespoon fish sauce
- 1 tablespoon lime juice
- 1 teaspoon palm sugar or brown sugar
- 2-3 Thai bird's eye chilies, thinly sliced (optional)
- Fresh cilantro leaves, for garnish
- Sliced red chili peppers, for garnish (optional)

- **Instructions:**

1. In a large pot, combine the chicken broth, coconut milk, lemongrass, galangal, and kaffir lime leaves. Bring to a gentle simmer over medium heat.
2. Add the sliced chicken breasts and mushrooms to the pot. Cook for 5-7 minutes, or until the chicken is cooked through and the mushrooms are tender.
3. Stir in the fish sauce, lime juice, palm sugar, and sliced Thai bird's eye chilies (if using). Taste and adjust seasoning as needed.
4. Remove the lemongrass stalks, galangal slices, and kaffir lime leaves from the soup before serving.
5. Ladle the soup into bowls and garnish with fresh cilantro leaves and sliced red chili peppers, if desired. Serve hot and enjoy!

Indonesian Beef Rendang with Galangal:

- **Ingredients:**

0. 1.5 lbs beef chuck, cut into bite-sized pieces
1. 2 tablespoons vegetable oil
2. 1 onion, finely chopped
3. 4 cloves garlic, minced
4. 3-4 slices galangal (about 1-inch each)
5. 2 lemongrass stalks, bruised and chopped into 2-inch pieces
6. 4 kaffir lime leaves
7. 1 can (13.5 oz) coconut milk
8. 1 cup beef broth
9. 2 tablespoons tamarind paste

10. 2 tablespoons palm sugar or brown sugar
11. Salt, to taste
12. Sliced red chili peppers, for garnish (optional)
13. Fresh cilantro leaves, for garnish

- **Instructions:**

1. Heat the vegetable oil in a large pot or Dutch oven over medium heat. Add the chopped onion and minced garlic, and cook until softened and fragrant.
2. Add the beef pieces to the pot and brown on all sides, about 5-7 minutes.
3. Stir in the sliced galangal, lemongrass stalks, and kaffir lime leaves. Cook for another 2-3 minutes.
4. Pour in the coconut milk and beef broth. Stir in the tamarind paste and palm sugar. Season with salt to taste.
5. Bring the mixture to a simmer, then reduce the heat to low. Cover and cook for 2-3 hours, or until the beef is tender and the sauce has thickened.
6. Remove the lemongrass stalks, galangal slices, and kaffir lime leaves from the pot before serving.
7. Garnish the beef rendang with sliced red chili peppers and fresh cilantro leaves. Serve hot with steamed rice or your favorite side dishes. Enjoy the rich and aromatic flavors of this Indonesian classic!

These recipes showcase the unique flavor and versatility of galangal, adding depth and complexity to dishes from different cuisines. Whether you're craving a comforting soup or a hearty beef stew, galangal is sure to elevate your culinary creations with its aromatic charm.

Incorporating Galangal into Your Life

Whether used in cooking, herbal medicine, or as a dietary supplement, galangal offers a myriad of benefits for health and well-being. You can find fresh galangal rhizomes, dried galangal slices, galangal powder, and galangal supplements in specialty grocery stores, Asian markets, and health food stores.

Incorporate galangal into your culinary creations to add depth of flavor and aromatic complexity to your dishes or brew a cup of galangal tea to soothe digestion and boost immunity. With its rich history, tantalizing flavor, and potent health benefits, galangal is truly a treasure worth exploring in both the kitchen and the medicine cabinet.

If you have specific health concerns, allergies, or conditions, it's advisable to consult with a healthcare professional or a registered dietitian before making significant changes to your diet.

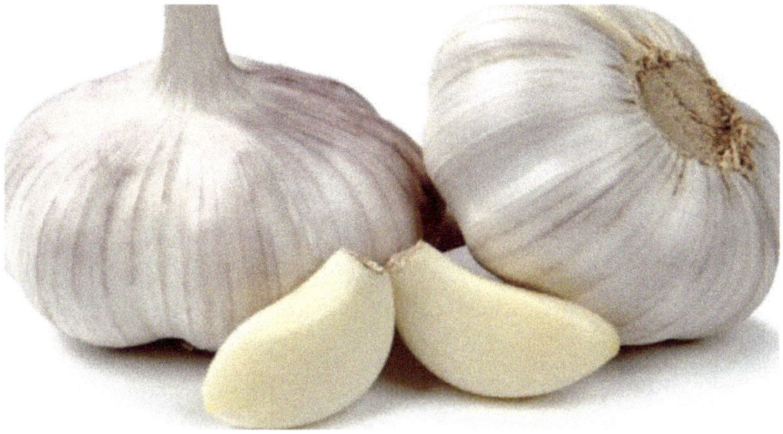

Garlic

Unveiling the Golden Clove: Exploring the Benefits and Versatility of Garlic

Garlic (Allium sativum), a bulbous flowering plant in the genus Allium, with its pungent aroma and distinctive flavor, has been cherished for centuries not only as a culinary staple but also as a powerhouse of health benefits. From ancient remedies to modern gourmet cuisine, garlic has maintained its status as a versatile and revered ingredient across cultures worldwide. Let's peel back the layers and uncover the myriad benefits and uses of this humble yet extraordinary herb.

Nutritional Powerhouse

Beyond its culinary appeal, garlic boasts an impressive nutritional profile. Rich in vitamins C and B6, manganese, and selenium, garlic provides essential nutrients that support overall health and well-being. Moreover, garlic contains potent sulfur compounds, including allicin, which exhibit antioxidant, anti-inflammatory, and antimicrobial properties. These bioactive compounds are believed to contribute to many of garlic's health benefits.

Vitamins:

Vitamin C: Garlic contains vitamin C, which is an essential nutrient known for its immune-boosting properties. It helps strengthen the immune system, promotes collagen production for healthy skin, and acts as a powerful antioxidant that protects cells from damage caused by free radicals.

Vitamin B6 (Pyridoxine):

Benefits:

- Plays a crucial role in brain development and function by aiding the synthesis of neurotransmitters such as serotonin and dopamine.
- Supports energy metabolism by helping convert food into energy.

- Contributes to the production of red blood cells and helps regulate homocysteine levels, which may reduce the risk of cardiovascular disease.
- Supports immune function and may help alleviate symptoms of premenstrual syndrome (PMS).

Vitamin B1 (Thiamine):

Benefits:

- Plays a vital role in energy metabolism by converting carbohydrates into energy.
- Supports nerve function and helps maintain a healthy nervous system.
- Required for the production of adenosine triphosphate (ATP), the primary energy currency of cells.
- May help improve cognitive function and protect against age-related cognitive decline.

Vitamin B5 (Pantothenic Acid):

Benefits:

- Essential for the synthesis of coenzyme A (CoA), which is involved in numerous metabolic pathways, including the production of energy from fats, proteins, and carbohydrates.
- Supports adrenal function and helps regulate the body's response to stress.
- Contributes to the synthesis of hormones and cholesterol, as well as the formation of red blood cells.

Vitamin B3 (Niacin):

Benefits:

- Plays a crucial role in energy metabolism by facilitating the conversion of carbohydrates, fats, and proteins into usable energy.
- Helps maintain healthy skin, nerves, and digestive system.
- Supports cardiovascular health by helping to lower LDL cholesterol levels and raise HDL cholesterol levels.
- May help improve joint mobility and alleviate symptoms of osteoarthritis.

Minerals:

Manganese: Garlic is a good source of manganese, a trace mineral that plays a role in bone health, metabolism, and antioxidant defense mechanisms. It also supports the formation of connective tissues and may contribute to wound healing.

Calcium: While not present in significant amounts, garlic does contain small amounts of calcium, which is crucial for bone health, muscle function, nerve transmission, and blood clotting.

Phosphorus: Garlic provides phosphorus, another essential mineral that supports bone and teeth health, helps in energy metabolism, and is involved in the formation of DNA and cell membranes.

Selenium: Garlic contains selenium, an important antioxidant mineral that helps protect cells from oxidative damage, supports thyroid function, and contributes to a healthy immune system.

Antioxidants:

Allicin: One of the key bioactive compounds in garlic, allicin, is formed when garlic is crushed or chopped. Allicin is known for its potent antimicrobial and antioxidant properties, helping to combat infections, reduce inflammation, and protect against oxidative stress.

Sulfur Compounds: Garlic contains sulfur compounds such as diallyl sulfide, diallyl disulfide, and diallyl trisulfide, which contribute to its distinct aroma and numerous health benefits. These compounds have been linked to potential anticancer effects, cardiovascular health, and detoxification processes in the body.

Flavonoids: Garlic contains flavonoids like quercetin and kaempferol, which have antioxidant and anti-inflammatory properties. Flavonoids may help reduce the risk of chronic diseases such as heart disease and certain types of cancer, as well as support overall health and well-being.

Health Benefits:

Garlic has long been revered for its potential health-promoting properties. Here are some of the key benefits supported by scientific research:

Heart Health: Garlic may help support cardiovascular health by promoting healthy cholesterol levels, regulating blood pressure, and reducing the risk of blood clot formation. Its ability to improve circulation and lower levels of LDL cholesterol ("bad" cholesterol) makes it a valuable ally in maintaining heart health.

Immune Support: Garlic's antimicrobial properties make it a popular natural remedy for fighting infections, including the common cold and flu. It has been shown to enhance immune function, helping the body defend against pathogens and reduce the severity and duration of illness.

Antioxidant Activity: The sulfur compounds in garlic act as potent antioxidants, scavenging free radicals and protecting cells from oxidative damage. By neutralizing harmful molecules that contribute to aging and disease, garlic may help reduce the risk of chronic conditions such as cancer and neurodegenerative diseases.

Digestive Health: Garlic has been traditionally used to promote digestive health and alleviate gastrointestinal discomfort. It may help stimulate digestion, support beneficial gut bacteria, and alleviate symptoms of bloating and indigestion.

Anti-inflammatory Effects: Chronic inflammation is linked to various health issues, including arthritis, cardiovascular disease, and autoimmune disorders. Garlic's anti-inflammatory properties may help reduce inflammation in the body, potentially offering relief from inflammatory conditions and supporting overall health.

Antibiotic Potential:

Diallyl sulfide, a garlic compound, outperformed popular antibiotics against the Campylobacter bacterium, showcasing potential antibiotic power.

Culinary Marvel

One of garlic's most celebrated attributes is its culinary versatility. Whether minced, sliced, crushed, or roasted, garlic adds depth and complexity to a wide range of dishes. From savory sauces and marinades to soups, stir-fries, and roasted vegetables, its robust flavor elevates the taste profile of countless recipes. Additionally, garlic can be infused into oils, pickled, or even fermented to create uniquely flavored condiments and spreads.

Incorporating Garlic into Your Diet: Adding garlic to your daily diet is easy and delicious. Here are some simple ways to incorporate this flavorful herb into your meals:

- **Sautéed or roasted:** Add minced or sliced garlic to stir-fries, sautéed vegetables, or roasted meats for an extra burst of flavor.
- **Raw:** Enjoy garlic raw in salads, dips, and dressings for a potent dose of its health-promoting compounds.
- **Infused oils and spreads:** Create infused garlic oils or spreads to drizzle over bread, pasta, or grilled vegetables.
- **Soups and stews:** Enhance the flavor of soups, stews, and sauces by adding crushed or chopped garlic during cooking.
- **Pickled or fermented:** Experiment with pickled or fermented garlic to add tangy flavor and probiotic benefits to your meals.

Here are two delicious recipes that feature garlic as a key ingredient:

Garlic Butter Shrimp:

Ingredients:

- 1 pound (about 450g) large shrimp, peeled and deveined
- 4 cloves garlic, minced
- 4 tablespoons unsalted butter
- 2 tablespoons olive oil

- 2 tablespoons fresh parsley, chopped
- Salt and pepper to taste
- Lemon wedges for serving

Instructions:

1. In a large skillet, heat the olive oil and 2 tablespoons of butter over medium-high heat.
2. Add the minced garlic to the skillet and sauté for about 1 minute until fragrant.
3. Add the shrimp to the skillet and season with salt and pepper. Cook the shrimp for 2-3 minutes on each side until they turn pink and opaque.
4. Once the shrimp are cooked through, add the remaining 2 tablespoons of butter to the skillet and stir until melted.
5. Remove the skillet from heat and sprinkle chopped parsley over the shrimp. Toss gently to coat the shrimp with the garlic butter sauce.
6. Serve the garlic butter shrimp hot with lemon wedges on the side. Enjoy as a main dish or serve over pasta, rice, or crusty bread.

Roasted Garlic Hummus:

Ingredients:

- 1 can (15 ounces) chickpeas (garbanzo beans), drained and rinsed
- 1/4 cup tahini (sesame paste)
- 3 tablespoons extra virgin olive oil
- 2 cloves garlic, roasted
- Juice of 1 lemon
- 1/2 teaspoon ground cumin
- Salt to taste
- 2-4 tablespoons water (as needed for desired consistency)
- Optional toppings: drizzle of olive oil, sprinkle of paprika, chopped fresh parsley

Instructions:

1. Preheat the oven to 400°F (200°C). Slice the top off a head of garlic to expose the cloves, drizzle with olive oil, wrap in foil, and roast in the oven for about 30-40 minutes until soft and golden brown.
2. In a food processor, combine the drained chickpeas, tahini, olive oil, roasted garlic cloves (squeeze them out of the skins), lemon juice, ground cumin, and salt.

3. Process the mixture until smooth, scraping down the sides of the bowl as needed. If the hummus is too thick, add water, one tablespoon at a time, until you reach your desired consistency.
4. Taste the hummus and adjust the seasoning as needed, adding more salt or lemon juice if desired.
5. Transfer the hummus to a serving bowl and drizzle with a little extra virgin olive oil. Sprinkle with paprika and chopped fresh parsley for garnish, if desired.
6. Serve the roasted garlic hummus with pita bread, vegetable sticks, or crackers. Enjoy as a healthy snack or appetizer!

These recipes showcase the versatility and deliciousness of garlic in both savory and healthy dishes. Enjoy cooking and savoring these flavorful creations!

Some ways to Use Garlic

Garlic and Honey

Garlic and honey are super foods when combined form an excellent natural remedy to combat conditions such as colds, flu, and other illnesses. The sulfur compounds in garlic and the nutrients in honey exert an anticoagulant and toning effect on the veins, preventing the formation of thrombosis and varicose veins.

Garlic, Ginger and Lemon

Ginger's anti-inflammatory and antioxidant effects, garlic's antimicrobial and immune-stimulating properties, and lemon's vitamin C content work harmoniously to fortify your immune system. This trio can help enhance your body's defense mechanisms, increase resistance to infections, and promote overall wellness.

Garlic and Ginger Tea

This tea is a yummy, healthy way to warm up while preventing and eradicating a sore throat. It only takes a few minutes to prepare, and the sliced ginger and garlic can be reused up to three times. You may not immediately like the taste of this tea, but the taste and benefits of it can grow on you over time!

A Word of Caution: While garlic offers numerous health benefits, it's essential to consume it in moderation, especially for individuals with certain medical conditions or sensitivities. Some people may experience digestive discomfort or allergic reactions to garlic. Additionally, garlic supplements may interact with certain medications, so it's advisable to consult with a healthcare professional before starting any new dietary regimen.

Conclusion:

Garlic's remarkable flavor and health-promoting properties have earned it a well-deserved place in kitchens and medicine cabinets around the world. Whether you're seeking to add depth to your culinary creations or harnessing its therapeutic potential, garlic stands as a shining example of nature's bounty. So go ahead, embrace the golden clove, and savor its many delights as you embark on a journey of flavor and wellness.

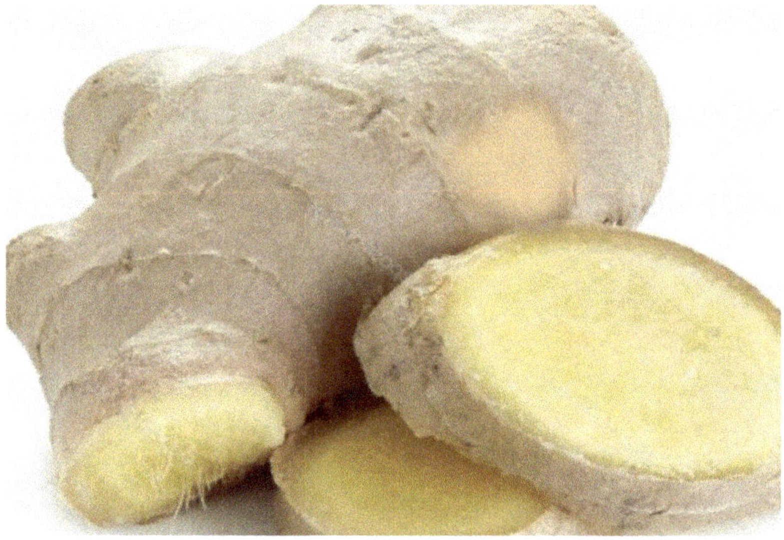

Ginger

A Culinary and Medicinal Marvel

Ginger, a flowering plant renowned for its rhizome, commonly known as ginger root, stands as a versatile spice and a revered component in folk medicine. This herbaceous perennial boasts annual pseudostems reaching a height of about one meter, adorned with slender leaf blades.

The applications of ginger extend far beyond mere culinary delight, finding a place in an array of food items, including vegetables, candy, soda, pickles, and alcoholic beverages. With its enticing aroma, ginger serves as a fragrant kitchen spice, with young ginger rhizomes offering a succulent and mildly flavored experience.

Beyond its culinary prowess, ginger brings forth a myriad of health benefits in various forms, enriching both the taste of your food and your overall well-being. In the annals of history, ginger has also served as an alternative form of medicine.

Nutritional Powerhouse

Ginger is rich in essential nutrients and bioactive compounds that contribute to its numerous health benefits. Here are some key nutrients found in ginger and their associated benefits:

Gingerol:

- **Benefits:** Gingerol is the primary bioactive compound in ginger, responsible for its distinctive flavor and many of its medicinal properties. It possesses potent anti-inflammatory and antioxidant properties, which may help reduce inflammation, oxidative stress, and the risk of chronic diseases such as heart disease, cancer, and neurodegenerative disorders. Gingerol also has antimicrobial properties that may help fight infections.

Vitamin C:

- **Benefits:** Vitamin C is a powerful antioxidant that supports immune function, helps protect cells from damage caused by free radicals, and promotes collagen production for healthy skin, hair, and connective tissues. Including ginger in your diet can contribute to your daily vitamin C intake and support overall health and well-being.

Magnesium:

- **Benefits:** Magnesium plays a crucial role in over 300 biochemical reactions in the body, including energy metabolism, muscle and nerve function, blood pressure regulation, and protein synthesis. Consuming ginger, which contains small amounts of magnesium, can help support these vital functions and contribute to overall health.

Potassium:

- **Benefits:** Potassium is an essential mineral that helps regulate fluid balance, muscle contractions, nerve signals, and blood pressure. Adequate potassium intake is important for maintaining cardiovascular health, muscle function, and overall electrolyte balance. While ginger contains only small amounts of potassium, every bit helps contribute to your daily intake.

Manganese:

- **Benefits:** Manganese is a trace mineral that plays a role in bone health, metabolism, antioxidant defense mechanisms, and the synthesis of connective tissues and sex hormones. Ginger provides small amounts of manganese, which can support these functions and contribute to overall well-being.

Dietary Fiber:

- **Benefits:** Ginger contains dietary fiber, which is important for digestive health, regulating bowel movements, and promoting feelings of fullness and satiety. Fiber also helps stabilize blood sugar levels, lower cholesterol levels, and support a healthy gut microbiome.

Ginger Essential Oil:

- **Benefits:** Ginger essential oil, derived from the rhizome of the ginger plant, contains concentrated amounts of gingerol and other bioactive compounds. It is used in aromatherapy and topical applications for its anti-inflammatory, analgesic, and digestive properties. Ginger essential oil may help alleviate muscle pain, arthritis symptoms, nausea, and indigestion when used properly and under guidance.

Incorporating ginger into your diet or using ginger supplements can provide a range of health benefits due to its rich nutrient profile and bioactive compounds. Whether consumed fresh, dried, as a spice, in teas, or as an extract, ginger has been celebrated for centuries for its culinary and medicinal virtues.

Unlocking the Health Potentials of Ginger

Gingerol, a natural constituent of ginger root, transcends its delicious taste to offer tangible benefits to gastrointestinal motility, facilitating the efficient passage of food through the digestive process. By promoting effective digestion, ginger prevents food from lingering excessively in the gut.

Boosting Immunity: Gingerol, a bioactive compound found in raw ginger, bolsters immunity with its antimicrobial and antifungal properties, alongside being a source of antioxidants and anti-inflammatory agents. These combined properties play a pivotal role in alleviating symptoms associated with common colds and the flu, such as coughs, fevers, headaches, and infections.

Relieving Nausea and Upset Stomach: Ginger's renowned ability to alleviate nausea, stemming from various causes such as motion sickness or morning sickness, extends to providing relief during cancer treatment, where it effectively counters symptoms like nausea and dizziness. This effect is achieved through anti-inflammatory properties, enhanced digestive responsiveness, and regulation of blood pressure.

Pregnancy and Morning Sickness: Through generations, ginger has been a trusted remedy for easing morning sickness and queasiness during pregnancy, acknowledged even by the American Academy of Obstetrics and Gynecology.

Potential Anti-Cancer Properties: While not a panacea, studies suggest that gingerol in ginger may offer preventative benefits against certain cancers, thanks to its antioxidant and anti-inflammatory characteristics.

Enhancing Digestion: Ginger accelerates the digestion process, benefiting those with digestive issues like indigestion, ulcers, constipation, and IBS. Studies show that ginger consumers digest food twice as fast, promoting movement in the digestive tract and fostering the action of enzymes that aid in food breakdown.

Alleviating PMS Symptoms: Incorporating ginger during the initial days of the menstrual cycle provides relief from menstrual pain and addresses bloating, thanks to its anti-inflammatory properties.

Cellular Protection and Healthier Skin: Ginger's antioxidant content helps manage free radicals, safeguarding cells from damage. Additionally, ginger enhances skin health by increasing blood circulation, offering antiseptic properties that improve acne symptoms, and aiding in the healing of irritated skin.

Pain Reduction: As a natural pain reliever, gingerol serves as a viable alternative to over-the-counter medications, especially for arthritis sufferers, reducing inflammation and increasing joint mobility.

Improving Brain Function: Ginger's anti-inflammatory properties protect the brain from free radicals, potentially mitigating cognitive decline and mental health issues. It also enhances memory function and releases neurotransmitters responsible for memory, focus, and reaction time.

Culinary Uses:

Beyond its medicinal properties, ginger adds depth and flavor to a wide range of culinary creations:

Spice in Cooking: Fresh ginger adds a zesty, slightly spicy flavor to savory dishes, soups, stir-fries, and marinades. It pairs exceptionally well with garlic, soy sauce, and citrus flavors, enhancing the taste of both meat and vegetable dishes.

Baking and Desserts: Ground ginger is a common ingredient in baking, imparting warmth and depth to cookies, cakes, bread, and desserts. It complements sweet flavors such as cinnamon, cloves, and molasses, creating delightful treats with a hint of spice.

Beverages: Ginger is a popular addition to teas, infusions, and beverages, lending its invigorating flavor and healthful properties to hot and cold drinks alike. Ginger tea is particularly soothing and comforting, offering a warming sensation on chilly days.

Condiment and Preserves: Ginger can be pickled, candied, or made into savory condiments like ginger paste, ginger chutney, or ginger-infused oils and vinegars. These versatile preparations add a punch of flavor to sandwiches, salads, and marinades.

Creative Ways to Incorporate Ginger

Ginger Tea: A popular choice, ginger tea can be prepared by steeping chopped or sliced ginger in water, with options to enhance flavor using honey or lemon.

Ginger Juice: A convenient daily shot of ginger juice, incorporating lime or lemon, honey, or natural cane sugar to taste, provides a simple yet effective way to enjoy ginger's benefits.

Add to Daily Meals: Incorporate minced ginger into various meals such as stir-fries, soups, curries, desserts, or smoothies, offering both health benefits and an extra burst of flavor.

Pickled Ginger: This sweet-tart-spicy condiment, commonly served with sushi, not only provides the healthy components of ginger but also offers probiotic benefits without excessive sodium content.

Here are two delicious recipes featuring ginger:

Ginger Garlic Chicken Stir-Fry:

Ingredients:

- 1 lb (450g) boneless, skinless chicken breasts, thinly sliced
- 2 tablespoons soy sauce
- 1 tablespoon oyster sauce
- 1 tablespoon cornstarch
- 1 teaspoon sesame oil
- 2 tablespoons vegetable oil
- 4 cloves garlic, minced
- 1 tablespoon fresh ginger, minced
- 1 bell pepper, thinly sliced
- 1 cup broccoli florets
- 1 carrot, julienned
- 2 green onions, sliced
- Cooked rice, for serving

Instructions:

1. In a bowl, combine the soy sauce, oyster sauce, cornstarch, and sesame oil. Add the sliced chicken and toss to coat. Let it marinate for at least 15 minutes.
2. Heat 1 tablespoon of vegetable oil in a large skillet or wok over medium-high heat. Add the marinated chicken and stir-fry until cooked through, about 4-5 minutes. Remove the chicken from the skillet and set aside.
3. In the same skillet, add the remaining tablespoon of vegetable oil. Add the minced garlic and ginger, and stir-fry for about 30 seconds until fragrant.
4. Add the sliced bell pepper, broccoli florets, and julienned carrot to the skillet. Stir-fry for 2-3 minutes until the vegetables are tender-crisp.
5. Return the cooked chicken to the skillet. Stir everything together and cook for another minute to heat through.
6. Garnish with sliced green onions and serve the ginger garlic chicken stir-fry hot over cooked rice.

Ginger Lemon Honey Tea:

Ingredients:

- 1-inch piece of fresh ginger, thinly sliced
- 1 lemon, thinly sliced
- 2 tablespoons honey (adjust to taste)
- 4 cups water

Instructions:

1. In a saucepan, bring the water to a boil over medium heat.
2. Add the sliced ginger and lemon to the boiling water. Reduce the heat to low and let the mixture simmer for about 5 minutes.
3. Remove the saucepan from the heat and let the tea steep for an additional 5 minutes.
4. Strain the tea to remove the ginger and lemon slices.
5. Stir in honey to taste, adjusting the sweetness as desired.
6. Pour the ginger lemon honey tea into mugs and serve hot. Enjoy the soothing and refreshing flavors of this comforting beverage!

These recipes showcase the versatility of ginger, adding flavor and depth to both savory dishes and beverages. Enjoy these culinary delights infused with the zesty goodness of ginger!

Cultural Significance:

In addition to its culinary and medicinal uses, ginger holds cultural significance in many societies:

- In Asian cultures, ginger is often incorporated into traditional medicine, herbal remedies, and ceremonial rituals. It symbolizes prosperity, good fortune, and vitality.
- In Indian Ayurvedic medicine, ginger is revered as a "universal medicine" that balances the body's doshas (energies) and promotes holistic wellness.
- In Jamaican and Caribbean cuisine, ginger is a key ingredient in spicy dishes, beverages like ginger beer, and herbal remedies known as "bush teas."

Growing Your Own:

Ginger is a tropical plant that thrives in warm, humid environments. It typically takes about 8 to 10 months for ginger to grow from planting to harvest. However, the exact time may vary depending on various factors such as growing conditions, ginger variety, and climate.

Here's a general timeline of ginger growth stages:

1. **Planting:** Ginger is usually planted from rhizomes, which are sections of the ginger root. The rhizomes are planted in shallow trenches or pots with well-draining soil, usually in the spring after the last frost date. The rhizomes should be planted with the buds facing upward and covered lightly with soil.
2. **Sprouting:** After planting, ginger rhizomes will begin to sprout shoots and develop roots. This stage typically occurs within a few weeks of planting, depending on soil temperature and moisture levels.
3. **Vegetative Growth:** Once sprouted, ginger plants will continue to grow vegetatively, producing foliage in the form of tall, green stems with lance-shaped leaves. During this stage, ginger requires regular watering and fertilization to support healthy growth.
4. **Rhizome Development:** As the ginger plant matures, it will allocate energy towards rhizome development underground. The rhizomes will gradually swell and develop the characteristic knobby appearance of ginger roots.
5. **Maturation:** Ginger rhizomes typically reach maturity around 8 to 10 months after planting. At this stage, the leaves may begin to yellow and die back, indicating that the rhizomes are ready for harvest. However, ginger can be harvested earlier if desired, but the rhizomes will be smaller.
6. **Harvesting:** To harvest ginger, carefully dig up the rhizomes using a garden fork or shovel, being careful not to damage them. Shake off excess soil and trim the foliage, leaving a few inches of stem attached to the rhizomes. After harvesting, ginger can be stored fresh, dried, or processed for culinary use.

Overall, growing ginger requires patience and attention to environmental conditions, but with proper care, you can enjoy a bountiful harvest of this versatile and flavorful spice.

Understanding Ginger's Side Effects

While research deems ginger safe in normal culinary quantities, caution is advised for those with diabetes, as large doses may impact insulin and lower blood sugar. Individuals with allergies should consult a physician before incorporating ginger into their diet.

Conclusion:

Integrating ginger into your daily routine can contribute to improved digestion, reduced inflammation, enhanced immunity, relief from nausea, cardiovascular health support, diabetes management, brain health, weight management, menstrual pain relief, and fortification against infections.

Ginger stands as a testament to nature's bounty, offering a treasure trove of health benefits, culinary delights, and cultural significance. Whether used to soothe an upset stomach, spice up a meal, or infuse warmth into a beverage, ginger continues to captivate our senses and enrich our lives. Embrace the wonders of ginger, and let its remarkable qualities inspire your culinary adventures and wellness journey.

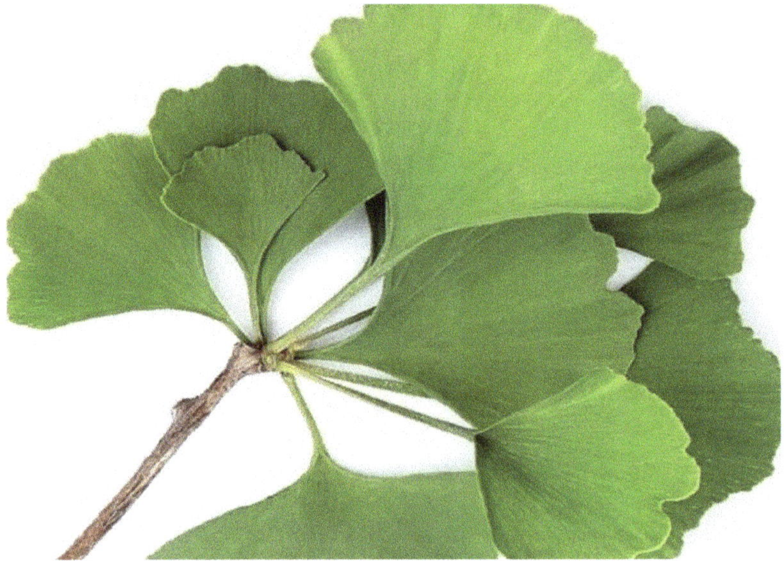

Ginkgo

Ginkgo Biloba: Unveiling the Timeless Herb's Benefits and Versatile Uses

Ginkgo biloba, a unique and ancient tree species, has been revered for centuries for its medicinal properties. Also known as the maidenhair tree, ginkgo is celebrated for its fan-shaped leaves and has found a significant place in traditional medicine. In this article, we'll explore the various benefits and versatile uses of ginkgo, shedding light on its enduring popularity.

Historical Significance:

Ginkgo biloba is considered a living fossil, with a lineage dating back millions of years. Native to China, ginkgo has been cultivated for both its ornamental beauty and medicinal value. The use of ginkgo extracts in traditional Chinese medicine can be traced back over a thousand years, where it was believed to enhance memory and cognitive function.

Key Components and Benefits:

Flavonoids and Terpenoids:

- **Benefits:**
    - **Antioxidant Action:** Ginkgo is rich in flavonoids and terpenoids, powerful antioxidants that help combat oxidative stress and reduce the damage caused by free radicals.
    - **Anti-Inflammatory Properties:** The anti-inflammatory effects of these compounds contribute to ginkgo's potential in managing conditions related to inflammation.

Ginkgolides and Bilobalides:

- **Benefits:**
    - **Blood Flow Enhancement:** Ginkgolides and bilobalides have been associated with improved blood flow, particularly in the brain. This makes ginkgo a popular choice for promoting cognitive health and addressing conditions related to poor circulation.

Terpene Lactones:

- **Benefits:**
    - **Cognitive Function:** Ginkgo is often linked to cognitive benefits, including improved memory and concentration. It is frequently used to support mental clarity and focus.

Versatile Uses:

Cognitive Support:

- Ginkgo biloba is widely recognized for its potential in supporting cognitive function. It is often used to address memory-related issues and promote overall brain health. Supplements containing ginkgo extract are popular choices for those seeking cognitive support.

Peripheral Circulation:

- The ability of ginkgo to enhance blood flow extends to peripheral circulation, making it beneficial for conditions such as intermittent claudication, where individuals experience pain in the legs due to poor circulation.

Vision Health:

- Ginkgo's antioxidant properties contribute to its potential in supporting vision health. It is believed to protect the eyes from oxidative damage and may be used as a complementary approach to maintaining eye health.

Anti-Anxiety and Antidepressant Effects:

- Some studies suggest that ginkgo biloba may have mild anti-anxiety and antidepressant effects. It is thought to modulate neurotransmitters in the brain, contributing to mood regulation.

Tinnitus Management:

- Ginkgo has been explored for its potential in managing tinnitus (ringing in the ears). While results vary, some individuals report a reduction in the severity of tinnitus symptoms with ginkgo supplementation.

Culinary Uses:

Ginkgo nuts are commonly used in traditional Asian cuisine, particularly in Chinese, Japanese, and Korean dishes.

Here are two recipes that incorporate ginkgo nuts:

Stir-Fried Ginkgo Nuts with Vegetables:

Ingredients:

- 1 cup fresh or frozen ginkgo nuts, shelled and peeled
- 2 cups mixed vegetables (such as bell peppers, broccoli, carrots, snap peas)
- 2 cloves garlic, minced
- 1 tablespoon vegetable oil
- 1 tablespoon soy sauce
- 1 teaspoon sesame oil
- Salt and pepper to taste
- Sesame seeds for garnish (optional)

Instructions:

1. If using fresh ginkgo nuts, shell and peel them. If using frozen ginkgo nuts, thaw them according to package instructions.
2. Blanch the ginkgo nuts in boiling water for 5 minutes to remove any bitterness. Drain and set aside.
3. Heat vegetable oil in a large skillet or wok over medium-high heat. Add minced garlic and stir-fry until fragrant, about 30 seconds.
4. Add the mixed vegetables to the skillet and stir-fry for 3-4 minutes until they are tender-crisp.
5. Add the blanched ginkgo nuts to the skillet and continue to stir-fry for another 2-3 minutes.
6. Season with soy sauce, sesame oil, salt, and pepper to taste. Stir to combine all ingredients evenly.
7. Transfer the stir-fried ginkgo nuts and vegetables to a serving dish. Garnish with sesame seeds if desired.
8. Serve hot as a side dish or as part of a larger meal. Enjoy the unique flavor and texture of ginkgo nuts in this nutritious stir-fry!

Ginkgo Nut Congee (Rice Porridge):

Ingredients:

- 1/2 cup white rice
- 4 cups water or chicken broth
- 1/2 cup fresh or frozen ginkgo nuts, shelled and peeled
- Salt to taste
- Sliced green onions or cilantro for garnish (optional)

Instructions:

1. Rinse the white rice under cold water until the water runs clear. Drain well.
2. In a large pot, combine the rinsed rice and water or chicken broth. Bring to a boil over high heat.
3. Once boiling, reduce the heat to low and simmer the rice, partially covered, for 30-40 minutes, stirring occasionally, until the rice is soft and creamy.
4. Add the shelled and peeled ginkgo nuts to the congee during the last 10-15 minutes of cooking. Stir to incorporate the ginkgo nuts into the congee.
5. Season the congee with salt to taste, adjusting the seasoning as needed.
6. Ladle the ginkgo nut congee into bowls. Garnish with sliced green onions or cilantro if desired.
7. Serve hot as a comforting and nourishing breakfast or light meal. Enjoy the creamy texture and nutty flavor of this traditional Asian congee with the addition of ginkgo nuts!

These recipes highlight the unique flavor and texture of ginkgo nuts and demonstrate how they can be incorporated into a variety of dishes for both taste and nutritional benefits.

Historical Uses:

Ginkgo biloba has a rich history of use in traditional medicine, particularly in Chinese and Japanese herbal practices. Here are a few historical uses of ginkgo:

Traditional Chinese Medicine:

- Ginkgo biloba has been a fundamental component of traditional Chinese medicine for over a thousand years. In this system, ginkgo leaves and seeds have been used to address various health concerns, including respiratory issues, digestive problems, and enhancing blood circulation. It was believed that ginkgo biloba could promote overall well-being and longevity.

Memory and Cognitive Enhancement:

- Ginkgo biloba has been historically associated with cognitive benefits, particularly in improving memory and concentration. In traditional Chinese medicine, ginkgo was believed to support mental clarity and enhance cognitive function. This historical use laid the foundation for contemporary interest in ginkgo as a potential cognitive enhancer.

Aesthetic and Ornamental Purposes:

- Beyond its medicinal uses, ginkgo biloba has been cultivated for its aesthetic appeal. The distinctive fan-shaped leaves of the ginkgo tree make it a popular ornamental tree in gardens and public spaces. The tree is often planted for its beauty, resilience, and symbolic significance, representing endurance and longevity.

While ginkgo biloba's historical uses are deeply rooted in traditional medicine, it gained widespread global attention in more recent times for its potential cognitive benefits. Today, ginkgo supplements are commonly consumed for cognitive support, and ongoing research explores its various applications in modern healthcare.

Conclusion:

Ginkgo biloba, with its rich historical legacy and diverse therapeutic properties, continues to captivate the interest of both traditional medicine practitioners and modern researchers. Whether sought for cognitive support, improved circulation, or other potential benefits, ginkgo remains a timeless herb that has stood the test of time. As with any supplement or herbal remedy, it's advisable to consult with a healthcare professional before incorporating ginkgo into your wellness routine to ensure safe and appropriate usage.

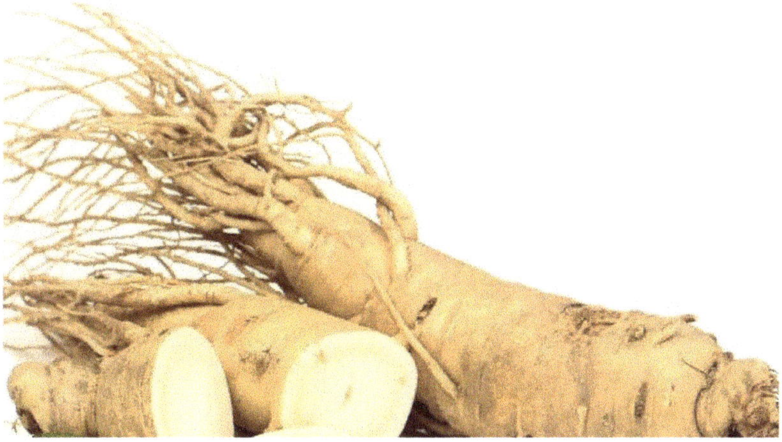

Ginseng

Power of Ginseng: A Comprehensive Exploration of Benefits and Uses

Ginseng, an ancient herb deeply rooted in traditional medicine, has been revered for centuries for its potential health benefits and adaptogenic properties. Known for its distinctively shaped roots and adaptability to various climates, ginseng belongs to the Panax genus and is prized for its ability to support overall well-being. In this article, we will delve into the rich history, nutritional components, and diverse uses of ginseng that make it a sought-after herbal remedy.

History and Origin:

Ginseng has a storied history that dates back thousands of years, with its roots deeply embedded in traditional Chinese medicine. The term "Panax" is derived from the Greek word meaning "all-healing," reflecting the high regard in which ginseng has been held. Ginseng has been traditionally used in Asia, particularly in China and Korea, where it was believed to enhance vitality, boost energy, and promote longevity.

Ginseng thrives in shaded woodland environments with well-drained soil. The plant is characterized by its compound leaves and small, inconspicuous flowers that develop into bright red berries. However, it is the fleshy, forked root of the ginseng plant that holds the key to its medicinal value.

Ginseng is classified into different species, such as Panax ginseng (Asian or Korean ginseng) and Panax quinquefolius (American ginseng), each prized for its unique qualities. Cultivation of ginseng requires patience, as the plant typically takes several years to reach maturity. The root is harvested for its beneficial compounds, known as ginsenosides, which contribute to the herb's adaptogenic and antioxidant properties. The growth and cultivation of ginseng involves careful attention to environmental conditions to ensure optimal development and potency of its prized roots.

Nutritional Profile:

Ginseng contains a variety of bioactive compounds that contribute to its medicinal properties. Some key components include ginsenosides, polysaccharides, and polyacetylenes. These compounds are believed to play a role in the adaptogenic and antioxidant effects of ginseng.

Health Benefits:

Adaptogenic Properties:

- Ginseng is classified as an adaptogen, meaning it may help the body adapt to stress and restore balance. Adaptogens are believed to have a normalizing effect on bodily functions, helping to reduce the impact of stressors.

Boosting Energy and Stamina:

- Traditional uses of ginseng include its reputation as an energy booster and stamina enhancer. Consuming ginseng may help combat fatigue, increase endurance, and improve overall physical performance.

Cognitive Function:

- Ginseng has been studied for its potential cognitive benefits. Some research suggests that ginsenosides, the active compounds in ginseng, may have neuroprotective effects and could support cognitive function, including memory and concentration.

Immune System Support:

- Ginseng is believed to have immune-modulating effects. Regular consumption may help support the immune system, potentially reducing the risk of infections and enhancing the body's natural defense mechanisms.

Common Uses:

Herbal Teas and Infusions:

- Ginseng roots or extracts are commonly used to prepare herbal teas and infusions. These beverages are consumed for their potential health benefits, including stress reduction and energy enhancement.

Ginseng Tea:

Ingredients: Dried ginseng slices, water

Instructions: Steep dried ginseng slices in hot water for about 15-20 minutes to make ginseng tea. Optionally, add honey or lemon for flavor. This soothing tea can be consumed regularly to experience the potential benefits of ginseng.

Ginseng Infused Honey:

Ingredients: Dried ginseng, honey

Instructions: Combine dried ginseng with honey in a jar and let it infuse for a week or longer. The result is a ginseng-infused honey that can be used as a natural sweetener in teas, drizzled over desserts, or added to various culinary creations.

Ginseng Tincture:

Ingredients: Dried ginseng root, alcohol (e.g., vodka or brandy)

Instructions: Create a ginseng tincture by placing dried ginseng root in a glass jar and covering it with alcohol. Let it steep in a dark place for several weeks, shaking the jar occasionally. Strain the mixture, and the resulting tincture can be consumed by adding a few drops to water or juice.

Supplements:

- Ginseng supplements, available in various forms such as capsules, powders, or liquid extracts, are widely used to incorporate ginseng into daily wellness routines. These supplements are often taken to support energy levels, combat fatigue, and promote overall vitality.

Traditional Medicine Practices:

- In traditional Chinese medicine and other herbal traditions, ginseng is used in formulations to address specific health concerns. It may be included in herbal remedies tailored to individual needs, such as tonics for improving stamina or addressing stress-related issues.

Culinary Uses:

Ginseng is often used in traditional Asian cuisine for its unique flavor and potential health benefits. Here are two recipes that incorporate ginseng:

Ginseng Chicken Soup (Samgyetang):

Ingredients:

- 1 whole chicken (about 3-4 pounds)
- 4 ginseng roots (fresh or dried)
- 8 dried jujubes (Korean red dates)
- 1 cup glutinous rice (sweet rice)
- 8 cloves garlic, peeled
- 8 cups water

- Salt and pepper to taste
- Optional garnishes: sliced green onions, sliced ginger, sesame seeds

Instructions:

1. Rinse the glutinous rice and soak it in water for about 30 minutes.
2. Wash the chicken thoroughly, removing any excess fat and giblets. Pat dry with paper towels.
3. Stuff the cavity of the chicken with the soaked glutinous rice, ginseng roots, dried jujubes, and garlic cloves.
4. Place the stuffed chicken in a large pot and add water until it covers the chicken completely.
5. Bring the water to a boil over high heat, then reduce the heat to low and simmer for about 1.5 to 2 hours, or until the chicken is fully cooked and tender.
6. Season the soup with salt and pepper to taste.
7. Ladle the soup into bowls, making sure to include some of the ginseng roots, jujubes, and garlic with each serving.
8. Garnish with sliced green onions, sliced ginger, and sesame seeds if desired.
9. Serve hot as a nourishing and comforting meal. Enjoy the rich flavors and healthful properties of this traditional Korean ginseng chicken soup!

Ginseng Tea:

Ingredients:

- 4 cups water
- 2-3 ginseng roots (fresh or dried)
- Honey or sweetener of choice (optional)

Instructions:

1. In a small saucepan, bring the water to a boil over high heat.
2. Rinse the ginseng roots under cold water to remove any dirt or debris.
3. Add the ginseng roots to the boiling water and reduce the heat to low.
4. Simmer the ginseng roots for about 30 minutes to 1 hour, depending on desired strength.
5. Remove the saucepan from the heat and let the ginseng tea steep for an additional 10-15 minutes.

6. Strain the tea to remove the ginseng roots.
7. Sweeten the tea with honey or your preferred sweetener if desired.
8. Serve the ginseng tea hot or chilled, depending on preference.
9. Enjoy the invigorating and healthful properties of this traditional ginseng tea!

These recipes showcase the versatility of ginseng and how it can be incorporated into both savory dishes and beverages for its unique flavor and potential health benefits.

Historical Uses:

Ancient Chinese Medicine:

- **Benefit:** Ginseng has been a cornerstone in traditional Chinese medicine for over 2,000 years. Ancient Chinese practitioners valued ginseng for its adaptogenic properties, believing it could restore balance to the body, enhance vitality, and combat fatigue. Ginseng was used to address a variety of health concerns, including promoting energy, supporting digestion, and improving overall well-being.

Native American Traditional Medicine:

- **Benefit:** Native American tribes, particularly those in North America, also recognized the value of ginseng. The root was used in traditional medicine to address conditions such as fatigue, headaches, and digestive issues. Additionally, Native Americans believed that ginseng had spiritual significance, viewing it as a powerful herb with rejuvenating properties.

Korean Ginseng in Ancient Korea:

- **Benefit:** Korean ginseng (Panax ginseng) has a rich history in ancient Korea, where it was considered a valuable medicinal herb. Historical records indicate its use in promoting physical stamina, improving mental clarity, and supporting overall resilience. Korean ginseng was often reserved for royalty and the elite due to its esteemed status.

European Herbal Traditions:

- **Benefit:** Ginseng found its way into European herbal traditions, where it was adopted for its perceived health benefits. In medieval Europe, ginseng was associated with various healing properties, including enhancing cognitive function, alleviating stress, and acting as a general tonic for overall health.

These historical uses of ginseng underscore its enduring reputation as a revered herbal remedy across diverse cultures. Whether in ancient China, Native American traditions, ancient Korea, or medieval Europe, ginseng consistently held a place of significance for its perceived adaptogenic and revitalizing properties. While modern research continues to explore the scientific basis for these historical uses, ginseng's legacy as a valued herb remains firmly rooted in centuries of traditional wisdom.

Conclusion:

Ginseng's enduring popularity is a testament to its historical significance and the potential benefits it offers. As a versatile herb with adaptogenic properties, ginseng continues to be embraced for its potential to support energy, enhance cognitive function, and promote overall well-being. Whether enjoyed in herbal teas, taken as supplements, or incorporated into traditional remedies, ginseng remains a valued herbal ally in the pursuit of optimal health. As with any herbal remedy, it's advisable to consult with a healthcare professional before incorporating ginseng into your routine, especially if you have underlying health conditions or are taking medications.

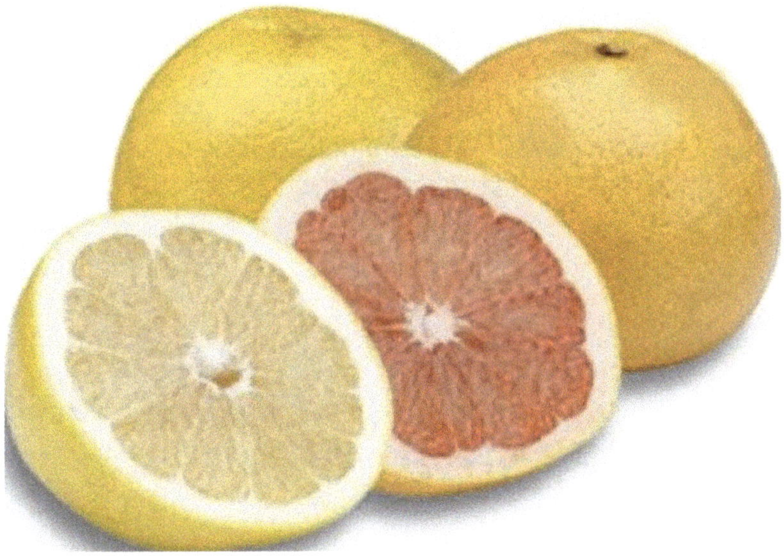

Grapefruit

The Zesty Marvel: Exploring the Benefits and Uses of Grapefruit

Grapefruit, with its vibrant taste and invigorating aroma, stands as a citrus gem renowned for more than just it's refreshing flavor. Packed with essential nutrients and versatile applications, this citrus fruit has earned its place as a nutritional powerhouse. Let's delve into the world of grapefruit, uncovering its numerous benefits and diverse uses.

Nutrient-Rich Composition:

Grapefruit is a low-calorie fruit that packs a punch when it comes to essential nutrients. Here's a breakdown of its nutritional composition:

Fiber:

With a notable fiber content, grapefruit contributes to digestive health, helps regulate blood sugar levels, and promotes a feeling of fullness.

Antioxidants:

Various antioxidants in grapefruit, such as flavonoids and carotenoids, contribute to reducing oxidative stress and inflammation in the body.

Flavonoids:

Benefits:

- Have antioxidant and anti-inflammatory properties.
- Contribute to heart health by improving blood vessel function.
- May have potential anticancer effects.

Naringenin:

Benefits:

- Exhibits antioxidant and anti-inflammatory effects.
- May have potential anti-cancer properties.
- Contributes to cardiovascular health by reducing cholesterol levels.

Carotenoids:

Benefits:

- Beta-carotene is a precursor to vitamin A, supporting vision and immune function.
- Lycopene has antioxidant properties and may contribute to cardiovascular health.

Cryptoxanthin:

Benefits:

- Functions as a provitamin A carotenoid, supporting immune function and vision.
- Exhibits antioxidant properties.

Quercetin:

Benefits:

- Has antioxidant and anti-inflammatory effects.
- May contribute to cardiovascular health by improving blood vessel function.
- Exhibits potential anticancer properties.

Kaempferol:

Benefits:

- Displays antioxidant and anti-inflammatory properties.
- May have potential anticancer effects.
- Contributes to cardiovascular health.

Limonoids:

Benefits:

- Exhibit antioxidant and anti-inflammatory effects.
- May have potential anticancer properties.

Pectin:

Benefits:

- Acts as a soluble fiber, promoting digestive health.
- May help lower cholesterol levels.
- Exhibits antioxidant properties.

Tannins:

Benefits:

- Exhibit antioxidant and anti-inflammatory properties.
- May contribute to cardiovascular health.
- Have potential antimicrobial effects.

Vitamins:

Vitamin C: Grapefruit is rich in vitamin C, an antioxidant that supports the immune system, promotes skin health, and aids in collagen synthesis.

Vitamin A: Grapefruit contains vitamin A, important for vision, immune function, and skin health.

Vitamin B1 (Thiamine): Thiamine is a B-vitamin involved in energy metabolism, and it is present in small amounts in grapefruit.

Vitamin B5 (Pantothenic Acid): Pantothenic acid is another B-vitamin found in grapefruit, playing a role in energy metabolism and hormone synthesis.

Vitamin B6 (Pyridoxine): Pyridoxine is a B-vitamin that supports brain development, metabolism, and the production of neurotransmitters.

Folate (Vitamin B9): Grapefruit contains folate, which is crucial for DNA synthesis and cell division.

Minerals:

Potassium: Grapefruit provides potassium, an electrolyte that supports heart health and helps regulate blood pressure.

Copper: While present in smaller amounts, copper is a trace mineral found in grapefruit that plays a role in various physiological processes.

Iron: Grapefruit contains small amounts of iron, an essential mineral for the formation of hemoglobin and oxygen transport in the blood.

Magnesium: Magnesium is a mineral found in grapefruit that plays a role in muscle and nerve function, blood glucose control, and bone health.

Phosphorus: Grapefruit contains phosphorus, an essential mineral that contributes to bone health and energy metabolism.

Zinc: Zinc is a trace mineral found in grapefruit, playing a role in immune function, wound healing, and DNA synthesis.

It's important to note that the specific content of vitamins and minerals in grapefruit can vary based on factors such as the variety of grapefruit and its growing conditions. Additionally, while grapefruit provides various nutrients, it's crucial to include a variety of foods in your diet to ensure a well-rounded intake of essential vitamins and minerals. If you have specific dietary concerns or health conditions, it's advisable to consult with a healthcare professional or a registered dietitian for personalized guidance.

Health Benefits:

Weight Management: The fiber content in grapefruit can aid in weight management by promoting satiety and reducing overall calorie intake.

Heart Health: Potassium in grapefruit supports heart health by helping regulate blood pressure. The fruit's antioxidants may also contribute to reducing the risk of cardiovascular diseases.

Immune Support: Vitamin C is known for its immune-boosting properties, and including grapefruit in your diet can help fortify your body's defenses against infections and illnesses.

Skin Health: The combination of vitamin C and antioxidants promotes healthy skin by supporting collagen production and protecting against free radical damage.

Blood Sugar Regulation: Some studies suggest that compounds in grapefruit may help improve insulin sensitivity, contributing to better blood sugar control.

Cancer Prevention: Certain compounds found in grapefruit, including limonoids and beta-carotene, have been studied for their potential anti-cancer properties. However, more research is needed to establish definitive links.

Nutritional Content

The nutritional content of 1 cup (about 230 grams) of grapefruit can vary slightly depending on the variety and specific size of the fruit, but here is a general approximation:

- Carbohydrates: Approximately 17 grams
- Protein: Approximately 1 gram
- Fiber: Approximately 2-3 grams
- Fat: Negligible (virtually zero grams)
- Sugar: Approximately 8-9 grams

It's worth noting that grapefruit is relatively low in calories, making it a nutritious choice for those looking to manage their weight or improve their overall diet. Additionally, grapefruit is an excellent source of vitamin C and contains various other vitamins, minerals, and antioxidants that contribute to its health benefits.

Versatile Culinary Uses:

Grapefruit's versatility extends beyond simply peeling and enjoying the segments. Here are various ways to incorporate grapefruit into your culinary endeavors:

Fresh Juices: Squeeze fresh grapefruit juice to create refreshing beverages. Mix it with other fruit juices, blend it into smoothies, or simply enjoy it on its own.

Salads: Add grapefruit segments to salads for a burst of citrus flavor. They pair well with greens, avocados, and nuts.

Desserts: Incorporate grapefruit zest or juice into desserts, such as sorbets, cakes, and fruit salads, to add a zesty and tangy element.

Salsas and Relishes: Create vibrant salsas or relishes with diced grapefruit, jalapeños, onions, and herbs. This can be a delightful accompaniment to grilled fish or tacos.

Breakfast: Top your morning cereal or yogurt with grapefruit segments for a refreshing and nutritious start to the day.

Here are two refreshing and delicious recipes that incorporate grapefruit:

Grapefruit and Avocado Salad:

Ingredients:

- 2 pink grapefruits, segmented
- 2 ripe avocados, diced
- 1 small red onion, thinly sliced
- 1 cup cherry tomatoes, halved
- 1/4 cup fresh cilantro, chopped
- 1/4 cup extra-virgin olive oil
- 2 tablespoons fresh lime juice
- Salt and pepper to taste
- Optional: Feta or goat cheese for topping

Instructions:

1. In a large bowl, combine the grapefruit segments, diced avocados, sliced red onion, cherry tomatoes, and chopped cilantro.
2. In a small bowl, whisk together the olive oil and lime juice to create the dressing.
3. Pour the dressing over the salad and gently toss to combine.
4. Season with salt and pepper to taste.
5. If desired, crumble feta or goat cheese on top before serving.
6. Chill in the refrigerator for at least 30 minutes before serving to allow the flavors to meld.

Sparkling Grapefruit Mint Cooler:

Ingredients:

- 2 pink grapefruits, juiced
- 1/4 cup fresh mint leaves
- 2 tablespoons agave syrup or honey (adjust to taste)
- Sparkling water
- Ice cubes
- Grapefruit slices and mint sprigs for garnish

Instructions:

1. In a blender, combine the fresh grapefruit juice, mint leaves, and agave syrup or honey. Blend until the mint is finely chopped.
2. Strain the mixture to remove the mint leaves and any pulp.
3. Fill glasses with ice cubes and pour the grapefruit-mint mixture over the ice.
4. Top each glass with sparkling water, adjusting the ratio to your preference.
5. Stir gently to combine.
6. Garnish with grapefruit slices and mint sprigs.
7. Serve immediately and enjoy this refreshing grapefruit mint cooler.

These recipes showcase the versatility of grapefruit, whether used in a vibrant salad or a refreshing beverage. Feel free to customize these recipes based on your taste preferences and enjoy the bright and citrusy flavors of grapefruit!

Cautionary Notes:

While grapefruit offers numerous health benefits, it's important to note that it can interact with certain medications. Grapefruit can interfere with enzymes in the liver, affecting the way some drugs are metabolized. If you are allergic or on medication, consult with your healthcare provider to determine whether grapefruit consumption is suitable for you.

Conclusion:

Grapefruit stands out not only as a zesty and flavorful fruit but also as a nutritional powerhouse offering a spectrum of health benefits. Whether enjoyed fresh, juiced, or incorporated into a variety of dishes, grapefruit has rightfully earned its place as a versatile and delicious addition to a balanced and healthy diet.

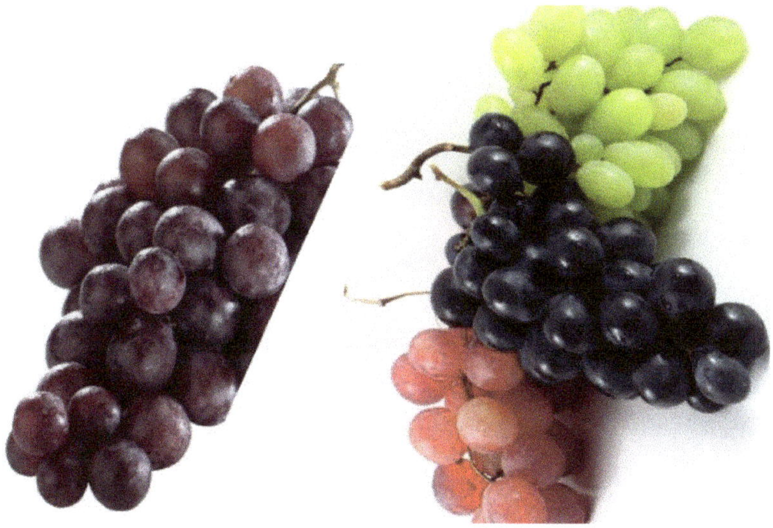

Grapes

The Healthful Bounty of Grapes: Benefits and Versatile Uses

Grapes, the succulent and versatile fruits, have been cherished for centuries for their delectable taste and numerous health benefits. Whether enjoyed fresh, dried, or in the form of juice or wine, grapes have made their mark as a delightful addition to our diets. In this article, we will explore the various benefits of grapes and their versatile uses.

Health Benefits of Grapes:

Rich in Antioxidants:

Grapes are packed with antioxidants, including resveratrol, flavonoids, and quercetin. These compounds help combat oxidative stress, reducing the risk of chronic diseases and promoting overall well-being.

Heart Health:

The high levels of resveratrol in grapes have been linked to heart health. Resveratrol is believed to lower blood pressure, reduce inflammation, and improve overall cardiovascular function.

Cancer Prevention:

Some studies suggest that the antioxidants in grapes may help prevent certain types of cancers. Resveratrol, in particular, has shown promising anti-cancer properties in research.

Improved Digestion:

Grapes contain fiber, which aids in digestion and promotes a healthy gut. The fiber content helps prevent constipation and supports the growth of beneficial gut bacteria.

Vitamins, Minerals and Immune System:

Grapes are a nutritious fruit that contain various vitamins, minerals, and antioxidants, each offering unique health benefits. The vitamins and minerals in grapes, such as vitamin C and manganese, contribute to a strengthened immune system. Regular consumption may help ward off common illnesses.

Here's a list of some key vitamins and minerals found in grapes, along with their benefits:

Vitamin C:

- **Benefits:** Vitamin C is a powerful antioxidant that supports immune function, promotes collagen synthesis for healthy skin, helps protect cells from damage caused by free radicals, and enhances iron absorption.

Vitamin K:

- **Benefits:** Vitamin K plays a crucial role in blood clotting, bone metabolism, and cardiovascular health. It helps maintain bone density and may reduce the risk of osteoporosis and fractures.

Vitamin B6 (Pyridoxine):

- **Benefits:** Vitamin B6 is involved in over 100 enzymatic reactions in the body, including protein metabolism, neurotransmitter synthesis, and immune function. It supports brain health, mood regulation, and may help reduce the risk of cardiovascular disease.

Potassium:

- **Benefits:** Potassium is an essential mineral that helps regulate fluid balance, muscle contractions, nerve signals, and blood pressure. Adequate potassium intake is important for heart health, muscle function, and overall electrolyte balance.

Copper:

- **Benefits:** Copper plays a role in energy metabolism, iron metabolism, and the synthesis of connective tissues and neurotransmitters. It supports immune function, antioxidant defense mechanisms, and may help maintain healthy skin and hair.

Manganese:

- **Benefits:** Manganese is a trace mineral that contributes to bone health, metabolism, antioxidant defense, and the synthesis of connective tissues and sex hormones. It supports collagen production, blood sugar regulation, and may help reduce inflammation.

Riboflavin (Vitamin B2):

- **Benefits:** Riboflavin is involved in energy metabolism, antioxidant defense, and the metabolism of carbohydrates, fats, and proteins. It supports healthy vision, skin, and mucous membranes, and may help reduce the frequency of migraine headaches.

Thiamine (Vitamin B1):

- **Benefits:** Thiamine is essential for energy metabolism, nerve function, and the synthesis of neurotransmitters and DNA. It supports heart health, brain function, and may help reduce the risk of neurodegenerative diseases.

Iron:

- **Benefits:** Iron is necessary for the production of hemoglobin, which carries oxygen in the blood, and myoglobin, which stores oxygen in muscles. It supports energy metabolism, immune function, and cognitive development.

Magnesium:

- **Benefits:** Magnesium is involved in over 300 enzymatic reactions in the body, including energy metabolism, muscle and nerve function, blood sugar regulation, and bone health. It supports heart health, muscle relaxation, and may help reduce the risk of migraine headaches.

Including grapes in your diet can provide a range of essential vitamins, minerals, and antioxidants that contribute to overall health and well-being. These nutrients work synergistically to support various physiological processes and may help reduce the risk of chronic diseases when consumed as part of a balanced diet.

Antioxidants

Grapes are rich in antioxidants, which are compounds that help protect cells from damage caused by free radicals and oxidative stress. Here are some key antioxidants found in grapes, along with their benefits:

1. **Resveratrol:**
    - **Benefits:** Resveratrol is a polyphenolic compound found in grape skins, particularly in red and purple grapes. It has potent antioxidant and anti-inflammatory properties and is associated with various health benefits, including heart health, improved insulin sensitivity, and potential anti-cancer effects. Resveratrol may also support brain health, protect against age-related cognitive decline, and promote longevity.
2. **Quercetin:**
    - **Benefits:** Quercetin is a flavonoid antioxidant found in the skin of grapes and other fruits and vegetables. It has anti-inflammatory and anti-allergic properties and may help protect against cardiovascular disease by reducing inflammation, improving

blood vessel function, and lowering blood pressure. Quercetin also supports immune function, promotes healthy aging, and may have anticancer effects.

3. **Anthocyanins:**

    - **Benefits:** Anthocyanins are a group of pigmented antioxidants found in the skins of red and purple grapes. They give grapes their vibrant color and are associated with various health benefits, including improved heart health, reduced inflammation, and enhanced cognitive function. Anthocyanins may also help protect against age-related cognitive decline, support eye health, and promote healthy aging.

4. **Flavonols (Kaempferol, Myricetin, and Quercetin):**

    - **Benefits:** Flavonols are a group of flavonoid antioxidants found in grape skins, seeds, and leaves. They have anti-inflammatory, antioxidant, and anti-cancer properties and may help protect against cardiovascular disease, improve blood vessel function, and lower the risk of certain cancers. Flavonols also support cognitive function, promote healthy aging, and may help protect against neurodegenerative diseases.

5. **Proanthocyanidins (Procyanidins):**

    - **Benefits:** Proanthocyanidins are a group of polyphenolic antioxidants found in grape seeds and skins. They have potent antioxidant and anti-inflammatory properties and may help protect against cardiovascular disease by reducing inflammation, improving blood vessel function, and lowering blood pressure. Proanthocyanidins also support skin health, promote wound healing, and may help reduce the risk of certain cancers.

6. **Vitamin C (Ascorbic Acid):**

    - **Benefits:** Vitamin C is a water-soluble antioxidant found in grapes and other fruits and vegetables. It helps protect cells from oxidative damage, supports immune function, promotes collagen synthesis for healthy skin, and enhances iron absorption. Vitamin C may also help reduce the risk of chronic diseases, including heart disease, cancer, and neurodegenerative disorders.

Including grapes in your diet can provide a rich source of these antioxidants, which work synergistically to promote overall health and protect against chronic diseases. Incorporating a variety of colorful fruits and vegetables, including grapes, can help ensure you receive a wide range of beneficial antioxidants and nutrients.

Skin Health:

The antioxidants in grapes play a role in maintaining healthy skin by fighting free radicals. Additionally, resveratrol may contribute to anti-aging effects, keeping the skin youthful and vibrant.

Nutritional Content

One cup (about 151 grams) of grapes typically contains the following approximate nutritional values:

- Carbohydrates: Approximately 27-28 grams
- Protein: Approximately 1 gram
- Fiber: Approximately 1-2 grams
- Fat: Negligible (virtually zero grams)
- Sugar: Approximately 23-24 grams

Grapes are naturally low in fat and protein but are a good source of carbohydrates, primarily in the form of natural sugars such as glucose, fructose, and sucrose. They also provide a small amount of dietary fiber, which contributes to digestive health and helps regulate blood sugar levels. Keep in mind that the exact nutritional content may vary slightly depending on the specific variety of grapes.

Versatile Uses of Grapes:

Fresh Consumption: Enjoying fresh grapes is a simple and delightful way to experience their natural sweetness. Red, green, or black, grapes make for a convenient and healthy snack.

Dried Grapes (Raisins): Drying grapes concentrates their natural sugars, resulting in raisins. Raisins are a convenient and nutritious addition to cereals, salads, or enjoyed on their own.

Grape Juice: Freshly squeezed grape juice is a refreshing beverage that not only quenches thirst but also provides essential vitamins and minerals. It serves as a healthier alternative to sugary drinks.

Wine Production: Grapes are the primary ingredient in wine production. The fermentation process transforms the sugars in grapes into alcohol, creating a wide variety of wines with distinct flavors and characteristics.

Culinary Applications:

Grapes can be incorporated into both sweet and savory dishes. They add a burst of flavor to salads, pair well with cheese, and can be used in desserts, sauces, and chutneys.

Here are two delicious recipes that incorporate grapes:

Chicken and Grape Salad:

Ingredients:

- 2 cups cooked chicken breast, shredded or diced

- 1 cup red grapes, halved
- 1 cup green grapes, halved
- 1/2 cup celery, finely chopped
- 1/4 cup red onion, finely chopped
- 1/4 cup mayonnaise
- 1/4 cup plain Greek yogurt
- 1 tablespoon Dijon mustard
- 1 tablespoon honey
- Salt and pepper to taste
- Lettuce leaves, for serving
- Chopped walnuts or pecans (optional)

Instructions:

1. In a large mixing bowl, combine the cooked chicken, red grapes, green grapes, celery, and red onion.
2. In a small bowl, whisk together the mayonnaise, Greek yogurt, Dijon mustard, honey, salt, and pepper until well combined.
3. Pour the dressing over the chicken and grape mixture and toss gently until everything is evenly coated.
4. Refrigerate the salad for at least 30 minutes to allow the flavors to meld.
5. To serve, line plates with lettuce leaves and spoon the chicken and grape salad on top.
6. Optionally, sprinkle chopped walnuts or pecans over the salad for added crunch.
7. Enjoy this refreshing and flavorful chicken and grape salad as a light lunch or dinner option!

Roasted Grape and Brie Crostini:

Ingredients:

- Baguette, thinly sliced
- Brie cheese, sliced
- Red and/or green grapes
- Olive oil
- Honey

- Fresh thyme leaves
- Salt and pepper

Instructions:

1. Preheat your oven to 375°F (190°C).
2. Place the baguette slices on a baking sheet and lightly brush each slice with olive oil.
3. Top each baguette slice with a slice of Brie cheese.
4. Place a few grapes on top of the Brie cheese on each crostini.
5. Drizzle a little honey over the grapes and cheese.
6. Sprinkle fresh thyme leaves, salt, and pepper over the crostini.
7. Place the baking sheet in the preheated oven and bake for about 10-12 minutes, or until the cheese is melted and bubbly, and the baguette slices are lightly toasted.
8. Remove from the oven and let cool slightly before serving.
9. Arrange the roasted grape and Brie crostini on a platter and serve as an elegant appetizer or snack option for parties or gatherings.
10. Enjoy the delightful combination of sweet roasted grapes, creamy Brie cheese, and crusty baguette in these delicious crostini!

These recipes showcase the versatility of grapes, whether they're used in a savory salad or as a sweet topping for crostini. Enjoy experimenting with these flavors in your kitchen!

Conclusion:

Grapes are not just a delightful treat for the taste buds but also a nutritional powerhouse with a myriad of health benefits. From promoting heart health to enhancing skin radiance, the humble grape has earned its place as a versatile and wholesome addition to our diets. So, whether enjoyed fresh, dried, juiced, or in the form of a fine wine, let the goodness of grapes enrich your culinary experiences and contribute to your well-being.

It's advisable to consult with healthcare professionals before making significant changes to one's diet, allergies or lifestyle based on specific compounds in foods.

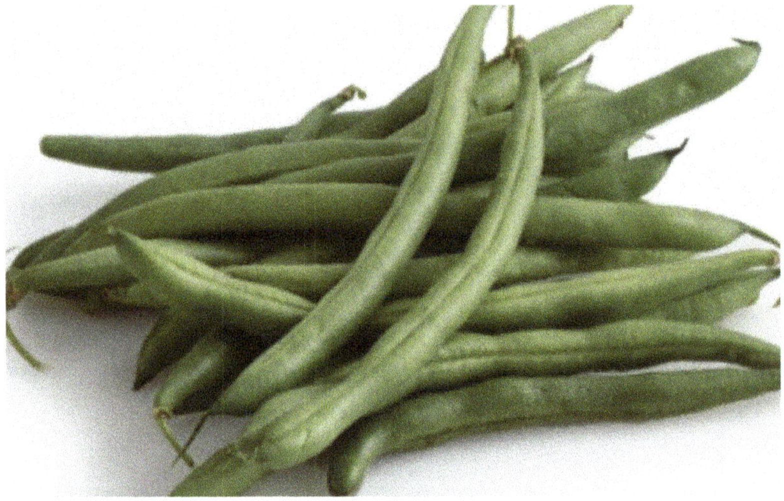

Green Beans

A Crisp and Nutrient-Packed Delight with Health Benefits and Culinary Versatility

Green beans, also known as string beans or snap beans, are a popular and versatile vegetable that graces tables across the globe. These vibrant, crisp pods not only contribute to the visual appeal of dishes but also offer a range of health benefits. In this article, we'll explore the nutritional advantages of green beans and the various creative ways in which they can be used in the kitchen.

Nutrient-Rich Composition:

Green beans are renowned for their impressive nutritional profile, providing a wealth of vitamins, minerals, and other essential nutrients. Here are some key components that make green beans a nutritious addition to your diet:

Vitamins:

Green beans, also known as snap beans or string beans, are a nutritious vegetable that provides various vitamins essential for health. Here's a list of vitamins found in green beans:

Vitamin C:

- Green beans are a good source of vitamin C, an antioxidant that supports the immune system, helps the body absorb iron, and promotes healthy skin.

Vitamin K:

- Green beans contain vitamin K, which is crucial for blood clotting and bone health. It plays a role in bone mineralization and contributes to overall bone density.

Vitamin A:

- Green beans provide vitamin A in the form of carotenoids, such as beta-carotene. Vitamin A is important for vision, immune function, and skin health.

Vitamin B1 (Thiamine):

- Thiamine is present in green beans and is essential for energy metabolism, nerve function, and the conversion of food into usable energy.

Vitamin B2 (Riboflavin):

- Green beans contain riboflavin, which is involved in energy production and supports the metabolism of fats, drugs, and steroids.

Vitamin B3 (Niacin):

- Niacin is found in green beans and plays a role in energy metabolism, DNA repair, and the functioning of the nervous system.

Vitamin B5 (Pantothenic Acid):

- Pantothenic acid is present in green beans and is involved in the synthesis of essential molecules in the body, including fatty acids and cholesterol.

Vitamin B6 (Pyridoxine):

- Green beans provide vitamin B6, which is important for the metabolism of amino acids, the synthesis of neurotransmitters, and immune function.

Including green beans in your diet can contribute to meeting your daily vitamin needs and provide a variety of essential nutrients that support overall health and well-being. As with any food, it's important to consume a variety of nutrient-rich foods to ensure a balanced intake of vitamins and other essential nutrients.

Minerals:
Green beans are a good source of various minerals, contributing to their nutritional value. Here's a list of minerals found in green beans:

Potassium:

- Green beans are rich in potassium, an essential mineral that helps regulate blood pressure, balance fluids in the body, and support proper muscle and nerve function.

Manganese:

- Green beans contain manganese, a trace mineral that plays a role in bone formation, blood clotting, and reducing inflammation.

Calcium:

- While not as high as in some other vegetables, green beans do provide a small amount of calcium, important for bone health, nerve function, and muscle contraction.

Magnesium:

- Magnesium in green beans supports muscle and nerve function, regulates blood pressure, and contributes to bone health.

Phosphorus:

- Phosphorus is present in green beans and is essential for bone and teeth formation, DNA synthesis, and energy metabolism.

Iron:

- Green beans provide iron, which is important for the formation of hemoglobin, the protein responsible for carrying oxygen in the blood.

Copper:

- Green beans contain copper, a trace mineral that is essential for the formation of red blood cells, maintenance of healthy bones and nerves, and immune system function.

Zinc:

- While present in smaller amounts, green beans provide zinc, a trace mineral important for immune function, wound healing, and DNA synthesis.

Including green beans in your diet can help ensure a diverse intake of minerals, supporting various physiological functions and promoting overall health. As with any food, it's important to consume a variety of nutrient-rich foods to ensure a broad spectrum of minerals and other essential nutrients.

Dietary Fiber:

- Green beans are rich in dietary fiber, promoting digestive health, regulating blood sugar levels, and aiding in weight management.

Antioxidants:

Green beans contain various antioxidants, including carotenoids and flavonoids, which help combat oxidative stress and inflammation.

Carotenoids:

- **Beta-carotene:** A precursor to vitamin A, beta-carotene gives green beans their vibrant color and is known for its antioxidant properties.
- **Lutein and Zeaxanthin:** These carotenoids are important for eye health and may help reduce the risk of age-related macular degeneration.

Flavonoids:

- **Quercetin:** A flavonoid with anti-inflammatory and antioxidant properties, quercetin is found in green beans and may contribute to various health benefits.
- **Kaempferol:** Another flavonoid present in green beans, kaempferol has antioxidant and anti-inflammatory effects.

Vitamin C:

- Green beans are a good source of vitamin C, a powerful antioxidant that supports the immune system, promotes skin health, and helps protect cells from oxidative damage.

Polyphenols:

- Green beans contain various polyphenols, including caffeic acid, ferulic acid, and chlorogenic acid, which have antioxidant and anti-inflammatory properties.

Minerals with Antioxidant Properties:

- Some minerals found in green beans, such as manganese and copper, also play a role in antioxidant defense systems within the body.

Consuming a diet rich in antioxidant-containing foods, like green beans, can contribute to overall health and may help protect against certain chronic diseases. Including a variety of colorful fruits and vegetables in your diet ensures a diverse intake of antioxidants and other essential nutrients.

Health Benefits:

Heart Health:

- The combination of fiber, potassium, and antioxidants in green beans contributes to heart health by regulating blood pressure, reducing cholesterol levels, and supporting overall cardiovascular function.

Bone Health:

- The presence of vitamin K and manganese in green beans is beneficial for bone health, aiding in bone mineralization and reducing the risk of osteoporosis.

Digestive Health:

- The fiber content in green beans promotes a healthy digestive system, preventing constipation and supporting optimal bowel function.

Weight Management:

- Low in calories and high in fiber, green beans provide a satisfying and nutritious addition to weight management plans, promoting a feeling of fullness.

Nutritional Content

One cup (about 125 grams) of cooked green beans typically contains the following approximate nutritional values:

- Carbohydrates: Approximately 10 grams
- Protein: Approximately 2 grams
- Fiber: Approximately 4 grams
- Fat: Approximately 0 grams
- Sugar: Approximately 4 grams

These values can vary slightly depending on factors such as cooking method and specific variety of green beans. Green beans are low in calories and fat, making them a nutritious addition to a balanced diet. They are a good source of dietary fiber, which promotes digestive health and helps maintain regular bowel movements. Additionally, green beans provide essential vitamins and minerals such as vitamin C, vitamin K, folate, and manganese.

Culinary Uses:

Sautéed Green Beans:

- Sauté green beans in olive oil with garlic, herbs, and a splash of lemon juice for a quick and flavorful side dish.

Green Bean Salad:

- Blanch green beans and toss them with cherry tomatoes, feta cheese, and a light vinaigrette for a refreshing salad.

Green Bean Stir-Fry:

- Include green beans in stir-fries with other colorful vegetables and your choice of protein for a vibrant and nutritious meal.

Green Bean Casserole:

- A classic dish during holiday seasons, green bean casserole combines green beans with creamy mushroom soup and crispy fried onions.

Green beans can be a versatile and tasty addition to a variety of dishes. Here are two delicious recipes featuring green beans:

Green Bean Almondine:

Ingredients:

- 1 lb fresh green beans, trimmed
- 2 tablespoons butter
- 2 tablespoons olive oil
- 2 cloves garlic, minced
- 1/3 cup sliced almonds
- 1 tablespoon lemon juice
- Salt and pepper to taste
- Fresh parsley for garnish

Instructions:

Blanch the Green Beans:

- Bring a large pot of salted water to a boil. Add the green beans and cook for 2-3 minutes until they are bright green and slightly tender. Immediately transfer them to an ice water bath to stop the cooking process. Drain and set aside.

Toast the Almonds:

- In a large skillet, melt butter and olive oil over medium heat. Add sliced almonds and toast them until golden brown, stirring frequently to prevent burning.

Sauté the Green Beans:

- Add minced garlic to the skillet and sauté for about 1 minute until fragrant. Add the blanched green beans and toss to coat in the almond and garlic mixture.

Finish and Serve:

- Drizzle lemon juice over the green beans, season with salt and pepper to taste, and toss everything together. Cook for an additional 2-3 minutes until the green beans are heated through.
- Garnish with fresh parsley and serve the Green Bean Almondine as a delightful side dish.

Chicken and Green Bean Stir-Fry:

Ingredients:

- 1 lb boneless, skinless chicken breasts, thinly sliced
- 1 lb fresh green beans, trimmed and cut into bite-sized pieces
- 3 tablespoons soy sauce
- 1 tablespoon oyster sauce
- 1 tablespoon sesame oil
- 2 tablespoons vegetable oil
- 2 cloves garlic, minced
- 1 tablespoon fresh ginger, grated
- Cooked rice for serving

Instructions:

1. **Marinate the Chicken:**
    - In a bowl, mix soy sauce, oyster sauce, and sesame oil. Add the sliced chicken and let it marinate for at least 15-20 minutes.
2. **Stir-Fry Chicken:**
    - Heat vegetable oil in a wok or large skillet over high heat. Add the marinated chicken and stir-fry until cooked through and slightly browned. Remove the chicken from the pan and set aside.
3. **Sauté Green Beans:**
    - In the same pan, add a bit more oil if needed. Sauté minced garlic and grated ginger until fragrant. Add the green beans and stir-fry for about 5-7 minutes until they are crisp-tender.
4. **Combine and Serve:**
    - Return the cooked chicken to the pan with the green beans. Toss everything together until well combined and heated through.
    - Serve the Chicken and Green Bean Stir-Fry over cooked rice for a delicious and balanced meal.

These recipes showcase the versatility of green beans, whether they are the star of a flavorful side dish or part of a delicious stir-fry. Enjoy incorporating these nutritious and vibrant vegetables into your culinary repertoire!

Tips on Growing Green Beans

The time it takes for green beans to grow from planting to harvest varies depending on the specific variety of green beans and growing conditions. However, in general, green beans typically take about 50 to 65 days from planting to harvest.

Here's a general timeline of the growth stages of green beans:

1. **Planting:** Green beans are usually planted directly into the soil after the danger of frost has passed and the soil has warmed up. Depending on your climate, this is typically done in the spring, once temperatures are consistently above freezing.
2. **Germination:** After planting, green bean seeds will germinate and begin to sprout within 7 to 14 days, depending on soil temperature and moisture levels.
3. **Vegetative Growth:** Once germinated, green bean plants enter a period of vegetative growth, during which they develop leaves, stems, and roots. They will continue to grow and produce more foliage as they mature.
4. **Flowering:** After several weeks of vegetative growth, green bean plants will begin to produce flowers. These flowers will eventually be pollinated, leading to the formation of bean pods.
5. **Pod Development:** Once pollinated, the flowers on green bean plants will develop into bean pods. Green beans typically reach maturity and are ready for harvest within 50 to 65 days after planting, depending on the variety.
6. **Harvesting:** Green beans are typically harvested when the pods are still young and tender, before the seeds inside have fully developed. Harvesting green beans regularly encourages the plants to produce more beans.
7. **Continuous Harvest:** Many green bean varieties are capable of producing multiple harvests throughout the growing season. By harvesting green beans regularly and providing proper care, you can enjoy a continuous supply of fresh beans throughout the summer months.

By following proper planting and care practices, you can grow your own green beans and enjoy a bountiful harvest of this versatile and nutritious vegetable.

Conclusion:

Green beans, with their vibrant color, crisp texture, and nutritional richness, deserve a regular place on your plate. Whether enjoyed as a simple side dish, added to salads, or incorporated into more complex recipes, green beans provide a burst of flavor and a myriad of health benefits. If you have specific health concerns, allergies, or conditions, it's advisable to consult with a healthcare professional or a registered dietitian before making significant changes to your diet. Embrace the versatility of green beans and savor the delicious and nutritious offerings they bring to your culinary adventures.

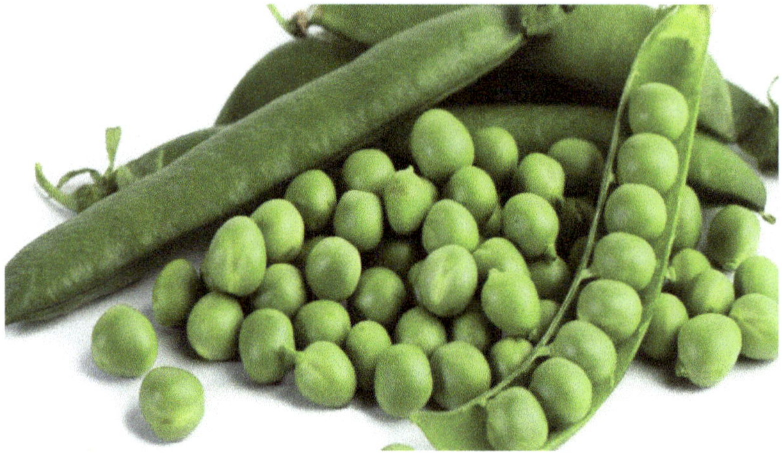

Green Peas

Tiny Gems Packed with Nutrition and Culinary Versatility

Green peas, the vibrant and versatile legumes, have been a beloved component of diets worldwide for centuries. Known for their sweet and delicate flavor, green peas are not only a delicious addition to a variety of dishes but also offer an impressive array of health benefits. In this article, we will explore the nutritional value, health benefits, and culinary uses that make green peas a nutrient-packed gem for both the palate and overall well-being.

Nutritional Powerhouse:

Green peas are a nutritional powerhouse, providing essential nutrients that contribute to a well-rounded and balanced diet. Key nutritional components of green peas include:

Protein:

- Despite their small size, green peas are a surprisingly good source of plant-based protein. Protein is essential for muscle repair, immune function, and overall growth and development.

Dietary Fiber:

- Green peas are rich in dietary fiber, both soluble and insoluble. Fiber supports digestive health, helps maintain a healthy weight by promoting a feeling of fullness, and contributes to heart health.

Vitamins:

Green peas are a good source of vitamins, including vitamin C, vitamin K, and several B-vitamins (folate, thiamine, and niacin). Vitamin C is an antioxidant that supports the immune system, while vitamin K is important for blood clotting.

Vitamin C:

- **Benefits:** As a potent antioxidant, vitamin C in green peas supports the immune system by protecting cells from damage caused by free radicals. It also aids in collagen synthesis, contributing to healthy skin, connective tissues, and wound healing.

Vitamin K:

- **Benefits:** Vitamin K is crucial for blood clotting and bone health. Green peas contribute to maintaining proper blood clotting, which is essential for wound healing, and support bone metabolism, reducing the risk of fractures.

Folate (Vitamin B9):

- **Benefits:** Folate is vital for DNA synthesis and repair, making it especially important during periods of rapid cell division, such as pregnancy. Adequate folate intake helps prevent neural tube defects in developing fetuses and supports overall cell function.

Thiamine (Vitamin B1):

- **Benefits:** Thiamine plays a crucial role in energy metabolism by aiding in the conversion of carbohydrates into energy. It also supports proper nerve function and is essential for the synthesis of neurotransmitters.

Minerals:

Green peas contain essential minerals such as iron, manganese, phosphorus, and potassium. Iron is crucial for oxygen transport in the blood, manganese plays a role in bone health, phosphorus supports energy metabolism, and potassium helps regulate blood pressure.

Iron:

- **Benefits:** Iron is a vital component of hemoglobin, the protein responsible for transporting oxygen in the blood. Adequate iron intake from green peas helps prevent iron-deficiency anemia and supports overall energy levels.

Manganese:

- **Benefits:** Manganese is essential for bone health, as it plays a role in the formation and maintenance of healthy bones. It also contributes to various enzyme systems involved in metabolism and antioxidant defenses.

Phosphorus:

- **Benefits:** Phosphorus is a structural component of DNA, RNA, and ATP (adenosine triphosphate), the primary energy carrier in cells. It is crucial for bone health, kidney function, and the metabolism of macronutrients.

Potassium:

- **Benefits:** Potassium is an electrolyte that plays a vital role in maintaining proper fluid balance, nerve impulses, and muscle contractions. It also supports heart health by helping to regulate blood pressure.

Health Benefits:

Heart Health:

- The combination of fiber, potassium, and antioxidants in green peas contributes to heart health. Fiber helps lower cholesterol levels, potassium regulates blood pressure, and antioxidants help reduce oxidative stress.

Blood Sugar Regulation:

- The fiber content in green peas slows down the absorption of sugars, contributing to better blood sugar control. This property makes green peas a suitable choice for individuals managing diabetes or those aiming to stabilize blood sugar levels.

Digestive Health:

- The fiber in green peas supports digestive health by promoting regular bowel movements and preventing constipation. It also contributes to a healthy gut microbiome.

Weight Management:

- The combination of protein and fiber in green peas promotes satiety, making them an excellent choice for those looking to manage their weight. The low-calorie content adds to their appeal as a nutritious and satisfying snack.

Nutritional Content

One cup (approximately 160 grams) of cooked green peas typically contains the following approximate nutritional values:

- Carbohydrates: Approximately 25 grams
- Protein: Approximately 8 grams
- Fiber: Approximately 9 grams
- Fat: Approximately 1 gram
- Sugar: Approximately 9 grams

These values can vary slightly depending on factors such as cooking method and specific variety of green peas. Green peas are a nutritious vegetable rich in carbohydrates, protein, dietary fiber, and various vitamins and minerals. They are low in fat and cholesterol and provide essential nutrients such as vitamin K, vitamin C, folate, and manganese.

Culinary Versatility:

Green peas are incredibly versatile in the kitchen, offering a burst of color, sweetness, and nutritional value to various dishes. Some common culinary uses include:

Pea Risotto:

- Incorporate green peas into a classic risotto for added sweetness, color, and nutritional value. The peas can be stirred in towards the end of the cooking process for a vibrant finish.

Minty Pea Soup:

- Create a refreshing and vibrant pea soup by blending cooked green peas with fresh mint, vegetable broth, and a touch of cream. This simple yet elegant soup can be served hot or cold.

Pea and Mint Pesto Pasta:

- Make a flavorful pesto by blending green peas, fresh mint, garlic, Parmesan cheese, and olive oil. Toss the pesto with cooked pasta for a light and summery dish.

Pea and Potato Mash:

- Combine green peas with boiled potatoes, a splash of milk, and a hint of butter to create a delicious and nutritious mashed potato alternative.

Here are two delicious and nutritious recipes featuring green peas:

Minty Pea and Avocado Toast:

Ingredients:

- 1 cup fresh or frozen green peas
- 1 ripe avocado
- 1 tablespoon fresh mint leaves, chopped
- 1 tablespoon lemon juice
- Salt and pepper to taste
- Whole grain bread slices
- Optional toppings: poached egg, feta cheese, chili flakes

Instructions:

1. Cook the green peas in boiling water for 2-3 minutes or until tender. Drain and set aside.
2. In a blender or food processor, combine the cooked green peas, ripe avocado, chopped mint leaves, lemon juice, salt, and pepper. Blend until smooth and creamy.

3. Toast whole grain bread slices to your liking.
4. Spread the minty pea and avocado mixture onto the toasted bread.
5. Top with optional ingredients such as a poached egg, crumbled feta cheese, or chili flakes for added flavor.
6. Serve immediately and enjoy a vibrant and nutritious toast.

Creamy Pea and Ham Risotto:

Ingredients:

- 1 cup Arborio rice
- 1 cup fresh or frozen green peas
- 1/2 cup cooked ham, diced
- 1 onion, finely chopped
- 2 cloves garlic, minced
- 4 cups chicken or vegetable broth, kept warm
- 1/2 cup dry white wine (optional)
- 1/4 cup Parmesan cheese, grated
- 2 tablespoons butter
- Salt and pepper to taste
- Fresh parsley, chopped (for garnish)

Instructions:

1. In a large pan, sauté the chopped onion in butter until softened. Add minced garlic and cook for an additional minute.
2. Add Arborio rice to the pan and cook, stirring, until the rice is lightly toasted.
3. If using wine, pour it into the pan and cook until it evaporates.
4. Begin adding warm broth to the rice one ladle at a time, stirring frequently. Allow the liquid to be absorbed before adding more.
5. When the rice is almost tender, stir in the green peas and diced ham.
6. Continue adding broth and stirring until the rice is creamy and cooked to your desired consistency.
7. Stir in grated Parmesan cheese and season with salt and pepper.
8. Garnish with fresh chopped parsley before serving.

9. Serve the creamy pea and ham risotto hot, savoring the rich flavors and creamy texture.

These recipes showcase the versatility of green peas, whether blended into a vibrant spread for toast or incorporated into a comforting and creamy risotto. Green peas not only add a burst of color but also contribute essential nutrients to these delightful dishes.

Tips on Growing Green Peas

Green peas, like many other vegetables, have different varieties with varying maturity times. However, in general, green peas typically take about 55 to 70 days from planting to harvest.

Here's a general timeline of the growth stages of green peas:

1. **Planting:** Green peas are usually planted directly into the soil in early spring, once the soil can be worked and the danger of frost has passed. They can also be planted in late summer for a fall harvest.
2. **Germination:** After planting, green pea seeds will germinate and begin to sprout within 7 to 14 days, depending on soil temperature and moisture levels.
3. **Vegetative Growth:** Once germinated, green pea plants enter a period of vegetative growth, during which they develop leaves, stems, and roots. They will continue to grow and produce more foliage as they mature.
4. **Flowering:** After several weeks of vegetative growth, green pea plants will begin to produce flowers. These flowers will eventually be pollinated, leading to the formation of pea pods.
5. **Pod Development:** Once pollinated, the flowers on green pea plants will develop into pea pods. Green peas typically reach maturity and are ready for harvest within 55 to 70 days after planting, depending on the variety.
6. **Harvesting:** Green peas are typically harvested when the pods are still young and tender, before the peas inside have fully developed. Harvesting green peas regularly encourages the plants to produce more peas.
7. **Continuous Harvest:** Many green pea varieties are capable of producing multiple harvests throughout the growing season. By harvesting green peas regularly and providing proper care, you can enjoy a continuous supply of fresh peas throughout the spring and early summer months.

By following proper planting and care practices, you can grow your own green peas and enjoy a bountiful harvest of this nutritious and versatile vegetable.

Conclusion:

Incorporating green peas into your diet is a delightful way to enhance both the taste and nutritional profile of your meals. Whether enjoyed as a standalone side dish or creatively incorporated into various recipes, green peas stand as tiny, nutrient-packed gems that contribute to a healthy and flavorful diet. While kidney beans are generally safe and healthy to consume as part of a balanced diet. As with any food, moderation is key. If you have specific health concerns, allergies, or conditions, it's advisable to consult with a healthcare professional or a registered dietitian before making significant changes to your diet.

With their appealing taste, versatility, and an abundance of health benefits, green peas deserve a special place in every kitchen.

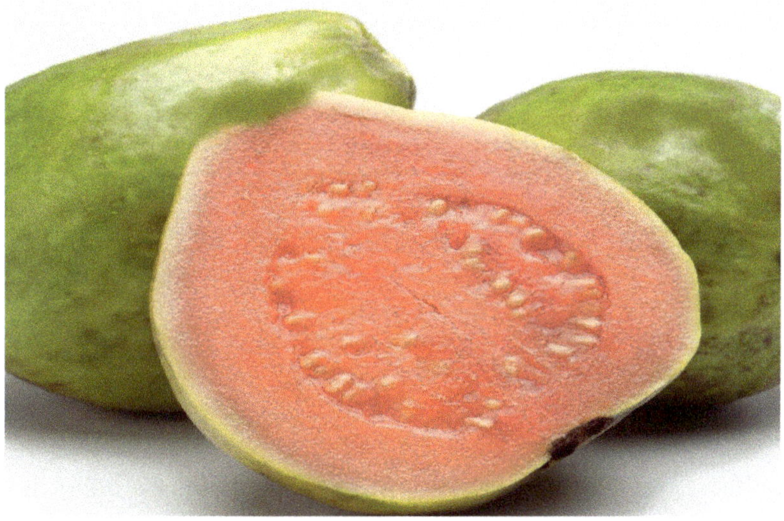

Guava

The Tropical Marvel: Guava - Benefits and Culinary Delights

Guava, a tropical fruit celebrated for its unique flavor and numerous health benefits, has been a culinary gem in various cultures around the world. This small, pear-shaped fruit is not only delicious but also packs a nutritional punch that contributes to overall well-being. In this article, we'll explore the benefits and versatile uses of guava, showcasing why it deserves a special place in your diet.

Nutrient-Rich Goodness:

Guava stands out as a nutrient-rich fruit, offering an impressive array of vitamins, minerals, and antioxidants. Here are some key nutritional components found in guava:

Vitamin C:

- **Benefits:** Boosts the immune system, supports skin health, acts as an antioxidant, aids in collagen production.

Dietary Fiber:

- **Benefits:** Promotes digestive health, helps regulate blood sugar levels, contributes to a feeling of fullness.

Vitamin A:

- **Benefits:** Essential for vision health, supports immune function, maintains healthy skin.

Potassium:

- **Benefits:** Helps regulate blood pressure, supports heart and muscle function, aids in fluid balance.

Folate (Vitamin B9):

- **Benefits:** Important for DNA synthesis and repair, aids in red blood cell formation.

Vitamin E:

- **Benefits:** Acts as an antioxidant, supports skin health, protects cells from damage.

Vitamin K:

- **Benefits:** Essential for blood clotting, contributes to bone health, helps regulate calcium in the body.

Calcium:

- **Benefits:** Important for bone and teeth health, supports muscle and nerve function.

Phosphorus:

- **Benefits:** Essential for bone and teeth health, involved in energy metabolism.

Magnesium:

- **Benefits:** Important for muscle and nerve function, supports bone health.

Iron:

- **Benefits:** Important for oxygen transport in the blood, supports energy metabolism.

Zinc:

- **Benefits:** Supports immune function, involved in wound healing, essential for DNA synthesis.

Sodium:

- **Benefits:** Plays a role in fluid balance, nerve function, and muscle contractions.

Manganese:

- **Benefits:** Contributes to bone formation, supports metabolism, acts as an antioxidant.

Copper:

- **Benefits:** Important for iron absorption, supports the formation of red blood cells.

B Vitamins (B1, B2, B3, B5, B6):

- **Benefits:** Essential for energy metabolism, support nerve function, and contribute to overall well-being.

Guava's impressive nutritional profile makes it a valuable addition to a well-balanced diet, offering a variety of vitamins and minerals that promote overall health and wellness.

Health Benefits:

Immune System Support:

- Guava's exceptionally high Vitamin C content supports the immune system, aiding the body in defending against infections and illnesses.

Digestive Health:

- The fiber in guava promotes healthy digestion, preventing constipation and supporting overall gut health.

Heart Health:

- Potassium in guava contributes to heart health by helping regulate blood pressure and supporting cardiovascular function.

Skin Health:

- The combination of Vitamin C and Vitamin E in guava supports skin health, promoting a youthful and radiant complexion.

Nutritional Content

The nutritional content of guava can vary slightly depending on factors like ripeness and variety, but here's a general idea of the nutritional breakdown for 1 cup (about 165 grams) of raw guava:

- Carbohydrates: Approximately 23 grams
- Protein: Roughly 4.2 grams
- Fiber: Around 9 grams
- Fat: Negligible, typically less than 1 gram
- Sugar: Approximately 12 grams

Guava is particularly known for its high fiber content, which can aid digestion and promote a feeling of fullness. It's also relatively low in calories and fat, making it a nutritious choice for a snack or addition to meals.

Versatile Culinary Uses:

Guava's versatility extends beyond its nutritional benefits, as it can be enjoyed in various culinary forms. Here are some popular uses:

Fresh Snacking:

- Peel and slice guava for a refreshing and nutritious snack. Its natural sweetness and juiciness make it an excellent alternative to less healthy snack options.

Smoothies and Juices:

- Blend guava into smoothies or juices to add a tropical flair. Combine it with other fruits, yogurt, or your favorite liquid for a delicious and vitamin-packed beverage.

Salads:

- Dice guava and add it to fruit salads or green salads for a burst of flavor and nutrition.

Desserts:

- Incorporate guava into desserts like sorbets, ice creams, and fruit salads for a unique and tropical twist.

Jams and Preserves:

- Utilize guava to make homemade jams or preserves. Its natural sweetness and aromatic flavor make for delightful spreads.

Here are two delicious recipes that showcase the unique flavor and nutritional benefits of guava:

Guava and Spinach Smoothie:

Ingredients:

- 1 cup fresh guava, peeled and seeded
- 1 cup fresh spinach leaves
- 1 banana
- 1/2 cup Greek yogurt
- 1 tablespoon chia seeds
- 1 cup coconut water or water
- Ice cubes (optional)
- Honey or agave syrup for sweetness (optional)

Instructions:

1. In a blender, combine fresh guava, spinach leaves, banana, Greek yogurt, chia seeds, and coconut water.
2. Blend until smooth and creamy. Add ice cubes if you prefer a colder smoothie.
3. Taste the mixture and add honey or agave syrup if additional sweetness is desired.
4. Pour into glasses and enjoy this nutrient-packed guava and spinach smoothie as a refreshing and wholesome beverage.

Guava and Mint Salad:

Ingredients:

- 2 cups fresh guava, peeled and diced
- 1 cucumber, peeled and diced
- 1/2 red onion, finely chopped
- 1/4 cup fresh mint leaves, chopped
- Juice of 1 lime
- 1 tablespoon extra-virgin olive oil
- Salt and pepper to taste
- Feta cheese, crumbled (optional)

Instructions:

1. In a large bowl, combine diced guava, cucumber, red onion, and chopped mint leaves.
2. In a small bowl, whisk together the lime juice and extra-virgin olive oil to create the dressing.
3. Drizzle the dressing over the guava mixture and toss gently to coat all ingredients.
4. Season with salt and pepper to taste. If desired, sprinkle crumbled feta cheese on top for an added burst of flavor.
5. Serve this guava and mint salad as a refreshing side dish for lunch or dinner. It's a perfect combination of sweet, savory, and citrusy flavors.

These recipes showcase the versatility of guava, whether blended into a nutritious smoothie or combined with fresh ingredients to create a vibrant salad. Enjoy the tropical goodness and unique taste of guava in these creative and healthy dishes!

Conclusion:

Guava is a tropical marvel that not only tantalizes the taste buds but also provides a wealth of health benefits. From its immune-boosting Vitamin C content to its digestive-friendly fiber, guava is a nutritious addition to any balanced diet. If you have specific health concerns, allergies, or conditions, it's advisable to consult with a healthcare professional or a registered dietitian before making significant changes to your diet.

Whether enjoyed fresh, blended into beverages, or incorporated into various culinary creations, guava invites you to savor the richness of tropical goodness while reaping the rewards of a nutrient-packed fruit. Embrace the unique benefits and culinary delights that guava brings to your table and enjoy the tropical goodness it has to offer.

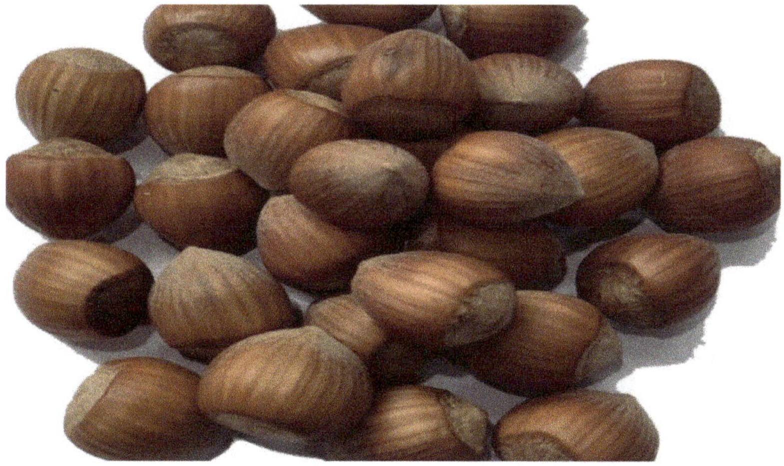

Hazelnuts

Nature's Nutrient-Rich Delight

Hazelnuts, often referred to as filberts, are not only a delicious addition to various culinary creations but also pack a nutritional punch. These small, flavorful nuts come from the Corylus avellana tree and have been enjoyed for centuries for their rich taste and versatile applications. Let's explore the benefits and diverse uses of hazelnuts that make them a delightful inclusion in a balanced and healthy diet.

Nutritional Powerhouse:

Hazelnuts are a nutrient-dense food, providing a wide array of essential vitamins, minerals, and antioxidants. Here's a breakdown of some key nutrients found in hazelnuts:

Healthy Fats:

Hazelnuts are rich in monounsaturated and polyunsaturated fats, particularly oleic acid and linoleic acid. These heart-healthy fats can contribute to better cardiovascular health.

Protein:

Hazelnuts are a good source of plant-based protein, making them an excellent option for those following vegetarian or vegan diets.

Vitamins:

Hazelnuts contain various vitamins, including vitamin E, vitamin B6, folate, thiamine, and riboflavin. Vitamin E, in particular, is a potent antioxidant that helps protect cells from damage caused by free radicals.

Vitamin E:

- **Benefits:** Vitamin E is a potent antioxidant that helps protect cells from oxidative stress and damage caused by free radicals. It is crucial for maintaining skin health, supporting the immune system, and promoting overall cellular function.

Vitamin B1 (Thiamine):

- **Benefits:** Thiamine is essential for energy metabolism. It helps convert food into energy and is crucial for the proper functioning of the nervous system.

Vitamin B2 (Riboflavin):

- **Benefits:** Riboflavin plays a key role in energy production and is essential for maintaining healthy skin, eyes, and nerve functions. It also acts as an antioxidant.

Vitamin B3 (Niacin):

- **Benefits:** Niacin is involved in energy metabolism, supporting the conversion of food into usable energy. It also plays a role in maintaining healthy skin and nervous system function.

Vitamin B6 (Pyridoxine):

- **Benefits:** Pyridoxine is crucial for brain development and function. It is involved in the synthesis of neurotransmitters and helps regulate mood. Vitamin B6 also plays a role in immune function and the metabolism of amino acids.

Folate (Vitamin B9):

- **Benefits:** Folate is essential for DNA synthesis and cell division. It is particularly important during periods of rapid cell growth, such as pregnancy. Adequate folate intake is crucial for preventing neural tube defects in developing fetuses.

Vitamin K:

- **Benefits:** Vitamin K is important for blood clotting and bone health. It helps in the synthesis of proteins involved in these processes, contributing to overall cardiovascular and skeletal well-being.

Vitamin C:

- **Benefits:** While hazelnuts are not particularly high in vitamin C, they still contain small amounts. Vitamin C is known for its antioxidant properties, supporting the immune system, promoting collagen synthesis for healthy skin, and aiding in the absorption of non-heme iron from plant-based sources.

These vitamins collectively contribute to the overall health and well-being of individuals, supporting functions ranging from energy metabolism to immune system function and skin health. Including hazelnuts in a balanced diet can be a delicious way to ensure a diverse intake of essential vitamins. However, it's important to note that the specific vitamin content can vary based on factors such as the variety of hazelnuts and the processing methods used.

Minerals:

These nuts provide essential minerals such as manganese, magnesium, phosphorus, potassium, and copper. These minerals play crucial roles in bone health, energy metabolism, and overall well-being.

Copper:

- **Benefits:** Copper plays a crucial role in the formation of collagen, the absorption of iron, and the development of connective tissues, bones, and blood vessels. It also acts as an antioxidant, helping to protect cells from damage.

Manganese:

- **Benefits:** Manganese is important for bone health, blood clotting, and reducing inflammation. It also plays a role in the metabolism of amino acids, cholesterol, and carbohydrates.

Magnesium:

- **Benefits:** Magnesium is essential for muscle and nerve function, energy production, and the maintenance of strong bones. It also contributes to regulating blood pressure and supporting the immune system.

Phosphorus:

- **Benefits:** Phosphorus is a vital component of DNA, RNA, and ATP (adenosine triphosphate), the primary energy carrier in cells. It also plays a crucial role in bone health, acid-base balance, and the synthesis of proteins.

Potassium:

- **Benefits:** Potassium is important for maintaining proper fluid balance, nerve signals, and muscle contractions. It also helps regulate blood pressure, supports heart health, and aids in the balance of electrolytes.

Zinc:

- **Benefits:** Zinc is involved in immune function, wound healing, DNA synthesis, and cell division. It also plays a role in maintaining the senses of taste and smell, as well as supporting reproductive health.

Iron:

- **Benefits:** While hazelnuts are not an exceptionally high source of iron, they do contain small amounts. Iron is crucial for the formation of hemoglobin, which carries oxygen in the blood. It also supports energy metabolism and overall vitality.

Calcium:

- **Benefits:** Calcium is vital for bone and teeth health, blood clotting, and muscle function. While hazelnuts are not a high-calcium food, they still contribute to overall dietary calcium intake.

Selenium:

- **Benefits:** Selenium acts as an antioxidant, protecting cells from oxidative damage. It is also involved in immune function, thyroid hormone metabolism, and reproduction.

Molybdenum:

- **Benefits:** Molybdenum is a cofactor for enzymes involved in the metabolism of certain amino acids and the detoxification of harmful substances in the body.

Including hazelnuts in your diet can provide a diverse array of essential minerals, supporting various physiological functions and contributing to overall health. It's important to note that the specific mineral content can vary based on factors such as the variety of hazelnuts and the growing conditions.

Dietary Fiber:

Hazelnuts are a good source of dietary fiber, promoting digestive health and helping to maintain a feeling of fullness, which can be beneficial for weight management.

Health Benefits:

Heart Health: The monounsaturated and polyunsaturated fats, coupled with vitamin E, contribute to heart health by reducing LDL cholesterol levels and promoting overall cardiovascular well-being.

Antioxidant Protection: Hazelnuts contain antioxidants such as vitamin E and phytochemicals that help neutralize free radicals, protecting cells from oxidative stress and inflammation.

Improved Digestive Health: The fiber content in hazelnuts supports digestive health by preventing constipation and promoting regular bowel movements.

Weight Management: The combination of healthy fats, protein, and fiber in hazelnuts can help control appetite and support weight management by promoting a feeling of fullness.

Bone Health: Minerals like manganese and phosphorus in hazelnuts contribute to maintaining strong and healthy bones.

Nutritional Content

The approximate nutritional breakdown for 1 cup (about 129 grams) of hazelnuts:

- Carbohydrates: Approximately 17 grams
- Protein: Roughly 17 grams
- Fiber: Around 11 grams
- Fat: Approximately 68 grams
- Sugar: About 4 grams

Hazelnuts are rich in healthy fats, particularly monounsaturated and polyunsaturated fats, which can be beneficial for heart health. They also provide a good amount of protein and fiber, making them a nutritious snack option.

Versatile Culinary Uses:

Hazelnuts enhance both sweet and savory dishes, providing a rich, nutty flavor and a satisfying crunch. Here are some ways to incorporate hazelnuts into your culinary repertoire:

Baking: Hazelnuts can be finely chopped or ground to add texture and flavor to cakes, cookies, and bread. They are a classic ingredient in popular treats like hazelnut chocolate spreads and pralines.

Salads: Toasted hazelnuts can be sprinkled over salads to add a delightful crunch. They pair well with leafy greens, fruits, and cheese.

Nut Butters: Homemade hazelnut butter is a nutritious and delicious alternative to commercial spreads. Simply roast and blend hazelnuts until smooth for a creamy and flavorful nut butter.

Trail Mix: Combine hazelnuts with other nuts, seeds, and dried fruits to create a wholesome and energizing trail mix.

Sauces and Dressings: Ground hazelnuts can be incorporated into sauces and dressings, adding depth and richness to the flavor profile.

Here are two delicious hazelnut recipes for you to try:

Chocolate Hazelnut Spread (Homemade Nutella):

Ingredients:

- 2 cups hazelnuts (roasted and peeled)
- 1 cup powdered sugar
- 1/2 cup unsweetened cocoa powder
- 1/4 cup vegetable oil
- 1 teaspoon vanilla extract
- 1/2 teaspoon salt

Instructions:

1. Preheat your oven to 350°F (175°C). Spread the hazelnuts on a baking sheet and roast for about 10-12 minutes or until the skins start to crack.
2. Allow the hazelnuts to cool slightly. Rub them in a clean kitchen towel to remove most of the skins.
3. In a food processor, blend the roasted hazelnuts until they form a smooth hazelnut butter. This process may take several minutes, depending on your food processor.
4. Add the powdered sugar, cocoa powder, vegetable oil, vanilla extract, and salt to the hazelnut butter. Continue processing until all the ingredients are well combined and the mixture is smooth.
5. Adjust sweetness and consistency by adding more sugar or oil if needed.
6. Transfer the homemade chocolate hazelnut spread to a jar or airtight container. Store in the refrigerator.

Roasted Brussels Sprouts with Hazelnuts and Balsamic Glaze:

Ingredients:

- 1 pound Brussels sprouts, trimmed and halved
- 2 tablespoons olive oil
- Salt and pepper, to taste
- 1/2 cup hazelnuts, toasted and chopped
- Balsamic glaze for drizzling

Instructions:

1. Preheat your oven to 400°F (200°C).
2. In a large bowl, toss the Brussels sprouts with olive oil, salt, and pepper until they are well coated.
3. Spread the Brussels sprouts on a baking sheet in a single layer.
4. Roast in the preheated oven for 20-25 minutes or until the Brussels sprouts are golden brown and crispy on the edges.
5. While the Brussels sprouts are roasting, toast the hazelnuts in a dry pan over medium heat until fragrant. Be careful not to burn them.
6. Once the Brussels sprouts are done, transfer them to a serving dish. Sprinkle the toasted hazelnuts on top.
7. Drizzle balsamic glaze over the roasted Brussels sprouts and hazelnuts.

8. Toss gently to combine and serve immediately.

These recipes showcase the versatility of hazelnuts, whether incorporated into a delightful spread or adding a crunchy, flavorful element to a savory dish. Enjoy!

Choosing and Storing Hazelnuts:

When selecting hazelnuts, look for those with intact, unblemished shells. Opt for fresh, plump nuts that feel heavy for their size. To store hazelnuts, keep them in an airtight container in a cool, dark place or in the refrigerator to maintain their freshness.

Conclusion:

Hazelnuts are more than just a tasty treat – they are a nutritional powerhouse offering a plethora of health benefits. If you have specific health concerns, allergies, or conditions, it's advisable to consult with a healthcare professional or a registered dietitian before making significant changes to your diet.

Whether enjoyed on their own as a snack, added to recipes, or transformed into delightful spreads, hazelnuts can be a versatile and delightful addition to a well-rounded, plant-based diet.

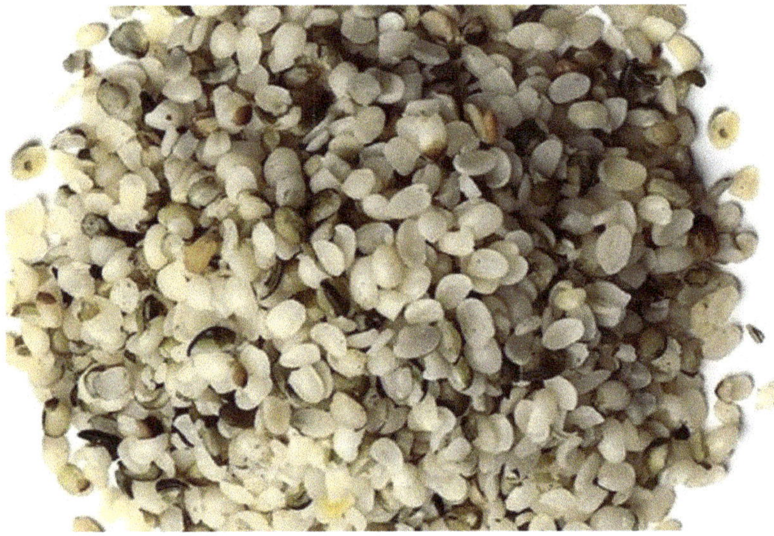

Hemp Seed

Harnessing the Power of Hemp Seeds: Exploring Their Benefits and Versatile Uses

Hemp seeds, derived from the Cannabis sativa plant species, have been revered for their nutritional value and versatility for centuries. Despite their association with cannabis, hemp seeds contain only trace amounts of THC (tetrahydrocannabinol), the psychoactive compound found in marijuana, and are prized for their rich array of nutrients and health-promoting properties. Let's delve into the world of hemp seeds and uncover their myriad benefits and uses.

Nutritional Powerhouse:

Hemp seeds are a nutritional powerhouse, packed with essential nutrients that support overall health and well-being. Here's a glimpse of what hemp seeds have to offer:

Complete Protein: Hemp seeds are a complete protein source, containing all nine essential amino acids that the body cannot produce on its own. This makes them particularly valuable for vegetarians, vegans, and individuals looking to boost their protein intake.

Healthy Fats: Hemp seeds are rich in healthy fats, including omega-3 and omega-6 fatty acids, in an optimal ratio for heart health and inflammation regulation. These fats are essential for brain function, cardiovascular health, and skin health.

Fiber: Hemp seeds are an excellent source of dietary fiber, which supports digestive health, promotes satiety, and helps regulate blood sugar levels.

Vitamins and Minerals:

Hemp seeds contain a variety of vitamins and minerals, including vitamin E, magnesium, phosphorus, potassium, iron, and zinc, which play essential roles in various physiological processes in the body.

Vitamins:

Vitamin E: Acts as a powerful antioxidant, protecting cells from damage caused by free radicals. Supports skin health, immune function, and cardiovascular health.

Vitamin B1 (Thiamine): Essential for energy metabolism, nerve function, and carbohydrate metabolism. Supports healthy brain function and may help reduce the risk of neurodegenerative diseases.

Vitamin B2 (Riboflavin): Supports energy production, metabolism of fats, carbohydrates, and proteins, and antioxidant activity. Important for healthy skin, eyes, and nerve function.

Vitamin B3 (Niacin): Plays a role in energy metabolism, DNA repair, and cell signaling. Supports cardiovascular health, brain function, and skin health.

Vitamin B6 (Pyridoxine): Necessary for amino acid metabolism, neurotransmitter synthesis, and immune function. Supports brain health, mood regulation, and hormone balance.

Vitamin B9 (Folate): Essential for DNA synthesis, cell division, and red blood cell formation. Supports fetal development during pregnancy and may help prevent neural tube defects.

Vitamin B5 (Pantothenic Acid): Plays a role in energy metabolism, hormone synthesis, and cholesterol synthesis. Supports healthy skin, hair, and nails.

Minerals:

Magnesium: Necessary for muscle function, nerve function, and energy metabolism. Supports bone health, cardiovascular health, and relaxation.

Phosphorus: Important for bone and teeth health, DNA synthesis, and energy metabolism. Supports kidney function and acid-base balance.

Potassium: Essential for nerve function, muscle contraction, and fluid balance. Helps regulate blood pressure and heart rhythm.

Iron: Necessary for oxygen transport in the blood and energy production. Supports immune function, cognitive function, and healthy skin.

Zinc: Important for immune function, wound healing, and DNA synthesis. Supports growth and development, reproductive health, and skin health.

Copper: Necessary for iron metabolism, antioxidant defense, and connective tissue formation. Supports brain health, immune function, and energy metabolism.

Manganese: Plays a role in bone formation, metabolism, and antioxidant activity. Supports wound healing, blood sugar regulation, and immune function.

Selenium: Acts as an antioxidant, supports thyroid function, and may have anti-inflammatory properties. Supports immune function, reproductive health, and cognitive function.

These vitamins and minerals found in hemp seeds are essential for various physiological processes in the body, including energy metabolism, immune function, bone health, and overall well-being. Incorporating hemp seeds into your diet can help ensure you're getting a wide range of nutrients to support optimal health.

Antioxidants:

Hemp seeds are rich in antioxidants, such as vitamin E and various phytonutrients, which help protect cells from damage caused by free radicals and oxidative stress.

Vitamin E: Acts as a potent antioxidant, protecting cell membranes from oxidative damage. Supports skin health, immune function, and cardiovascular health.

Gamma-Tocopherol: A form of vitamin E with unique antioxidant properties. May help reduce inflammation, protect against cardiovascular disease, and support brain health.

Phytosterols: Plant compounds with antioxidant and anti-inflammatory properties. May help lower cholesterol levels, support immune function, and reduce the risk of certain cancers.

Phospholipids: Found in cell membranes, phospholipids act as antioxidants and support cellular structure and function. May help improve cognitive function and liver health.

Carotenoids: Plant pigments with antioxidant properties. Beta-carotene, lutein, and zeaxanthin are carotenoids found in hemp seeds. They may help protect against age-related macular degeneration, support skin health, and boost immune function.

Phosphatidylserine: A type of phospholipid with antioxidant properties. Supports brain health, cognitive function, and memory.

Polyphenols: Plant compounds with antioxidant and anti-inflammatory properties. Found in varying amounts in hemp seeds, polyphenols may help reduce the risk of chronic diseases, such as heart disease and cancer, and support overall health.

Squalene: An antioxidant compound found in hemp seeds and other plant sources. May help protect against oxidative stress, support skin health, and improve cholesterol levels.

These antioxidants found in hemp seeds help neutralize free radicals, reduce inflammation, and protect cells from damage, contributing to overall health and well-being. Incorporating hemp seeds into your diet can be a valuable way to increase your intake of these beneficial antioxidants and support optimal health.

Health Benefits:

Incorporating hemp seeds into your diet can offer a wide range of health benefits, including:

Heart Health: The omega-3 and omega-6 fatty acids found in hemp seeds support cardiovascular health by reducing inflammation, lowering cholesterol levels, and improving blood vessel function.

Brain Function: The omega-3 fatty acids in hemp seeds are crucial for brain development, cognitive function, and mood regulation. They may also help reduce the risk of neurodegenerative diseases such as Alzheimer's and Parkinson's.

Digestive Health: The high fiber content of hemp seeds promotes regular bowel movements, prevents constipation, and supports a healthy gut microbiome.

Skin Health: The vitamin E and essential fatty acids in hemp seeds help nourish and moisturize the skin, reduce inflammation, and protect against damage from UV radiation and environmental pollutants.

Muscle Repair and Growth: The complete protein content of hemp seeds provides the building blocks necessary for muscle repair, growth, and recovery after exercise.

Versatile Uses:

Hemp seeds can be incorporated into a wide variety of dishes and recipes, adding a nutty flavor and a nutritional boost. Here are some popular ways to use hemp seeds in the kitchen:

Smoothies: Add hemp seeds to your favorite smoothie recipe for a creamy texture and an extra protein punch.

Salads: Sprinkle hemp seeds on top of salads for added crunch and nutritional value.

Baking: Use hemp seeds as a topping for bread, muffins, cookies, and other baked goods, or incorporate them into the batter for extra texture and flavor.

Granola and Cereal: Mix hemp seeds into homemade granola or sprinkle them over cereal for a nutritious breakfast option.

Yogurt and Oatmeal: Stir hemp seeds into yogurt or oatmeal for a protein-rich and satisfying snack or meal.

Dips and Spreads: Blend hemp seeds into hummus, pesto, or other dips and spreads for added creaminess and nutritional benefits.

Here are two delicious recipes featuring hemp seeds:

Hemp Seed Pesto:

Ingredients:

- 1 cup fresh basil leaves, packed
- 1/4 cup hemp seeds
- 2 cloves garlic, peeled
- 1/4 cup grated Parmesan cheese (or nutritional yeast for a vegan option)
- 1/4 cup extra virgin olive oil
- 1 tablespoon lemon juice
- Salt and pepper to taste

Instructions:

1. In a food processor, combine the basil leaves, hemp seeds, garlic, and Parmesan cheese.
2. Pulse until the ingredients are finely chopped.
3. With the food processor running, slowly drizzle in the olive oil and lemon juice until the mixture forms a smooth paste.
4. Season with salt and pepper to taste.
5. Serve the hemp seed pesto tossed with cooked pasta, spread on sandwiches or wraps, or used as a dip for vegetables.

Hemp Seed Energy Bites:

Ingredients:

- 1 cup rolled oats
- 1/2 cup hemp seeds
- 1/4 cup almond butter (or any nut butter of your choice)
- 1/4 cup honey or maple syrup
- 1/4 cup chopped nuts (such as almonds, walnuts, or pecans)
- 1/4 cup dried fruit (such as raisins, cranberries, or chopped dates)
- 1 teaspoon vanilla extract
- Optional add-ins: chocolate chips, shredded coconut, chia seeds

Instructions:

1. In a large mixing bowl, combine the rolled oats, hemp seeds, chopped nuts, and dried fruit.
2. In a small saucepan, heat the almond butter and honey (or maple syrup) over low heat until melted and well combined.
3. Remove the saucepan from the heat and stir in the vanilla extract.
4. Pour the almond butter mixture over the dry ingredients and stir until everything is evenly coated.
5. If desired, add any optional add-ins, such as chocolate chips or shredded coconut.
6. Using your hands, roll the mixture into bite-sized balls and place them on a parchment-lined baking sheet.
7. Refrigerate the energy bites for at least 30 minutes to firm up before serving.
8. Store the hemp seed energy bites in an airtight container in the refrigerator for up to one week.

These recipes showcase the versatility of hemp seeds and their ability to add nutrition and flavor to a wide variety of dishes. Enjoy these delicious and nutritious hemp seed recipes as part of a healthy diet!

Conclusion:

Hemp seeds are a versatile and nutrient-dense superfood that can be easily incorporated into a healthy diet. Whether you're looking to boost your protein intake, support heart health, or simply add a flavorful and nutritious ingredient to your meals, hemp seeds are a valuable addition to any kitchen pantry. Embrace the power of hemp seeds and reap the numerous benefits they have to offer for your health and well-being.

If you have specific health concerns, allergies, or conditions, it's advisable to consult with a healthcare professional or a registered dietitian before making significant changes to your diet.

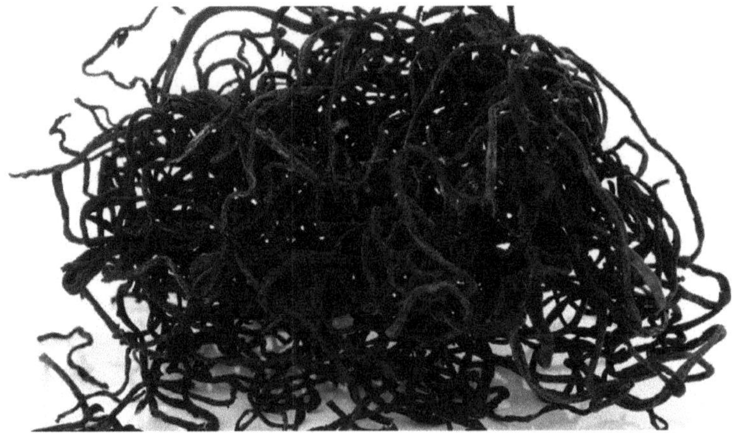

Hijiki

Unlocking the Health Benefits and Culinary Versatility of a Seaweed Superfood

Hijiki, a type of seaweed that has been a staple in Asian cuisine for centuries, is gaining popularity worldwide for its unique taste and impressive health benefits. Derived from the Sargassum fusiforme species of brown seaweed, hijiki is not only a culinary delight but also a nutritional powerhouse. In this article, we'll explore the many benefits of hijiki and discover its diverse uses in the kitchen.

Nutritional Powerhouse:

Hijiki is celebrated for its rich nutritional content, making it a valuable addition to a balanced and health-conscious diet. Here are some key nutrients found in hijiki:

Dietary Fiber:

Hijiki is an excellent source of dietary fiber, aiding in digestive health and promoting a feeling of fullness.

Minerals:

Rich in essential minerals such as calcium, iron, magnesium, and iodine, hijiki contributes to bone health, oxygen transport, and thyroid function.

Iodine:

- Crucial for thyroid function and the production of thyroid hormones, which play a role in regulating metabolism.

Calcium:

- Important for bone health, muscle function, and nerve transmission.

Iron:

- Essential for the formation of hemoglobin, which carries oxygen in the blood, and the prevention of iron-deficiency anemia.

Magnesium:

- Necessary for muscle and nerve function, energy production, and the maintenance of bone health.

Zinc:

- Important for immune function, wound healing, and DNA synthesis.

Potassium:

- Plays a role in maintaining proper heart and muscle function, regulating fluid balance, and supporting overall cardiovascular health.

Phosphorus:

- Vital for bone and teeth health, energy metabolism, and the synthesis of DNA and RNA.

Sodium:

- While sodium is typically present in seaweeds, including hijiki, it is important for maintaining fluid balance and nerve function.

Manganese:

- Contributes to bone formation, blood clotting, and reducing inflammation.

Copper:

- Important for the formation of red blood cells, maintenance of bones and nerves, and the functioning of the immune system.

It's important to note that the mineral content of hijiki can vary based on factors such as its origin, growing conditions, and preparation methods. While hijiki provides a rich source of minerals, it should be consumed in moderation due to its potential iodine content, as excessive iodine intake can have adverse effects on thyroid function. As with any food, it's recommended to incorporate hijiki into a well-balanced diet for optimal health benefits.

Vitamins:

Hijiki contains vitamins such as vitamin K, which plays a role in blood clotting, and vitamin B2 (riboflavin), important for energy metabolism.

Vitamin A:

- Important for vision, immune function, and skin health.

Vitamin C:

- An antioxidant that supports immune function, helps the body absorb iron, and promotes healthy skin.

Vitamin E:

- An antioxidant that helps protect cells from damage caused by free radicals.

Vitamin K:

- Essential for blood clotting and bone health.

Vitamin B1 (Thiamine):

- Crucial for energy metabolism and the proper functioning of the nervous system.

Vitamin B2 (Riboflavin):

- Plays a key role in energy production, cell growth, and the maintenance of healthy skin.

Vitamin B3 (Niacin):

- Essential for DNA repair, energy metabolism, and the proper functioning of the nervous system.

Vitamin B5 (Pantothenic Acid):

- Involved in the synthesis of fatty acids, amino acids, and other important molecules.

Vitamin B6 (Pyridoxine):

- Essential for brain development, the production of neurotransmitters, and the metabolism of amino acids.

Vitamin B9 (Folate):

- Important for DNA synthesis and cell division. Adequate folate intake is particularly important during pregnancy for fetal development.

Vitamin B12 (Cobalamin):

- While vitamin B12 is primarily found in animal products, some seaweeds may contain small amounts. However, it's important to note that hijiki is not a reliable source of vitamin B12.

The vitamin content of hijiki can vary based on factors such as its origin, growing conditions, and preparation methods. Incorporating hijiki into a well-balanced diet can provide a range of essential vitamins that contribute to overall health and well-being.

Protein:

While not as high in protein as some other sources, hijiki provides plant-based protein, making it a valuable option for vegetarians and vegans.

Health Benefits:

Iodine for Thyroid Health: Hijiki is a rich source of iodine, a crucial mineral for the proper functioning of the thyroid gland. Adequate iodine intake supports thyroid hormone production, which is essential for metabolism.

Bone Health: The calcium content in hijiki contributes to bone health and may help prevent conditions like osteoporosis.

Iron for Anemia Prevention: Hijiki is a good source of iron, which is important for the formation of hemoglobin and the prevention of iron-deficiency anemia.

Antioxidant Properties: Hijiki contains antioxidants that help neutralize free radicals, reducing oxidative stress and supporting overall health.

Nutritional Content

Hijiki is a type of seaweed commonly used in Japanese cuisine. Here's an approximate nutritional breakdown for 1 cup (about 136 grams) of cooked hijiki:

- Carbohydrates: Approximately 12 grams
- Protein: Roughly 2 grams
- Fiber: Around 3 grams
- Fat: Less than 1 gram
- Sugar: Less than 1 gram

Hijiki is low in fat and calories but a good source of dietary fiber. It also contains various vitamins and minerals such as calcium, magnesium, and iron. However, it's important to note that hijiki can absorb toxins from the sea, so it's recommended to consume it in moderation and from reputable sources. Additionally, due to its high iodine content, individuals with thyroid issues should consume hijiki cautiously.

Culinary Uses:

Hijiki's unique flavor and versatility make it a popular ingredient in various dishes. Here are some common culinary uses of hijiki:

Salads: Rehydrated hijiki can be added to salads, providing a chewy texture and a burst of umami flavor. Combine it with fresh vegetables and a light dressing for a nutritious side dish.

Stir-Fries: Hijiki works well in stir-fries, absorbing the flavors of other ingredients while maintaining its distinct taste and texture.

Sushi Rolls: In Japanese cuisine, hijiki is often used as a filling for sushi rolls, adding both nutritional value and depth of flavor.

Soups and Stews: Hijiki can be incorporated into soups and stews, enhancing the overall taste and providing a nutrient boost to the dish.

Rice Dishes: Mix hijiki into rice dishes for added nutrition and a touch of oceanic flavor. It pairs well with various grains and complements the natural sweetness of rice.

Hijiki, with its unique flavor and nutritional benefits, can be incorporated into various delicious recipes. ***Here are two recipes featuring hijiki:***

Hijiki Seaweed Salad:

Ingredients:

- 1/2 cup dried hijiki seaweed
- 1 carrot, julienned
- 1/2 cucumber, thinly sliced
- 1/4 cup thinly sliced red onion
- 2 tablespoons soy sauce
- 1 tablespoon rice vinegar
- 1 tablespoon sesame oil
- 1 tablespoon maple syrup or agave nectar
- 1 teaspoon grated fresh ginger
- Sesame seeds for garnish

Instructions:

1. **Rehydrate the Hijiki:**
    - Rinse the dried hijiki under cold water and soak it in warm water for about 15-20 minutes or until it becomes tender. Drain and set aside.
2. **Prepare Vegetables:**
    - In a large bowl, combine the rehydrated hijiki, julienned carrot, sliced cucumber, and red onion.
3. **Make the Dressing:**
    - In a small bowl, whisk together soy sauce, rice vinegar, sesame oil, maple syrup or agave nectar, and grated fresh ginger.
4. **Combine and Toss:**
    - Pour the dressing over the vegetables and hijiki. Toss everything together until well coated.

5. **Chill and Serve:**
    - Refrigerate the salad for at least 30 minutes to let the flavors meld.
    - Garnish with sesame seeds before serving.
6. **Enjoy this refreshing and nutritious Hijiki Seaweed Salad as a side dish or a light, standalone meal.**

Hijiki and Vegetable Stir-Fry:

Ingredients:

- 1/2 cup dried hijiki seaweed
- 1 cup broccoli florets
- 1 bell pepper, thinly sliced
- 1 carrot, julienned
- 1 tablespoon vegetable oil
- 2 tablespoons soy sauce
- 1 tablespoon mirin (Japanese sweet rice wine)
- 1 tablespoon sesame seeds
- Cooked rice for serving

Instructions:

1. **Rehydrate the Hijiki:**
    - Rinse the dried hijiki under cold water and soak it in warm water for about 15-20 minutes. Drain and set aside.
2. **Prepare Vegetables:**
    - In a wok or large skillet, heat vegetable oil over medium-high heat.
    - Add broccoli, bell pepper, and julienned carrot. Stir-fry for a few minutes until the vegetables are slightly tender.
3. **Add Hijiki:**
    - Add the rehydrated hijiki to the vegetables and continue stir-frying for another 2-3 minutes.
4. **Make the Sauce:**
    - In a small bowl, mix soy sauce and mirin. Pour the sauce over the vegetables and hijiki in the wok.

5. **Finish and Serve:**
    - Continue stir-frying until the vegetables are cooked to your liking and the hijiki is well-coated in the sauce.
    - Sprinkle sesame seeds on top and serve over cooked rice.
6. **Enjoy this savory and satisfying Hijiki and Vegetable Stir-Fry as a quick and nutritious meal.**

These recipes showcase the versatility of hijiki, allowing you to enjoy its distinct flavor and reap its health benefits in a variety of culinary creations.

Conclusion:

Hijiki stands as a testament to the culinary and nutritional treasures found in the sea. With its impressive array of health benefits and versatile applications in the kitchen, hijiki has rightfully earned its place as a superfood. Whether you're seeking to enhance the nutritional profile of your meals or explore new and flavorful culinary experiences, hijiki is a seaweed that deserves a spot on your plate. If you have specific health concerns, allergies, or conditions, it's advisable to consult with a healthcare professional or a registered dietitian before making significant changes to your diet.

Embrace the richness of hijiki and embark on a journey of taste and well-being inspired by the bounty of the ocean.

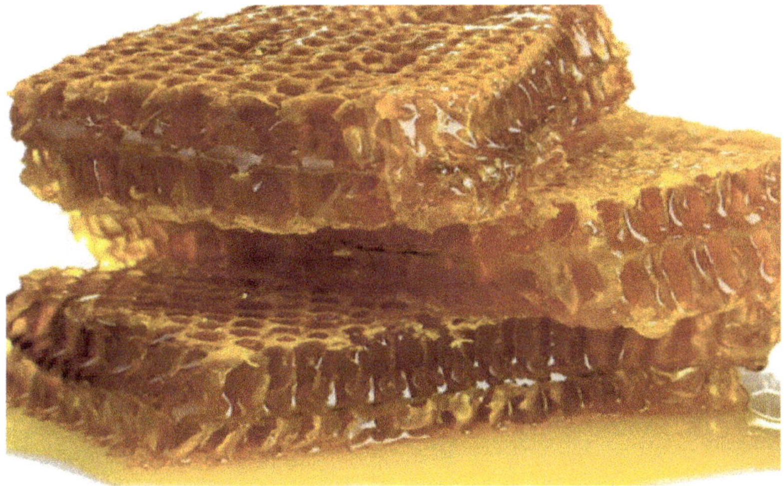

Honey

The Sweet Nectar of Nature

Honey, the golden elixir crafted by bees from the essence of flowers, has captivated human taste buds and fascinated healers for millennia. Beyond its irresistible sweetness, honey boasts a plethora of health benefits and versatile uses that have earned it a cherished place in culinary, medicinal, and even spiritual practices across cultures worldwide. From ancient civilizations to modern science, honey continues to unveil its remarkable properties, enriching both palate and well-being.

A Natural Nutrient Powerhouse:

Honey isn't just sugar; it's a complex blend of natural sugars, enzymes, antioxidants, vitamins, and minerals. While its precise composition may vary based on floral sources, honey typically contains glucose and fructose, providing a quick energy boost without the crash associated with refined sugars. Furthermore, honey contains trace amounts of essential nutrients like vitamin C, calcium, potassium, and iron, contributing to its nutritional profile.

Vitamins:

- **Vitamin C**: While present in small amounts, vitamin C in honey contributes to immune function, collagen synthesis, and wound healing.
- **Vitamin B2 (Riboflavin)**: Important for energy metabolism, riboflavin aids in breaking down carbohydrates, proteins, and fats, promoting overall energy production.
- **Vitamin B3 (Niacin)**: Supports nervous system function and plays a role in cholesterol management.

Minerals:

- **Calcium**: Essential for bone health, muscle function, and nerve transmission.

- **Iron**: Helps in the formation of hemoglobin, which carries oxygen in the blood, and supports energy production.
- **Magnesium**: Involved in hundreds of biochemical reactions in the body, including muscle and nerve function, blood glucose control, and blood pressure regulation.
- **Potassium**: Crucial for heart health, potassium helps maintain normal blood pressure levels and supports muscle and nerve function.
- **Phosphorus**: Important for bone health, energy production, and DNA synthesis.

Enzymes:

- **Glucose Oxidase**: An enzyme that, when combined with glucose and oxygen, produces hydrogen peroxide, which has antimicrobial properties and contributes to honey's ability to inhibit bacterial growth.
- **Diastase**: Supports the breakdown of complex carbohydrates into simple sugars, aiding in digestion and nutrient absorption.

Antioxidants:

- **Flavonoids**: These plant-based antioxidants help neutralize free radicals, reducing oxidative stress and inflammation in the body. Flavonoids are associated with a lower risk of chronic diseases such as heart disease and cancer.
- **Phenolic Compounds**: Including compounds like caffeic acid, gallic acid, and quercetin, these antioxidants have anti-inflammatory, antimicrobial, and anticancer properties.
- **Vitamin E**: A fat-soluble antioxidant that protects cells from oxidative damage and supports skin health.

Immune Support and Healing Properties:

One of honey's most celebrated attributes is its potential to support immune function and promote healing. Its antimicrobial properties, stemming from hydrogen peroxide and other compounds, make it an effective natural remedy for minor wounds, burns, and sore throats. Studies suggest that honey's antimicrobial activity may inhibit the growth of bacteria, fungi, and even some viruses, making it a valuable ally in combating infections.

Soothing and Protective for the Throat:

Honey's soothing effect on sore throats has been cherished for generations. Its viscous texture coats the throat, providing relief from irritation and coughing. When combined with warm water or herbal teas, honey becomes a comforting tonic that eases discomfort and promotes relaxation. Additionally, the antioxidant compounds in honey may help reduce inflammation and protect the delicate tissues of the throat.

Honey's antibiotic properties, recognized since the late 19th century, have been extensively studied. Its potential as a cough remedy is acknowledged by health authorities, with recommendations for children as a safer alternative to over-the-counter medications. Additionally, honey's mild laxative effect can be beneficial in alleviating constipation and bloating.

Research suggests honey's potential role in preventing acid reflux, with its ability to line the esophagus and stomach, reducing the upward flow of stomach acid. Moreover, honey's antiviral and antifungal effects have been explored, showcasing its inhibitory action on various pathogens.

Honey's applications in ophthalmology, as a carbohydrate source for athletes, and its potential positive effects in preventing cancer, managing chest pain, and aiding skin graft fixations add to its multifaceted nature.

Honey is used worldwide for the treatment of various ophthalmological conditions like blepharitis, keratitis, conjunctivitis, corneal injuries, chemical and thermal burns to eyes.

Honey's suitability for long-term storage, with preservation attributed to its composition and chemical properties, further underscores its versatility. However, preservation involves limiting access to humidity and avoiding rapid heating. Excessive heat can compromise honey's nutritional value.

Nutritional Content

The nutritional content in 1 tablespoon (about 21 grams) of honey typically includes:

- Carbohydrates: Approximately 17.3 grams
- Protein: Negligible, typically less than 0.1 grams
- Fiber: Negligible, typically less than 0.1 grams
- Fat: Negligible, typically less than 0.1 grams
- Sugar: Approximately 17.2 grams

Honey is primarily composed of carbohydrates, primarily in the form of sugars like glucose and fructose. It's low in protein, fiber, and fat but provides quick energy due to its high sugar content.

A Culinary Delight and Versatile Ingredient:

Beyond its medicinal properties, honey enriches culinary creations with its unique flavor profile and versatility. From drizzling over pancakes and yogurt to incorporating into marinades and salad dressings, honey adds depth and complexity to both sweet and savory dishes. Its natural sweetness can balance the acidity of dressings, enhance the richness of baked goods, or elevate the flavor of sauces and glazes.

Here are two recipes that use honey:

Honey Garlic Glazed Salmon:

Ingredients:

- 4 salmon fillets
- 4 cloves garlic, minced
- 1/4 cup soy sauce
- 3 tablespoons honey
- 1 tablespoon olive oil
- 1 tablespoon lemon juice
- Salt and pepper to taste
- Chopped green onions and sesame seeds for garnish (optional)

Instructions:

1. Preheat your oven to 375°F (190°C). Line a baking sheet with parchment paper or lightly grease it.
2. In a small bowl, whisk together the minced garlic, soy sauce, honey, olive oil, and lemon juice.
3. Place the salmon fillets on the prepared baking sheet. Season each fillet with salt and pepper to taste.
4. Brush the honey garlic sauce generously over the salmon fillets, reserving some sauce for later.
5. Bake the salmon in the preheated oven for 12-15 minutes, or until the salmon is cooked through and flakes easily with a fork.
6. Remove the salmon from the oven and brush with the remaining honey garlic sauce.
7. Garnish with chopped green onions and sesame seeds if desired and serve hot. Enjoy!

Honey Lemon Ginger Tea:

Ingredients:

- 2 cups water
- 1 tablespoon freshly grated ginger
- 2 tablespoons honey
- 2 tablespoons lemon juice

- Thinly sliced lemon and fresh mint leaves for garnish (optional)

Instructions:

1. In a small saucepan, bring the water to a simmer over medium heat.
2. Add the freshly grated ginger to the simmering water and let it steep for about 5 minutes.
3. After 5 minutes, remove the saucepan from the heat and strain out the ginger using a fine mesh strainer or cheesecloth.
4. Stir in the honey and lemon juice until well combined.
5. Pour the honey lemon ginger tea into mugs.
6. Garnish each mug with a slice of lemon and a sprig of fresh mint if desired.
7. Serve hot and enjoy the soothing and refreshing flavor of this honey lemon ginger tea!

These recipes showcase the versatility of honey in both savory and sweet dishes, adding a touch of natural sweetness and depth of flavor to your meals.

A Sweetener with Health Benefits:

Unlike refined sugars, which offer empty calories devoid of nutrients, honey provides sweetness along with potential health benefits. While it's important to consume honey in moderation due to its calorie content, its natural sugars are accompanied by antioxidants that may help reduce oxidative stress and inflammation in the body. Choosing honey as a sweetener can be a flavorful way to enhance dishes while supporting overall health.

Folk medicine

Traditions across various civilizations recognized honey's therapeutic properties. In ancient Greece, Egypt, Ayurveda, and traditional Chinese medicine, honey was applied orally and topically for ailments ranging from gastric disturbances to skin disorders. Ayurvedic experts considered honey a boon for weak digestion, an effective remedy for irritating coughs, and valuable for maintaining oral health. Egyptian medicine, enriched with honey, featured its use in embalming, wound healing, and as a topical ointment.

In ancient Greek practices, Oenomel, a beverage combining honey and unfermented grape juice, was employed as a folk remedy. Hippocrates, a prominent Greek scientist, recommended honey for diverse purposes, including pain relief, hydration, and as a treatment for various conditions. The historical use of honey for medicinal purposes continued, with recommendations from scientists like Avicenna for treating tuberculosis almost a millennium ago.

Medicinally, Ayurvedic practices encompass a wide array of uses for honey, addressing issues from hiccups and stress to gastrointestinal problems and arthritis. Laboratory and clinical investigations have also unveiled honey's antibacterial and anti-inflammatory properties, making it a versatile therapeutic agent.

Exploring Varietal Honeys:

Just as wine reflects the terroir of its grapes, honey captures the essence of its floral sources and geographical origins. Varietal honeys, such as acacia, clover, lavender, and manuka, offer distinct flavors, colors, and aromas based on the nectar gathered by bees. Each variety of honey carries its unique characteristics and potential health benefits, inviting exploration and appreciation of the diverse world of honey.

Preservation

Because of its composition and chemical properties, honey is suitable for long-term storage, and is easily assimilated even after long preservation. Honey, and objects immersed in honey, have been preserved for centuries. The key to preservation is limiting access to humidity.

Temperature

Honey should not be heated rapidly, over direct heat. Basically, the hotter you heat honey, the more potential for reducing nutritional value. Excessive heat can have detrimental effects on the nutritional value of honey. Heating up to 37°C (98.6 F) causes loss of nearly 200 components, part of which are antibacterial.

Adverse effects of honey

Honey is relatively free of adverse effects. Topical application of honey may lead to transient stinging sensation. Otherwise, it is described in different forms as soothing, relieving pain, to be non-irritating and a painless dressing change. Allergy to honey is rare, but there could be an allergic reaction to either pollen or bee proteins in honey. If you are allergic steer away from honey and consult your physician. Excessive application of honey may lead to dehydration of tissues which can however be restored by saline packs. Theoretical risk of rise in blood glucose levels may always be there when applied to large open wounds in diabetics.

Honey is a form of sugar, so a person's intake should be moderate.

Conclusion:

Honey stands as a testament to the harmonious relationship between nature and humanity, offering not only sweetness to the palate but also a myriad of health-promoting properties. From ancient remedies to modern culinary delights, honey continues to inspire and nourish, reminding us of the boundless wonders found in the natural world. Whether enjoyed straight from the hive or incorporated into culinary creations, honey remains a timeless treasure, enriching our lives with its golden glow and golden promise of well-being.

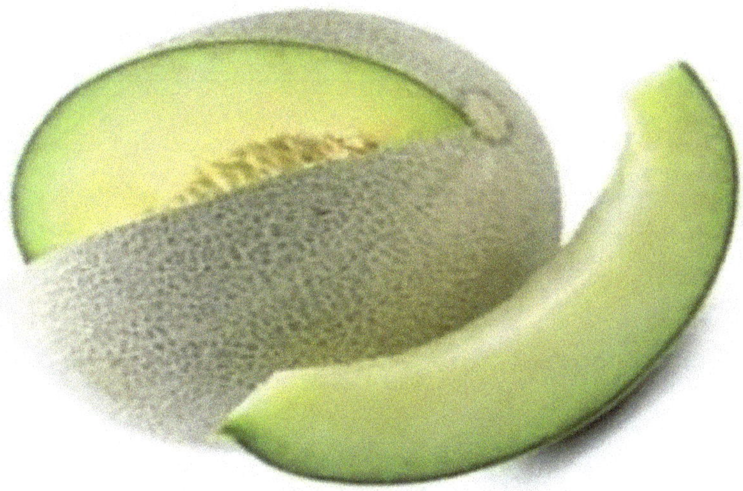

Honeydew

The Sweet Elegance of Honeydew: Benefits and Culinary Inspirations

Honeydew, a lusciously sweet and refreshing melon, is not only a summer delight but also a nutrient-packed addition to a wholesome diet. Known for its pale green flesh and succulent taste, honeydew offers a variety of health benefits and versatile culinary uses. In this article, we will explore the many virtues of honeydew, from its nutritional richness to its creative applications in the kitchen.

Nutritional Richness:

Honeydew, like other melons, is a hydrating and low-calorie fruit that brings a host of essential nutrients to the table. Here are some key components of honeydew's nutritional profile:

Vitamin C:

- **Benefits:** Boosts the immune system, supports skin health, acts as an antioxidant, aids in collagen production.

Potassium:

- **Benefits:** Helps regulate blood pressure, supports heart and muscle function, aids in fluid balance.

Fiber:

- **Benefits:** Promotes digestive health, helps regulate blood sugar levels, contributes to a feeling of fullness.

Vitamin K:

- **Benefits:** Essential for blood clotting, contributes to bone health, helps regulate calcium in the body.

Folate (Vitamin B9):

- **Benefits:** Important for DNA synthesis and repair, aids in red blood cell formation.

Vitamin B6 (Pyridoxine):

- **Benefits:** Important for brain development and function, helps the body convert food into energy, supports the nervous system.

Vitamin B3 (Niacin):

- **Benefits:** Supports energy metabolism, helps maintain skin health.

Vitamin B5 (Pantothenic Acid):

- **Benefits:** Essential for the synthesis of fatty acids, supports energy metabolism.

Vitamin B1 (Thiamine):

- **Benefits:** Essential for energy metabolism, supports nerve function.

Vitamin B2 (Riboflavin):

- **Benefits:** Important for energy production, supports normal vision and skin health.

Calcium:

- **Benefits:** Important for bone and teeth health, supports muscle and nerve function.

Magnesium:

- **Benefits:** Important for muscle and nerve function, supports bone health.

Copper:

- **Benefits:** Supports the formation of red blood cells, aids in iron absorption.

Zinc:

- **Benefits:** Supports immune function, involved in wound healing, essential for DNA synthesis.

Phosphorus:

- **Benefits:** Essential for bone and teeth health, involved in energy metabolism.

Iron:

- **Benefits:** Important for oxygen transport in the blood, supports energy metabolism.

These vitamins and minerals make honeydew a nutritious addition to a well-balanced diet, offering a range of health benefits. Including honeydew in your diet can help you meet your nutritional needs while enjoying a naturally sweet and hydrating fruit.

Health Benefits:

Hydration:

- With a high-water content, honeydew helps keep you hydrated, especially during hot weather.

Skin Health:

- The combination of Vitamin C and water content contributes to healthy and radiant skin.

Heart Health:

- Potassium in honeydew supports heart health by helping regulate blood pressure.

Digestive Health:

- The fiber in honeydew promotes digestive regularity and a healthy gut.

Nutritional Content

The nutritional content in 1 cup (about 177 grams) of honeydew melon typically includes:

- Carbohydrates: Approximately 15 grams
- Protein: Roughly 1.5 grams
- Fiber: Around 1.4 grams
- Fat: Less than 0.2 grams
- Sugar: Approximately 14 grams

Honeydew melon is low in calories and fat, making it a refreshing and nutritious choice for a snack or addition to meals. It's also a good source of vitamin C, potassium, and other essential nutrients.

Culinary Inspirations:

Honeydew's subtly sweet flavor and crisp texture make it a versatile ingredient in the kitchen. Here are some creative ways to incorporate honeydew into your culinary creations:

Fruit Salads:

- Combine honeydew with other fresh fruits like strawberries, blueberries, and mint for a vibrant and refreshing fruit salad.

Smoothies:

- Blend honeydew with Greek yogurt, cucumber, and a hint of mint for a hydrating and nutritious smoothie.

Sorbet and Ice Cream:

- Puree honeydew and freeze it to make a delightful honeydew sorbet. It can also be incorporated into homemade ice cream for a naturally sweet twist.

Salsas and Relishes:

- Dice honeydew and combine it with jalapeños, red onion, cilantro, and lime juice to create a unique salsa or relish. This pairs exceptionally well with grilled fish or chicken.

Here are two delicious and refreshing recipes that highlight the natural sweetness of honeydew:

Honeydew and Mint Gazpacho:

Ingredients:

- 1 medium-sized honeydew melon, peeled, seeded, and diced
- 1 cucumber, peeled and diced
- 1 green bell pepper, diced
- 1/2 red onion, finely chopped
- 2 cloves garlic, minced
- 1/4 cup fresh mint leaves, chopped
- 3 tablespoons lime juice
- 2 tablespoons extra-virgin olive oil
- Salt and pepper to taste
- 1 cup cold water
- Optional: Feta cheese for garnish

Instructions:

1. In a blender, combine honeydew melon, cucumber, green bell pepper, red onion, garlic, mint leaves, lime juice, and extra-virgin olive oil.
2. Blend until smooth, adding cold water gradually to achieve the desired consistency.
3. Season with salt and pepper to taste. Chill the gazpacho in the refrigerator for at least 1-2 hours.
4. Before serving, stir the gazpacho well and garnish with crumbled feta cheese if desired.
5. Serve this honeydew and mint gazpacho cold as a refreshing appetizer on a warm day.

Honeydew and Prosciutto Skewers:

Ingredients:

- 1 small honeydew melon, peeled, seeded, and cut into bite-sized cubes
- 10 slices of prosciutto, cut into strips
- 1 cup fresh mozzarella balls
- Fresh basil leaves
- Balsamic glaze for drizzling

Instructions:

1. Thread a piece of honeydew, a strip of prosciutto, a mozzarella ball, and a basil leaf onto small skewers or toothpicks.
2. Repeat the process until all the skewers are assembled.
3. Arrange the honeydew and prosciutto skewers on a serving platter.
4. Just before serving, drizzle balsamic glaze over the skewers for added flavor.
5. Serve these honeydew and prosciutto skewers as an elegant and refreshing appetizer at your next gathering.

These recipes showcase the versatility of honeydew, whether blended into a chilled soup with a hint of mint or paired with prosciutto, mozzarella, and basil for delightful skewers. Enjoy the unique and sweet flavors of honeydew in these creative and satisfying dishes!

Tips on Growing Honeydew Melons

The growth process of honeydew melons, like many other fruits, goes through several distinct stages. Here's a detailed explanation of each stage and the approximate time it takes for honeydew melons to grow:

1. **Germination (5-10 days):** The growth process begins with planting honeydew seeds in a suitable growing medium, such as soil or a seed-starting mix. Germination occurs when the seed absorbs water and begins to sprout. This stage typically takes 5 to 10 days, depending on factors like soil temperature and moisture levels.
2. **Seedling Stage (2-3 weeks):** After germination, the honeydew seedlings emerge from the soil. During this stage, the seedlings develop their first true leaves and establish a root system. Seedlings require consistent watering and adequate sunlight to support healthy growth. This stage usually lasts around 2 to 3 weeks.
3. **Vine Growth and Vegetative Stage (4-6 weeks):** As the honeydew plants mature, they enter a phase of vigorous vine growth and vegetative development. During this stage, the plants produce long trailing vines, additional leaves, and lateral branches. Adequate

spacing between plants is crucial to allow for proper vine expansion. This stage typically lasts around 4 to 6 weeks, depending on growing conditions.

4. **Flowering (1-2 weeks):** Honeydew melon plants begin to flower once they reach a certain level of maturity, typically around 6 to 8 weeks after planting. Honeydew plants produce both male and female flowers on the same vine. Bees and other pollinators play a vital role in transferring pollen from male to female flowers, leading to fruit set. Flowering usually lasts 1 to 2 weeks.
5. **Fruit Development (6-8 weeks):** After successful pollination, the fertilized flowers develop into young honeydew fruits. Initially, the fruits are small and green, gradually increasing in size as they mature. During this stage, the honeydew melons require consistent watering and nutrients to support healthy fruit development. Depending on the variety and growing conditions, fruit development typically takes around 6 to 8 weeks.
6. **Ripening (1-2 weeks):** As the honeydew melons near maturity, they undergo ripening, during which the fruits develop their characteristic flavor, aroma, and sweetness. The skin color changes from green to creamy yellow or pale white, and the fruit becomes slightly soft to the touch. Honeydew melons are typically harvested when they reach full maturity. Ripening usually takes around 1 to 2 weeks, depending on environmental conditions.

Overall, the entire growth process of honeydew melons, from seed to harvest, typically takes approximately 80 to 100 days under optimal growing conditions. However, variations in climate, soil quality, and cultural practices can influence the duration of each stage and the overall growth timeline. It's essential for growers to monitor their honeydew plants closely and provide appropriate care throughout each stage of growth to ensure healthy and productive crops.

Conclusion:

Honeydew is not only a deliciously sweet and hydrating fruit but also a nutritional powerhouse that can be enjoyed in a variety of ways. From fresh snacks to creative culinary experiments, honeydew adds a touch of elegance to your table while providing essential vitamins and minerals. If you have specific health concerns, allergies, or conditions, it's advisable to consult with a healthcare professional or a registered dietitian before making significant changes to your diet.

Embrace the benefits and versatility of honeydew as you savor its delightful taste and nourish your body with its health-promoting properties.

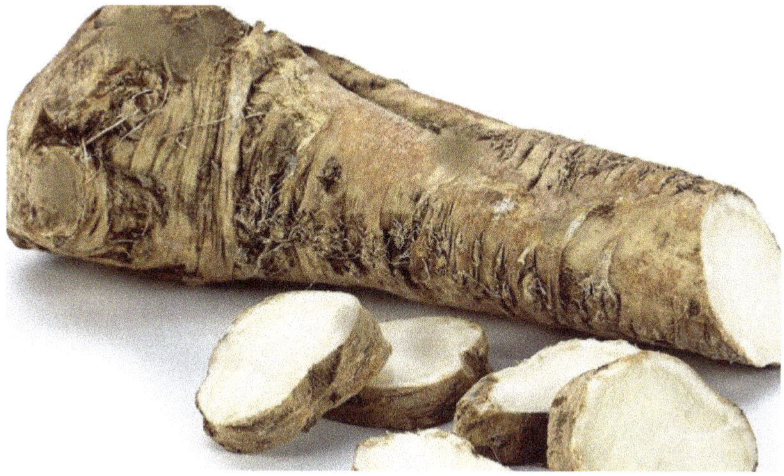

Horseradish

Exploring the Health Benefits and Culinary Wonders of Horseradish

Horseradish (Armoracia rusticana), a pungent root vegetable known for its bold flavor, has been cherished for centuries not only as a culinary delight but also for its numerous health benefits. From spicing up dishes to providing a range of therapeutic advantages, horseradish is a versatile root that deserves a place in both the kitchen and the medicine cabinet. In this article, we'll delve into the benefits and diverse uses of horseradish.

Nutritional Profile:

Horseradish is not only renowned for its distinctive taste but also for its nutritional richness. Some key nutrients found in horseradish include:

Vitamin C:

- **Boosts Immunity:** Vitamin C is an antioxidant that supports the immune system, helping the body fight off infections and illnesses.

Potassium:

- **Maintains Blood Pressure:** Potassium plays a role in regulating blood pressure, contributing to cardiovascular health.

Fiber:

- **Supports Digestive Health:** Horseradish is a good source of dietary fiber, promoting a healthy digestive system and regular bowel movements.

Glucosinolates:

- **Anticancer Properties:** Horseradish contains glucosinolates, compounds known for their potential anticancer properties. These compounds may help inhibit the growth of certain cancer cells.

Magnesium:

Benefits:

- **Muscle and Nerve Function:** Magnesium is essential for muscle and nerve function, contributing to overall neuromuscular health.
- **Bone Health:** Supports bone density and calcium absorption, promoting strong and healthy bones.

Calcium:

Benefits:

- **Bone Health:** Calcium is crucial for the formation and maintenance of strong bones and teeth.
- **Blood Clotting**: Essential for blood clotting processes, contributing to wound healing and preventing excessive bleeding.

Health Benefits:

Consuming horseradish can offer a range of health benefits:

Respiratory Health:

- **Decongestant Properties**: Horseradish is a natural decongestant and can help relieve respiratory issues by clearing nasal passages and reducing congestion.

Anti-Inflammatory Effects:

- Horseradish has anti-inflammatory properties that may provide relief from inflammatory conditions, such as arthritis or joint pain.

Digestive Aid:

- The fiber in horseradish supports digestive health by promoting regular bowel movements and preventing constipation.

Detoxification:

- Glucosinolates in horseradish may contribute to detoxification processes in the body, supporting the elimination of harmful substances.

Nutritional Content

Horseradish is a root vegetable known for its pungent flavor and culinary uses. Here's an approximate nutritional breakdown for 1 cup (about 130 grams) of grated horseradish:

- Carbohydrates: Approximately 17 grams
- Protein: Roughly 2 grams
- Fiber: Around 4 grams

- Fat: Less than 1 gram
- Sugar: Approximately 5 grams

Horseradish is low in calories and fat but contains a moderate amount of carbohydrates, primarily in the form of starches and dietary fiber. It's also a good source of vitamin C, potassium, calcium, and other nutrients. The pungent flavor of horseradish comes from compounds called isothiocyanates, which are released when the root is grated or crushed. These compounds are also responsible for some of the potential health benefits associated with horseradish, including its antimicrobial and anti-inflammatory properties.

Culinary Uses:

Horseradish's distinctive flavor makes it a popular addition to various culinary creations:

Condiment:

- Horseradish is commonly used as a condiment, either freshly grated or prepared as a sauce, to accompany dishes like roast beef, seafood, or sandwiches.

Ingredient in Sauces:

- It adds a zesty kick to sauces, dips, and dressings, enhancing the overall flavor profile of the dish.

Pickling:

- Horseradish can be used in pickling recipes, providing a unique flavor to pickled vegetables or condiments.

Marinades:

- Incorporating horseradish into marinades adds depth and spiciness to meats and vegetables.

Here are two delicious recipes that showcase the bold and zesty flavor of horseradish:

Horseradish-Crusted Salmon

Ingredients:

- 4 salmon fillets
- 2 tablespoons prepared horseradish
- 2 tablespoons Dijon mustard
- 1 tablespoon honey
- 1 cup breadcrumbs
- Salt and pepper to taste

- Lemon wedges for serving

Instructions:

1. Preheat the oven to 400°F (200°C).
2. In a small bowl, mix together the prepared horseradish, Dijon mustard, and honey.
3. Season the salmon fillets with salt and pepper.
4. Spread the horseradish mixture evenly over the top of each salmon fillet.
5. Press breadcrumbs onto the horseradish-coated side of the salmon, creating a crust.
6. Place the salmon fillets on a baking sheet lined with parchment paper.
7. Bake for 12-15 minutes or until the salmon is cooked through and the crust is golden brown.
8. Serve the horseradish-crusted salmon with lemon wedges for an extra burst of flavor.

Creamy Horseradish Mashed Potatoes

Ingredients:

- 4 large potatoes, peeled and cubed
- 1/2 cup butter
- 1/4 cup milk
- 2 tablespoons prepared horseradish
- Salt and pepper to taste
- Fresh chives for garnish (optional)

Instructions:

1. Boil the peeled and cubed potatoes in a large pot of salted water until fork-tender.
2. Drain the potatoes and return them to the pot.
3. Mash the potatoes with a potato masher or fork.
4. In a small saucepan, melt the butter and add the milk. Heat until warm but not boiling.
5. Pour the warm butter and milk mixture into the mashed potatoes and mix until smooth.
6. Stir in the prepared horseradish, adjusting the amount to your desired level of spiciness.
7. Season with salt and pepper to taste.
8. Garnish with fresh chives if desired and serve these creamy horseradish mashed potatoes as a delightful side dish.

Enjoy these recipes that showcase the versatility of horseradish, adding a delightful kick to both salmon and mashed potatoes.

Historical Uses:

Horseradish has a long history of use dating back centuries, valued for both its culinary and medicinal properties. Here are two historical uses of horseradish:

Medicinal Purposes: Horseradish has been used medicinally for its believed therapeutic properties. In ancient times, it was used as a remedy for various ailments, including respiratory issues, digestive disorders, and rheumatic conditions. Horseradish was often included in herbal remedies and poultices for its purported anti-inflammatory, decongestant, and antibacterial properties. It was also used as a diuretic and to stimulate appetite. While modern scientific research has not fully confirmed all historical medicinal uses, horseradish continues to be valued in traditional and alternative medicine practices.

Preservation and Flavoring: Historically, horseradish was prized for its ability to preserve food and enhance flavor. Before the advent of modern refrigeration techniques, horseradish was used as a natural preservative for meat and fish due to its antimicrobial properties. Grated horseradish root was often mixed with vinegar or salt to create a pungent condiment known as prepared horseradish. This condiment not only added flavor to dishes but also helped to extend their shelf life. Additionally, horseradish was used to flavor sauces, marinades, and pickles, adding a distinctive spicy kick to culinary preparations.

These historical uses of horseradish highlight its versatility and importance in traditional culinary and medicinal practices throughout history. Today, horseradish remains a popular ingredient in many cuisines worldwide, valued for its unique flavor and potential health benefits.

Tips on Growing Horseradish

Horseradish is a perennial plant primarily grown for its pungent root, which is used as a condiment and flavoring agent in various culinary dishes. The growth timeline of horseradish involves several stages, and it can take about 1 to 2 years to reach maturity. Here's a detailed explanation of how long it takes for horseradish to grow:

1. **Planting:** Horseradish can be propagated either from seeds or more commonly from root cuttings. Most gardeners prefer using root cuttings because they provide a quicker and more reliable method of establishing new plants. Root cuttings are typically 6 to 8 inches long and about the thickness of a pencil. They are planted horizontally in well-draining soil during the early spring or fall seasons. Planting horseradish from root cuttings allows for the development of a strong taproot, which is essential for the plant's growth and productivity.
2. **Initial Growth and Establishment (1st Year):** After planting, horseradish roots begin to establish themselves in the soil. During the first growing season, the plant primarily focuses on developing a robust root system and producing foliage. Horseradish leaves emerge from the soil and grow into large, coarse, dark green leaves with serrated edges. These leaves

capture sunlight and photosynthesize, providing energy for the developing root system. Throughout the first year, the horseradish plant continues to grow and expand, but it typically does not produce significant root growth during this time.

3. **Overwintering (1st Year):** In regions with cold winters, horseradish plants undergo a period of dormancy during the winter months. The foliage dies back as temperatures drop, and the plant enters a state of dormancy. Horseradish is cold-hardy and can withstand freezing temperatures, making it well-suited for overwintering in temperate climates. While the plant remains dormant during the winter, the root system continues to develop and store energy in preparation for the following growing season.
4. **Second Year Growth and Harvest (2nd Year):** In the second year of growth, horseradish plants resume active growth as temperatures warm up in the spring. The foliage regenerates from the dormant root system, and the plant begins to allocate more energy towards producing new leaves and expanding the root system. During the second growing season, the horseradish root undergoes significant enlargement and develops the characteristic pungent flavor and aroma for which it is prized. Harvesting of horseradish roots typically occurs in the fall of the second year, after the foliage has died back and the roots have reached their maximum size.
5. **Continued Growth and Maintenance (Subsequent Years):** Horseradish is a perennial plant that can continue to produce roots for several years under proper growing conditions. After the initial harvest in the second year, the plant can be left in the ground to produce additional crops in subsequent years. With proper care, including regular watering, fertilization, and weed control, horseradish plants can remain productive for many years, providing a steady supply of fresh roots for culinary use.

Overall, the complete growth cycle of horseradish from planting to harvest can take approximately 1 to 2 years, depending on factors such as climate, soil conditions, and cultural practices. Proper care and maintenance throughout each stage of growth are essential for maximizing the yield and quality of horseradish roots.

Conclusion:

Horseradish is more than just a flavorful spice; it's a nutritional powerhouse with potential health benefits. Whether you're looking to add a kick to your culinary creations or seeking natural remedies for respiratory or digestive issues, horseradish offers a unique solution. Embrace the boldness of horseradish, and let its multifaceted qualities elevate both your meals and your well-being.

If you have specific health concerns, allergies, or conditions, it's advisable to consult with a healthcare professional or a registered dietitian before making significant changes to your diet.

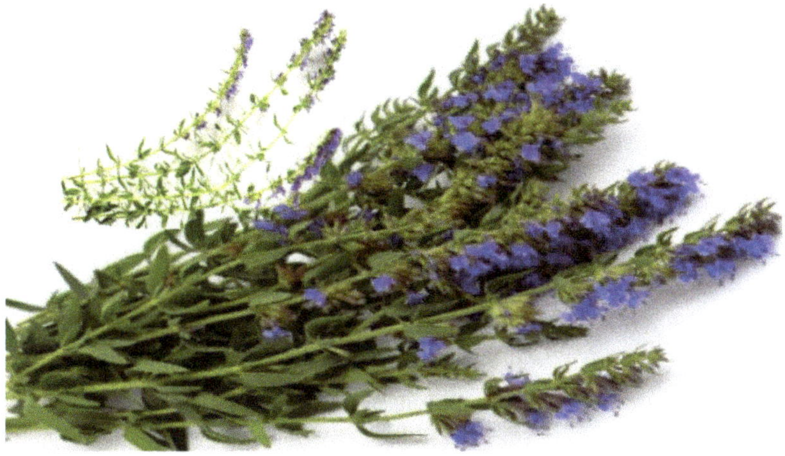

Hyssop

Healing Potential of Hyssop

Nestled within the annals of herbal medicine lies a humble yet powerful herb known as Hyssop. Revered for centuries for its medicinal properties, Hyssop (Hyssopus officinalis) has been celebrated across cultures for its plethora of health benefits and versatile applications. From ancient times to modern holistic practices, this botanical gem continues to captivate with its healing prowess. Let's delve into the world of Hyssop, exploring its benefits and diverse uses.

A Brief Introduction to Hyssop: Hyssop is a perennial herbaceous plant native to the Mediterranean region and parts of Asia. Belonging to the mint family (Lamiaceae), it boasts slender stems adorned with clusters of vibrant flowers, typically ranging from blue to violet. Not only valued for its ornamental appeal, but Hyssop also holds a rich history of culinary and medicinal use.

While it is primarily known for its aromatic qualities and its potential as a culinary herb, it also contains various vitamins, minerals, and antioxidants that contribute to its health benefits. Here's a list of some of the key nutrients found in hyssop and their associated benefits:

Vitamins:

- **Vitamin C:** Known for its immune-boosting properties, vitamin C also acts as an antioxidant, helping to protect cells from damage caused by free radicals.
- **Vitamin B6:** Essential for brain development and function, vitamin B6 also plays a role in the synthesis of neurotransmitters and the regulation of mood.
- **Vitamin A:** Important for vision, immune function, and skin health, vitamin A is a powerful antioxidant that supports overall wellbeing.

Minerals:

- **Calcium:** Essential for bone health, calcium also plays a role in muscle function, nerve transmission, and hormone secretion.

- **Magnesium:** Involved in over 300 biochemical reactions in the body, magnesium is crucial for energy production, muscle and nerve function, and maintaining heart health.
- **Potassium:** Helps regulate fluid balance, muscle contractions, and nerve signals. It also plays a role in maintaining healthy blood pressure levels.

Antioxidants:

- **Rosmarinic Acid:** Found in many aromatic herbs, including hyssop, rosmarinic acid possesses antioxidant and anti-inflammatory properties. It may help protect against oxidative stress and inflammation in the body.
- **Flavonoids:** Hyssop contains various flavonoids, such as quercetin and apigenin, which have antioxidant, anti-inflammatory, and immune-boosting effects. They may also support heart health and help reduce the risk of chronic diseases.

Health Benefits of Hyssop:

Respiratory Support: Hyssop has long been prized for its ability to promote respiratory health. Its expectorant properties help to ease congestion, alleviate coughs, and clear the respiratory passages, making it a valuable ally during colds, flu, and respiratory infections.

Anti-inflammatory Effects: Rich in antioxidants and anti-inflammatory compounds, Hyssop exhibits potent anti-inflammatory properties. It may help reduce inflammation associated with conditions such as arthritis, asthma, and inflammatory skin disorders.

Digestive Aid: Hyssop has been traditionally used to support digestive health. It may help relieve indigestion, bloating, and gas, while also stimulating appetite and promoting healthy digestion.

Immune Boosting: Packed with immune-boosting nutrients, Hyssop can fortify the body's defenses against pathogens. Regular consumption or use of Hyssop may help strengthen the immune system and ward off infections.

Antimicrobial Action: Hyssop possesses antimicrobial properties, which can inhibit the growth of harmful bacteria and fungi. It may be utilized topically to cleanse wounds, soothe skin irritations, and prevent infections.

Versatile Uses of Hyssop:

Herbal Infusions: Hyssop leaves and flowers can be steeped to create fragrant herbal teas. These teas are not only delicious but also serve as a soothing remedy for respiratory issues and digestive discomfort.

Aromatic Baths: Adding Hyssop essential oil to bathwater can create a relaxing and therapeutic experience. The aromatic steam helps to clear the airways, ease muscle tension, and promote relaxation.

Steam Inhalation: Inhaling steam infused with Hyssop essential oil can provide quick relief from congestion, sinusitis, and respiratory congestion. Simply add a few drops of Hyssop oil to hot water, cover your head with a towel, and inhale deeply.

Topical Preparations: Hyssop-infused oils, creams, and ointments can be applied topically to soothe skin irritations, alleviate muscle pain, and promote wound healing. Its antimicrobial properties make it an excellent addition to natural skincare formulations.

Culinary Delights:

In the kitchen, Hyssop leaves can be used to add flavor and aroma to a variety of dishes. Whether sprinkled fresh over salads, infused into soups, or used as a seasoning for meats and poultry, Hyssop lends a delightful culinary twist.

Here are two recipes that incorporate hyssop:

Hyssop Infused Honey:

Ingredients:

- 1 cup honey
- 2-3 sprigs of fresh hyssop

Instructions:

1. Rinse the hyssop sprigs under cold water to remove any dirt or debris. Pat them dry with a paper towel.
2. Place the hyssop sprigs in a clean, dry glass jar.
3. Heat the honey in a small saucepan over low heat until it becomes warm and fluid.
4. Pour the warm honey over the hyssop sprigs in the jar, ensuring they are fully submerged.
5. Let the mixture cool to room temperature, then seal the jar tightly.
6. Allow the hyssop to infuse in the honey for at least 24 hours, preferably longer, to develop its flavor.
7. Once infused, strain the honey through a fine-mesh sieve to remove the hyssop sprigs.
8. Transfer the infused honey to a clean jar or container with a tight-fitting lid.
9. Store the hyssop-infused honey in a cool, dry place. Use it as a sweetener for teas, drizzle it over yogurt or desserts, or enjoy it on toast.

Hyssop Tea:

Ingredients:

- 1-2 teaspoons dried hyssop leaves (or 2-3 fresh hyssop sprigs)
- 1 cup water
- Optional: honey, lemon slices

Instructions:

1. If using fresh hyssop, rinse the sprigs under cold water and pat them dry with a paper towel. If using dried hyssop leaves, measure out the desired amount.
2. Bring the water to a boil in a small saucepan or kettle.
3. Place the hyssop leaves or sprigs in a teapot or heatproof mug.
4. Once the water reaches a rolling boil, pour it over the hyssop in the teapot or mug.
5. Cover the teapot or mug and let the hyssop steep in the hot water for 5-10 minutes, depending on your preference for strength.
6. After steeping, strain the tea through a fine-mesh sieve to remove the hyssop leaves or sprigs.
7. If desired, sweeten the tea with honey and/or add a squeeze of lemon for extra flavor.
8. Serve the hyssop tea hot and enjoy its aromatic and soothing properties.

These recipes offer delightful ways to incorporate the unique flavor and potential health benefits of hyssop into your culinary repertoire. Enjoy experimenting with this versatile herb!

Historical uses:

Hyssop has a long history of both culinary and medicinal uses. Here are two historical and medicinal uses of hyssop:

Ancient Medicinal Herb:

- Hyssop has been used medicinally for centuries, with its origins dating back to ancient times. It was mentioned in various ancient texts, including the Bible and writings from ancient Egypt, Greece, and Rome.
- In ancient civilizations, hyssop was valued for its medicinal properties, often used to treat respiratory ailments such as coughs, colds, and bronchitis. It was also believed to have expectorant properties, helping to clear mucus from the respiratory tract.

- Additionally, hyssop was used topically as an antiseptic and wound healer. Its antimicrobial properties were thought to help prevent infections and promote wound healing.

Traditional Remedies:

- Throughout history, hyssop has been incorporated into traditional herbal remedies in various cultures around the world. It was often brewed into teas, tinctures, or infusions for its medicinal benefits.
- Hyssop tea was commonly used to alleviate symptoms of respiratory conditions, including congestion, sore throat, and cough. Its soothing and expectorant properties were believed to help loosen phlegm and ease breathing.
- In traditional herbal medicine, hyssop was also used to promote digestive health. It was believed to stimulate digestion, relieve bloating and gas, and soothe gastrointestinal discomfort.

While modern scientific research on hyssop's medicinal properties is ongoing, historical accounts and traditional uses suggest that this herb has been valued for its potential health benefits for centuries. However, it's essential to consult with a healthcare professional before using hyssop or any herbal remedy for medicinal purposes, especially if you are allergic, have underlying health conditions or are taking medications.

Tips on Growing Hyssop

Hyssop (Hyssopus officinalis) is a perennial herb that can be grown from seeds or propagated from cuttings. Here are the general details on how long it takes for hyssop to grow:

1. **Germination**: When growing hyssop from seeds, germination typically occurs within 7 to 21 days after sowing, depending on factors such as soil temperature, moisture levels, and seed quality.
2. **Seedling Stage**: After germination, hyssop seedlings will emerge and begin to grow. During this stage, they require consistent moisture and adequate sunlight or grow lights if grown indoors. Seedlings usually develop true leaves within 2 to 3 weeks after germination.
3. **Establishment**: Once hyssop seedlings have developed several sets of true leaves, they can be transplanted into their final growing location, whether it's a garden bed, container, or herb garden. At this point, they will continue to grow and establish their root systems.
4. **Maturity**: Hyssop plants typically reach maturity and full size within their first year of growth. By the end of the growing season, which can range from 3 to 6 months depending on the climate and growing conditions, hyssop plants can be harvested for their leaves and flowers.
5. **Optimal Growth Conditions**: Hyssop thrives in well-draining soil with full sun exposure. It is drought-tolerant once established but benefits from regular watering, especially during periods of prolonged dryness. Hyssop is hardy in USDA zones 4-9.

6. **Propagation**: Hyssop can also be propagated from stem cuttings, which can root and establish within a few weeks under optimal conditions. This method can expedite the growth process compared to growing from seeds.

Overall, from germination to maturity, hyssop typically takes several months to grow into a healthy, harvestable plant. With proper care and attention to its growing needs, you can enjoy a bountiful supply of this aromatic and versatile herb in your garden.

Conclusion:

Hyssop stands as a testament to the bountiful gifts offered by nature. From its healing properties to its myriad of uses, this botanical treasure continues to enrich our lives in profound ways. Whether sipped as a comforting tea, applied as a soothing balm, or savored in culinary creations, Hyssop invites us to embrace its therapeutic embrace and embark on a journey of holistic wellness.

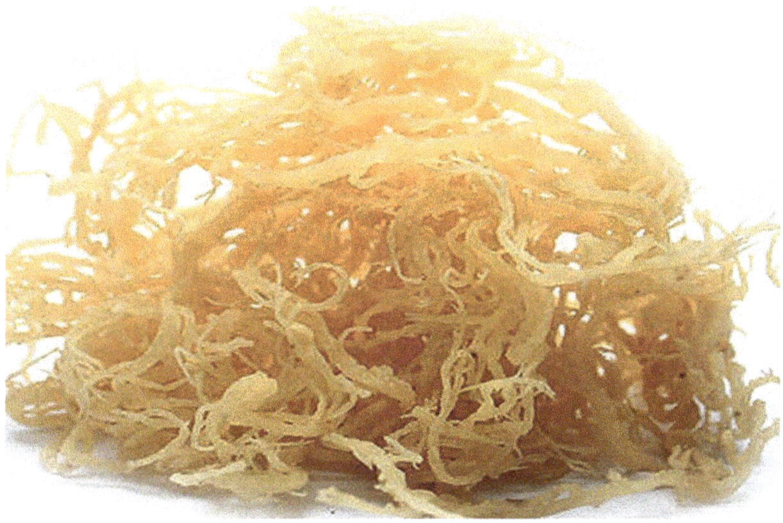

Irish Moss / Sea Moss

The Marvels of Chondrus Crispus

Sea moss, scientifically known as Chondrus crispus, but is also known as Irish moss or red seaweed is a type of red algae that has been gaining popularity for its numerous health benefits and versatile uses. Commonly found along the rocky shores of the Atlantic coastlines, especially in Ireland and the Caribbean, sea moss has been a staple in traditional medicine and culinary practices for centuries. In this article, we will explore the various benefits of sea moss and its diverse applications.

Nutritional Powerhouse:

One of the key reasons for the surge in sea moss popularity is its rich nutritional profile. Packed with essential vitamins and minerals, sea moss is a potent source of nutrients such as iodine, iron, calcium, magnesium, and vitamins A, C, and K. Additionally, it contains a unique blend of antioxidants and amino acids that contribute to its overall health-promoting properties.

Vitamins:

Vitamin A: Essential for vision health, immune function, and skin health.

Vitamin C: Boosts the immune system, promotes collagen production for skin health, and acts as an antioxidant to protect cells from damage.

Vitamin E: Provides antioxidant properties, supports skin health, and helps protect cells from oxidative stress.

Vitamin K: Important for blood clotting and bone health.

Minerals:

Iodine: Crucial for thyroid function and hormone regulation.

Calcium: Essential for bone health, muscle function, and nerve transmission.

Magnesium: Supports muscle and nerve function, regulates blood sugar levels, and contributes to bone health.

Potassium: Helps regulate blood pressure, fluid balance, and muscle contractions.

Sulfur: Important for joint health, detoxification, and collagen production.

Iron: Necessary for oxygen transport in the blood and energy production.

Zinc: Supports immune function, wound healing, and cell division.

Amino Acids:

Taurine: Supports cardiovascular health, vision health, and nervous system function.

Cysteine: Precursor to glutathione, a powerful antioxidant that helps protect cells from damage.

Glycine: Supports muscle growth, cognitive function, and detoxification processes.

Proline: Essential for collagen synthesis, which is important for skin, joint, and connective tissue health.

Alanine: Provides energy to muscles, supports immune function, and helps regulate blood sugar levels.

Antioxidants:

Flavonoids: Help reduce inflammation, support cardiovascular health, and protect cells from oxidative damage.

Phenolic Compounds: Have antioxidant properties that help neutralize free radicals and reduce the risk of chronic diseases.

Carotenoids: Act as antioxidants, supporting eye health, immune function, and skin health.

Sulfated Polysaccharides: Have anti-inflammatory and antioxidant properties, supporting immune function and cardiovascular health.

Nutritional Support during Famine:

In times of famine or scarcity, communities near coastal regions historically turned to sea moss as a valuable source of nutrition. With its abundance of vitamins, minerals, and essential nutrients, sea moss provided a reliable and easily accessible food source during periods when other crops might have been scarce. It played a crucial role in sustaining communities during challenging times.

Benefits for Health and Wellness:

Immune System Support:

Sea moss is known for its immune-boosting properties. The high concentration of antioxidants helps strengthen the immune system, making the body more resilient to infections and illnesses.

Traditional Respiratory Support:

Throughout history, sea moss has been used in traditional medicine to address respiratory conditions. Its mucilaginous nature is believed to have soothing properties, making it a remedy for respiratory issues such as coughs, colds, and respiratory infections. The mucilage may help coat the throat and alleviate irritation, providing relief to those with respiratory discomfort.

Thyroid Health:

Iodine, a crucial element for thyroid function, is abundant in sea moss. Regular consumption can contribute to maintaining a healthy thyroid, which plays a vital role in regulating metabolism.

Digestive Health:

Sea moss contains prebiotics, which promote the growth of beneficial gut bacteria. This, in turn, supports digestion and helps maintain a healthy gut microbiome.

Joint and Skin Health:

The collagen and amino acids found in sea moss contribute to the health of joints and skin. Many people incorporate sea moss into their routine to promote smoother skin and support joint flexibility.

Wound Healing and Skin Care:

Sea moss has been historically used externally for its potential benefits in wound healing and skincare. Its mucilaginous gel was applied topically to wounds or skin irritations to promote healing and soothe inflammation. The collagen content in sea moss may have contributed to its historical use in supporting skin health, potentially aiding in the repair of damaged tissues.

Nutritional Content

Sea moss, also known as Irish moss or carrageenan moss, is a type of seaweed commonly used in various culinary and dietary applications. Here's an approximate nutritional breakdown for 1 cup (about 82 grams) of dried sea moss before rehydration:

- Carbohydrates: Approximately 10 grams
- Protein: Roughly 1 gram
- Fiber: Around 3 grams

- Fat: Less than 1 gram
- Sugar: Less than 1 gram

It's important to note that the nutritional content of sea moss can vary slightly based on factors such as the specific species of seaweed and growing conditions. Additionally, the above values are for dried sea moss before it's rehydrated. Once rehydrated, sea moss will have a higher water content and may have slightly different nutritional values.

Sea moss is valued not only for its nutritional content but also for its potential health benefits, including its high mineral content (such as iodine, magnesium, and potassium) and its mucilaginous properties, which may support digestive health. It's often used in various recipes, including smoothies, soups, and desserts, to add texture and nutrition.

Culinary Uses:

Beyond its health benefits, sea moss has found its way into kitchens around the world due to its versatility. It can be used in various culinary applications, including:

Smoothies and Juices:

Adding sea moss gel to smoothies and juices is a popular way to incorporate its nutritional benefits into a daily diet. The gel provides a smooth texture and doesn't alter the taste significantly.

Soups and Stews:

Sea moss can be used as a thickening agent in soups and stews. Its mild flavor allows it to complement a wide range of savory dishes.

Desserts:

Sea moss can be transformed into a gel and used in desserts like puddings and ice creams. Its unique texture adds a delightful element to sweet treats.

Beverages:

Some people infuse sea moss into teas and other beverages to enjoy its benefits in a refreshing way.

Here are three recipes that use sea moss:

Sea Moss Smoothie:

Ingredients:

- 1 cup almond milk (or any preferred milk)
- 1 ripe banana
- 1 tablespoon sea moss gel
- 1 tablespoon honey or maple syrup (optional, for sweetness)
- 1/2 teaspoon vanilla extract
- 1/2 teaspoon ground cinnamon
- Handful of spinach (optional, for added nutrients)
- Ice cubes (optional, for a colder smoothie)

Instructions:

1. If your sea moss is dried, soak it in water for at least 4 hours until it expands and becomes soft. Rinse it thoroughly to remove any debris or salt.
2. In a blender, combine all the ingredients: almond milk, banana, sea moss gel, honey or maple syrup, vanilla extract, cinnamon, spinach, and ice cubes.
3. Blend until smooth and creamy. If the smoothie is too thick, you can add more almond milk to reach your desired consistency.
4. Pour into glasses and serve immediately. Enjoy your nutritious sea moss smoothie!

Sea Moss Gel Dessert:

Ingredients:

1. 1/4 cup dried sea moss
2. 2 cups water
3. 1/2 cup coconut milk
4. 2-3 tablespoons agave syrup or sweetener of choice
5. 1 teaspoon vanilla extract
6. Pinch of ground nutmeg (optional)
7. Fresh berries or fruit of choice for topping

Instructions:

1. Rinse the dried sea moss thoroughly to remove any debris or salt.
2. Soak the sea moss in water for at least 4 hours or overnight until it expands and becomes soft.
3. After soaking, rinse the sea moss again and drain.
4. In a blender, combine the soaked sea moss and 2 cups of fresh water. Blend until smooth and creamy.
5. In a saucepan, combine the sea moss puree, coconut milk, agave syrup, vanilla extract, and nutmeg. Cook over medium heat, stirring frequently, until the mixture thickens and bubbles slightly (about 10-15 minutes).
6. Remove from heat and let the mixture cool to room temperature.
7. Transfer the sea moss gel into serving bowls or glasses. Refrigerate for at least 2 hours or until set.
8. Once chilled and set, top the sea moss gel with fresh berries or fruit of your choice.
9. Serve and enjoy your delicious sea moss gel dessert as a healthy and refreshing treat!

Jamaican Irish Moss Drink:

Ingredients:

- 1/4 cup dried Irish moss
- 2 cups water (for boiling)
- 2 cups milk (or a dairy-free alternative like almond milk, coconut milk, etc.)
- 1/4 cup condensed milk (optional, adjust to taste)
- 1 teaspoon vanilla extract
- 1/4 teaspoon ground cinnamon
- 1/4 teaspoon grated nutmeg
- 1/4 cup sweetened fruit juice (optional, such as pineapple or mango)
- Sweetener of choice (honey, agave syrup, sugar) to taste

Instructions:

1. Rinse the dried Irish moss thoroughly to remove any debris or salt.
2. Soak the Irish moss in water for at least 4 hours or overnight until it expands and becomes soft.
3. After soaking, rinse the Irish moss again and drain.
4. In a pot, bring 2 cups of water to a boil. Add the soaked Irish moss to the boiling water and let it simmer for about 20-25 minutes until it becomes gelatinous and tender. Stir occasionally.
5. Once cooked, remove the pot from heat and let the Irish moss mixture cool to room temperature.
6. In a blender, combine the cooked Irish moss mixture, milk (or dairy-free alternative), condensed milk (if using), vanilla extract, ground cinnamon, grated nutmeg, and sweetened fruit juice (if using). Blend until smooth and creamy.
7. Taste the mixture and adjust sweetness if needed by adding your preferred sweetener.
8. Pour the Irish moss drink into glasses, sprinkle a little extra nutmeg or cinnamon on top for garnish if desired.
9. Serve chilled or over ice. Enjoy your refreshing Jamaican Irish Moss drink!

Note: This recipe is customizable, so feel free to adjust the ingredients and sweetness level according to your preference. Additionally, some people like to add other flavorings such as vanilla essence, almond essence, or Guinness for a richer taste.

Sea Moss Side Effects

It's important to note that individual responses to sea moss can vary, and while many people enjoy its health benefits without experiencing adverse effects, those with specific health concerns or conditions should seek professional advice before incorporating sea moss into their routine. As with any dietary supplement, moderation and informed consumption are key.

Conclusion:

Sea moss stands out as a nutritional powerhouse with a plethora of health benefits and versatile uses. Whether consumed for its immune-boosting properties, thyroid support, or as a culinary ingredient, sea moss has rightfully earned its place in the spotlight for promoting overall well-being. As interest in natural and holistic health solutions continues to grow, sea moss is likely to remain a fascinating subject of exploration and innovation.

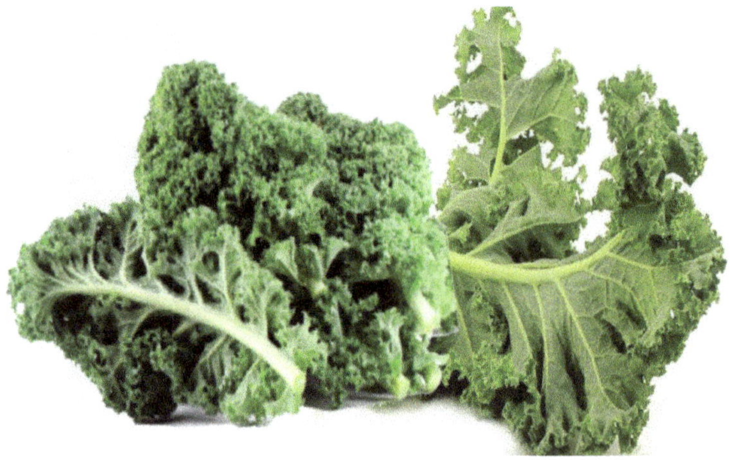

Kale

A Nutrient-Packed Green Superstar

Kale, a cruciferous vegetable, has gained widespread acclaim for its exceptional nutritional profile and versatile culinary uses. Originating from the Mediterranean region, Kale has evolved into a globally recognized superfood.

Historical Roots:

Dating back to ancient times, Kale has a rich history as a dietary staple. Its popularity surged in recent years due to its remarkable health benefits and adaptability in various cuisines.

Nutritional Powerhouse

This leafy green is a nutritional powerhouse, boasting an array of essential vitamins and minerals. A single serving provides a significant dose of Vitamin A, Vitamin K, Vitamin C, calcium, iron, and antioxidants.

Kale is a nutrient-dense leafy green vegetable packed with vitamins, minerals, and antioxidants that offer numerous health benefits. Here's a list of some key nutrients found in kale and their potential benefits:

Vitamins:

- **Vitamin A:** Supports vision health, immune function, and skin health.
- **Vitamin C:** Boosts immune function, promotes collagen synthesis, and acts as an antioxidant.
- **Vitamin K:** Essential for blood clotting, bone health, and may help prevent bone fractures.
- **Vitamin B6:** Supports brain health, energy metabolism, and nervous system function.

- **Vitamin B9 (Folate):** Important for DNA synthesis, cell division, and fetal development during pregnancy.
- **Vitamin E:** Acts as an antioxidant, protects cells from damage, and supports skin health.

Minerals:

- **Calcium:** Essential for bone health, muscle function, and nerve transmission.
- **Potassium:** Regulates blood pressure, supports heart health, and may reduce the risk of stroke.
- **Magnesium:** Important for muscle function, energy production, and bone health.
- **Iron:** Necessary for oxygen transport in the blood and energy metabolism.
- **Manganese:** Supports bone health, collagen production, and antioxidant defense.
- **Copper:** Essential for iron metabolism, connective tissue formation, and immune function.
- **Phosphorus:** Required for bone and teeth formation, energy metabolism, and cell structure.

Antioxidants:

- **Beta-carotene:** Converts to vitamin A in the body, acts as an antioxidant, and may protect against chronic diseases.
- **Lutein and zeaxanthin:** Support eye health, protect against age-related macular degeneration, and act as antioxidants.
- **Quercetin:** Exhibits anti-inflammatory and antioxidant properties, may help reduce blood pressure, and supports heart health.
- **Kaempferol:** Anti-inflammatory and antioxidant properties, may help protect against cancer and chronic diseases.
- **Sulforaphane:** Supports detoxification, may have anti-cancer properties, and promotes heart health.

Consuming kale regularly can contribute to overall health and well-being due to its rich nutrient profile. Incorporating kale into your diet through salads, smoothies, stir-fries, or soups can help you reap the benefits of these vitamins, minerals, and antioxidants.

Comparison with Peers:

In a nutritional face-off, Kale surpasses many common vegetables in terms of overall nutrient density. Its low calorie and high nutrient content make it a preferred choice for health-conscious individuals.

Health Benefits

Antioxidant Richness:

Kale's high antioxidant content contributes to its role in combating oxidative stress, reducing inflammation, and promoting overall well-being.

Heart Health and Cholesterol Management:

Studies suggest that regular consumption of Kale may contribute to cardiovascular health by lowering cholesterol levels and supporting heart function.

Bone Health Booster:

Abundant in Vitamin K, Kale plays a pivotal role in bone health. It aids in calcium absorption, contributing to the maintenance of strong and healthy bones.

The leafy vegetable is also a great reservoir of minerals such as calcium, potassium, and manganese, promoting not only bone health but blood pressure regulation, and optimal metabolic function.

Weight Management and Digestive Health:

The fiber content in Kale supports digestive health and weight management by promoting satiety and aiding in proper digestion.

With its low-calorie content and high fiber content, kale is an excellent choice for those seeking to maintain a healthy weight and support digestive health. Inclusion of kale in one's diet can contribute significantly to overall well-being and nutritional balance.

Culinary Delights and Growing Tips

Kale Varieties and Culinary Uses:

Explore the diverse world of Kale varieties, including Curly Kale, Lacinato Kale, and Red Russian Kale. From vibrant salads to hearty soups and savory stir-fries, Kale seamlessly integrates into a multitude of dishes.

Here is some ways Kale can be prepared:

Raw in Salads:

One of the simplest and healthiest ways to enjoy kale is by incorporating it into salads. Remove the tough stems, chop the leaves finely, and toss them with other fresh vegetables, fruits, nuts, and a flavorful dressing. Massaging the kale with the dressing helps soften its texture and enhances its taste.

Sauteed or Stir-Fried:

Sautéing or stir-frying kale is a quick and delicious method that imparts a slightly crispy texture. Heat some olive oil or a preferred cooking oil, add minced garlic or onions for extra flavor, and toss in chopped kale until it wilts and becomes tender. Season with salt, pepper, or herbs to taste.

Baked Kale Chips:

Transforming kale into crispy chips is a popular and nutritious snack option. After removing the stems, coat the kale leaves with a bit of olive oil, sprinkle with salt or desired seasonings, and bake until they become crisp. This provides a satisfying alternative to traditional potato chips.

Blended in Smoothies:

Kale can seamlessly be incorporated into smoothies, contributing a nutrient boost without altering the drink's flavor significantly. Combine kale leaves with fruits like bananas, berries, and a liquid base such as almond milk or yogurt for a refreshing and health-packed beverage.

In Soups and Stews:

Kale can add depth and nutrition to soups and stews. Simply chop the leaves and add them towards the end of the cooking process to maintain their vibrant color and nutrients. Kale complements various hearty soups, providing an extra layer of flavor and nutritional content.

Here are two delicious recipes using kale:

Kale and Quinoa Salad with Lemon Vinaigrette:

Ingredients:

- 1 bunch kale, stems removed and leaves chopped
- 1 cup cooked quinoa
- 1/2 cup cherry tomatoes, halved
- 1/4 cup red onion, thinly sliced
- 1/4 cup crumbled feta cheese (optional)
- 1/4 cup chopped walnuts or almonds
- Lemon Vinaigrette:
    - 1/4 cup extra virgin olive oil
    - 2 tablespoons fresh lemon juice
    - 1 teaspoon Dijon mustard
    - 1 teaspoon honey or maple syrup

- Salt and pepper to taste

Instructions:

1. In a large bowl, combine the chopped kale, cooked quinoa, cherry tomatoes, red onion, and crumbled feta cheese (if using).
2. In a small bowl, whisk together the ingredients for the lemon vinaigrette: olive oil, lemon juice, Dijon mustard, honey or maple syrup, salt, and pepper.
3. Pour the lemon vinaigrette over the kale mixture and toss until well coated.
4. Sprinkle chopped walnuts or almonds on top for added crunch.
5. Serve immediately or refrigerate for later. The flavors will meld together even more if allowed to sit for a while before serving.

Sautéed Kale with Garlic and Lemon:

Ingredients:

- 1 bunch kale, stems removed and leaves chopped
- 2 cloves garlic, minced
- 2 tablespoons olive oil
- 1 tablespoon fresh lemon juice
- Salt and pepper to taste
- Red pepper flakes (optional)

Instructions:

1. Heat olive oil in a large skillet over medium heat.
2. Add minced garlic to the skillet and sauté for about 1 minute until fragrant.
3. Add the chopped kale to the skillet and toss to coat with the garlic-infused oil.
4. Cook the kale, stirring occasionally, for about 5-7 minutes until wilted and tender.
5. Drizzle fresh lemon juice over the sautéed kale and season with salt, pepper, and red pepper flakes (if using). Toss to combine.
6. Remove from heat and transfer to a serving dish.
7. Serve hot as a nutritious side dish or as a topping for grains or proteins.

These recipes showcase the versatility of kale and how it can be incorporated into delicious and nutritious meals. Enjoy!

Cultivation Tips:

For those with green thumbs, cultivating Kale is a rewarding endeavor. Discover the ideal growing conditions, planting techniques, and harvesting tips to ensure a bountiful yield. Be mindful of common pests and diseases that may affect Kale plants.

Garden Cultivation:

The time it takes for kale to grow from seed to harvest varies depending on several factors, including the variety of kale, environmental conditions, and cultivation practices. However, here's a detailed breakdown of the typical growth timeline for kale:

1. **Seed Germination (5-10 days):** Kale seeds are planted in well-draining soil, either directly in the garden or started indoors in seed trays. Germination typically occurs within 5 to 10 days, although it can vary depending on factors such as soil temperature and moisture levels.

2. **Seedling Stage (2-4 weeks):** After germination, kale seedlings emerge from the soil. During this stage, they develop their first true leaves and establish a strong root system. Seedlings require consistent moisture, adequate sunlight, and proper spacing to support healthy growth. This stage usually lasts 2 to 4 weeks.

3. **Vegetative Growth (4-6 weeks):** As kale plants mature, they enter a phase of vigorous vegetative growth. During this stage, the plants continue to develop additional leaves and increase in size. Adequate spacing between plants is essential to allow for proper air circulation and minimize competition for nutrients. Vegetative growth typically lasts 4 to 6 weeks, depending on the variety and growing conditions.

4. **Maturity and Harvest (8-12 weeks):** Kale is typically ready for harvest when the leaves reach a suitable size and texture for consumption. The exact time to harvest depends on the desired maturity level and whether you prefer baby kale or mature leaves. Baby kale can be harvested as early as 4 to 6 weeks after planting, while mature kale may take 8 to 12 weeks or longer. Harvesting individual leaves from the outer portions of the plant encourages continued growth and prolongs the harvest period.

5. **Bolting and Flowering (varies):** In some cases, kale plants may bolt, or send up flower stalks, especially in response to heat stress or long daylight hours. Bolting can negatively impact leaf quality and taste, so it's generally best to harvest kale before this occurs. However, some varieties are more resistant to bolting than others.

Overall, the entire growth cycle of kale, from seed to harvest, typically takes approximately 8 to 12 weeks under optimal growing conditions. Proper care and maintenance throughout each stage of growth, including adequate watering, fertilization, and pest control, are essential for successful kale cultivation. Additionally, harvesting kale regularly encourages continued production and ensures a steady supply of fresh, nutritious leaves.

Container Gardening:

Kale is well-suited for container gardening, making it accessible for individuals with limited space. Choose a large container with good drainage, fill it with nutrient-rich potting soil, and sow kale seeds or transplant seedlings. Place the container in a sunny location and water regularly to keep the soil consistently moist. Container gardening allows for flexibility in moving the kale to optimal sunlight conditions and provides easy access for harvesting. Regularly trim outer leaves to encourage continuous growth.

Embracing Kale in Your Lifestyle

Kale has experienced a notable surge in popularity in recent years, becoming a staple in health-conscious diets and a symbol of the wellness movement. Recognized for its exceptional nutrient content, kale has transitioned from a humble leafy green to a culinary and cultural phenomenon.

This nutritional vegetable has become synonymous with a healthy lifestyle, influencing food choices and contributing to a broader shift toward plant-based and nutrient-dense diets. Its versatility, combined with a robust nutrient profile, has solidified kale's place not only on the dinner plate but also in the cultural fabric of contemporary health and wellness trends.

Conclusion:

Kale stands as a nutritional powerhouse with myriad health benefits. Its versatility in the kitchen, combined with its easy cultivation, makes it a valuable addition to any diet. Whether you're a culinary enthusiast or a health-conscious individual, Kale offers a delicious and nutritious way to enhance your well-being. Embrace the wonders of Kale and savor the journey to a healthier lifestyle!

If you have specific health concerns, allergies, or conditions, it's advisable to consult with a healthcare professional or a registered dietitian before making significant changes to your diet.

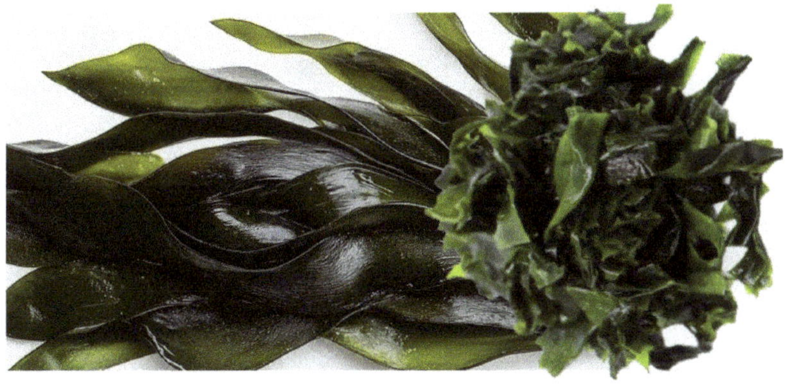

Kelp (Kombu)

An Oceanic Superfood Packed with Nutrients and Versatility

Kelp, a type of large brown seaweed, has long been a staple in various cuisines and traditional medicine due to its impressive nutritional profile and numerous health benefits. Harvested from underwater kelp forests, this marine vegetable offers a unique combination of vitamins, minerals, and bioactive compounds. In this article, we will explore the benefits and diverse uses of kelp, showcasing its importance as an oceanic superfood.

Nutrient-Rich Composition:

Kelp is celebrated for its rich array of essential nutrients, making it a valuable addition to a balanced diet. Here are some key components that make kelp a nutritional powerhouse:

Iodine:

- Kelp is an exceptionally rich source of iodine, a vital mineral essential for thyroid function. Adequate iodine intake is crucial for the synthesis of thyroid hormones that regulate metabolism.

Vitamins:

Kelp contains various vitamins, including vitamin K, vitamin A, vitamin C, and several B vitamins. These vitamins contribute to immune function, bone health, and overall well-being.

Vitamin K:

- Kelp is a good source of vitamin K, which plays a crucial role in blood clotting and contributes to bone health by aiding in bone mineralization.

Vitamin A:

- Kelp provides vitamin A in the form of carotenoids. Vitamin A is essential for vision, immune function, and skin health.

Vitamin C:

- Kelp contains vitamin C, an antioxidant that supports the immune system, promotes healthy skin, and aids in the absorption of iron.

Vitamin E:

- While present in smaller amounts, kelp also provides vitamin E, an antioxidant that helps protect cells from oxidative damage.

Vitamin B1 (Thiamine):

- Kelp contains thiamine, an essential B-vitamin that plays a role in energy metabolism and the proper functioning of the nervous system.

Vitamin B2 (Riboflavin):

- Riboflavin is found in kelp, contributing to energy production and the metabolism of fats, drugs, and steroids.

Vitamin B3 (Niacin):

- Niacin is present in kelp and is involved in energy metabolism, DNA repair, and the functioning of the nervous system.

Vitamin B5 (Pantothenic Acid):

- Kelp provides pantothenic acid, a B-vitamin important for the synthesis of essential molecules, including fatty acids and cholesterol.

Vitamin B6 (Pyridoxine):

- Kelp contains vitamin B6, which is important for the metabolism of amino acids, the synthesis of neurotransmitters, and immune function.

Vitamin B9 (Folate):

- Folate, also known as vitamin B9, is found in kelp and is essential for DNA synthesis and cell division.

Vitamin B12:

- Kelp contains a form of vitamin B12, although its bioavailability for humans is debated. Vitamin B12 is crucial for nerve function and red blood cell formation.

Including kelp in your diet can contribute to a diverse intake of vitamins, supporting various physiological functions and promoting overall health. As with any food, it's important to consume a variety of nutrient-rich foods to ensure a balanced intake of vitamins and other essential nutrients.

Minerals:

Rich in minerals such as calcium, magnesium, potassium, and iron, kelp supports bone health, muscle function, and helps maintain proper electrolyte balance.

Calcium:

- Kelp contains calcium, an essential mineral for bone health, muscle function, and nerve transmission.

Potassium:

- Potassium is found in kelp and plays a role in regulating blood pressure, balancing fluids in the body, and supporting proper muscle and nerve function.

Magnesium:

- Magnesium in kelp contributes to muscle and nerve function, regulates blood pressure, and supports overall cardiovascular health.

Sodium:

- While seaweed, including kelp, naturally contains sodium, its sodium content is generally lower compared to traditional table salt.

Phosphorus:

- Phosphorus is present in kelp and is essential for bone and teeth formation, energy metabolism, and DNA synthesis.

Iron:

- Kelp provides iron, an important mineral for the formation of hemoglobin, the protein responsible for carrying oxygen in the blood.

Zinc:

- Zinc, a trace mineral, is found in kelp and is important for immune function, wound healing, and DNA synthesis.

Copper:

- Copper is present in kelp and plays a role in the formation of red blood cells, maintenance of healthy bones and nerves, and immune system function.

Manganese:

- Manganese, a trace mineral, is found in kelp and is involved in bone formation, blood clotting, and reducing inflammation.

Selenium:

- Kelp contains selenium, a trace element with antioxidant properties that supports the immune system and protects against oxidative stress.

Including kelp in your diet can contribute to a diverse intake of minerals, supporting various physiological functions and promoting overall health. It's important to note that excessive consumption of iodine-rich foods, including kelp, should be avoided, as it may lead to iodine toxicity. As with any food, moderation and a balanced diet are key for optimal health.

Dietary Fiber:

- Kelp is a good source of dietary fiber, promoting digestive health and contributing to a feeling of satiety.

Antioxidants:

Kelp contains antioxidants, including carotenoids and flavonoids, which help neutralize harmful free radicals and reduce oxidative stress.

Carotenoids:

- Kelp contains carotenoids, including beta-carotene, which is a precursor to vitamin A. Carotenoids have antioxidant properties that help neutralize free radicals in the body.

Flavonoids:

- Flavonoids are a group of polyphenolic compounds found in kelp with antioxidant and anti-inflammatory properties. They contribute to the overall health benefits of kelp.

Chlorophyll:

- Chlorophyll, the green pigment in plants and algae, is present in kelp. It has antioxidant properties and is involved in the process of photosynthesis.

Phlorotannins:

- Kelp is particularly rich in phlorotannins, unique polyphenolic compounds specific to brown seaweeds. Phlorotannins have been studied for their antioxidant, anti-inflammatory, and potential anti-cancer properties.

Vitamin E:

- While present in smaller amounts, kelp provides vitamin E, which is an antioxidant that protects cells from oxidative stress.

Selenium:

- Selenium, present in kelp, is an essential trace element that functions as part of antioxidant enzymes, helping to neutralize free radicals.

Zinc:

- Zinc, a trace mineral found in kelp, plays a role in the function of antioxidant enzymes, contributing to the body's defense against oxidative stress.

Manganese:

- Manganese in kelp is involved in the activation of antioxidant enzymes, supporting the body's antioxidant defense mechanisms.

These antioxidants work together to help combat oxidative stress, reduce inflammation, and contribute to overall health. Including kelp in your diet can provide a unique combination of these bioactive compounds, promoting a well-rounded approach to antioxidant support. As with any food, it's essential to consume a variety of nutrient-rich foods to ensure a diverse intake of antioxidants and other essential nutrients.

Health Benefits:

Thyroid Function:

- The high iodine content in kelp supports thyroid health, helping to prevent iodine deficiency and related thyroid disorders.

Heart Health:

- Kelp's rich mineral content, including potassium and magnesium, contributes to heart health by regulating blood pressure and supporting cardiovascular function.

Bone Health:

- The combination of calcium, magnesium, and vitamin K in kelp is beneficial for maintaining strong and healthy bones.

Weight Management:

- Kelp's dietary fiber content promotes a feeling of fullness, making it a valuable addition to weight management plans.

Nutritional Content

Kelp, a type of seaweed commonly used in various cuisines, particularly in Asian dishes, is highly nutritious and offers several health benefits. Here's an approximate nutritional breakdown for 1 cup (about 67 grams) of raw kelp:

- Carbohydrates: Approximately 4 grams
- Protein: Roughly 1 gram

- Fiber: Around 1 gram
- Fat: Less than 1 gram
- Sugar: Less than 1 gram

It's important to note that the nutritional content of kelp can vary slightly depending on factors such as the species of seaweed, growing conditions, and preparation methods. Additionally, kelp is often consumed in dried or rehydrated forms, which can affect its nutritional profile.

Kelp is particularly prized for its high mineral content, including iodine, calcium, magnesium, and potassium. It's also a good source of vitamins, such as vitamin K and various B vitamins. The fiber content in kelp primarily consists of soluble fiber, which can support digestive health and promote feelings of fullness.

Due to its low calorie and carbohydrate content, kelp is often included in weight loss and low-carb diets. However, it's essential to consume kelp in moderation, as excessive intake of iodine-rich foods like kelp can lead to thyroid issues in some individuals.

Overall, incorporating kelp into your diet can provide a variety of essential nutrients and contribute to overall health and well-being. It's commonly used in dishes like soups, salads, sushi rolls, and stir-fries, adding a unique flavor and nutritional boost to meals.

Culinary Uses:

Seaweed Salad:

- Kelp can be incorporated into a refreshing seaweed salad by rehydrating it and combining it with sesame oil, soy sauce, and other seasonings.

Kelp Noodles:

- Kelp noodles, made from the inner portion of the kelp plant, provide a low-calorie and gluten-free alternative to traditional noodles. They can be used in various dishes like stir-fries and salads.

Smoothie Booster:

- Adding powdered kelp to smoothies enhances nutritional content, providing an extra boost of vitamins and minerals.

Broth Base:

- Kelp can be used as a base for savory broths, imparting a rich umami flavor and enhancing the nutritional value of the broth.

Kelp's unique flavor and nutritional benefits make it a versatile ingredient in various dishes. Here are two recipes featuring kelp:

Kelp Noodle Salad:

Ingredients:

- 1 package kelp noodles
- 1 cup shredded cabbage
- 1 carrot, julienned
- 1 cucumber, thinly sliced
- 1 bell pepper, thinly sliced
- 1/4 cup chopped scallions
- 2 tablespoons sesame oil
- 3 tablespoons soy sauce or tamari
- 1 tablespoon rice vinegar
- 1 tablespoon maple syrup or honey
- Sesame seeds for garnish
- Optional: Grilled tofu or shrimp for added protein

Instructions:

1. **Prepare Kelp Noodles:**
    - Rinse kelp noodles under cold water and set aside.
2. **Prepare Vegetables:**
    - In a large bowl, combine shredded cabbage, julienned carrot, sliced cucumber, bell pepper, and chopped scallions.
3. **Make Dressing:**
    - In a small bowl, whisk together sesame oil, soy sauce, rice vinegar, and maple syrup. Adjust quantities to taste.
4. **Combine and Toss:**
    - Add the kelp noodles to the bowl of vegetables. Pour the dressing over the salad and toss until well combined.
5. **Garnish and Serve:**
    - Garnish with sesame seeds and, if desired, top with grilled tofu or shrimp.

- Serve chilled and enjoy this refreshing and nutrient-packed kelp noodle salad.

Seaweed and Mushroom Soup:

Ingredients:

- 1 oz dried kelp (kombu)
- 4 cups vegetable or mushroom broth
- 1 cup shiitake mushrooms, sliced
- 1 cup enoki mushrooms, trimmed
- 1 cup tofu, cubed
- 2 tablespoons soy sauce
- 1 tablespoon sesame oil
- 1 teaspoon grated ginger
- 2 cloves garlic, minced
- Green onions for garnish
- Red pepper flakes (optional)

Instructions:

1. **Prepare Kelp Broth:**
    - In a pot, combine dried kelp and vegetable or mushroom broth. Bring to a simmer over low heat for about 15-20 minutes. Do not boil.
2. **Remove Kelp and Add Ingredients:**
    - Remove the kelp from the broth and discard. Add sliced shiitake mushrooms, enoki mushrooms, tofu, soy sauce, sesame oil, grated ginger, and minced garlic to the pot.
3. **Simmer:**
    - Allow the soup to simmer for an additional 10-15 minutes until the mushrooms are tender and flavors are well combined.
4. **Garnish and Serve:**
    - Garnish with chopped green onions and red pepper flakes if you like a bit of heat.
    - Serve this nourishing seaweed and mushroom soup hot, and savor the umami-rich flavors.

These recipes showcase the versatility of kelp in creating delicious and nutritious meals. Whether in a refreshing salad or a comforting soup, kelp adds a unique and healthful twist to your culinary repertoire.

Tips Incorporating Kelp into your Diet

Incorporating kelp into your diet can seem daunting at first, especially if you're unfamiliar with cooking with seaweed. However, with a bit of knowledge and creativity, you can easily transition to enjoying the benefits of kelp in your meals. Here's a guide to help you overcome any challenges and seamlessly integrate kelp into your diet:

1. Start with Familiar Dishes: Begin by incorporating kelp into dishes that you already enjoy. For example, if you love soups and stews, try adding a strip of kelp to your broth to enhance its flavor and nutritional value. Kelp can also be added to salads, stir-fries, and pasta dishes for a unique twist.

2. Experiment with Different Forms: Kelp is available in various forms, including dried, powdered, and fresh. Experiment with different forms to find what works best for your taste preferences and cooking style. Dried kelp is convenient and can be easily rehydrated, while powdered kelp can be sprinkled onto dishes as a seasoning.

3. Educate Yourself: Take the time to learn about the nutritional benefits of kelp and how it can contribute to a healthy diet. Understanding its health-promoting properties may motivate you to incorporate it into your meals more regularly.

4. Start Slowly: If you're new to eating kelp, start by incorporating small amounts into your meals and gradually increase the quantity as you become more accustomed to its flavor and texture.

5. Experiment with Flavors: Kelp has a unique umami flavor that can enhance the taste of a wide range of dishes. Experiment with different flavor combinations by pairing kelp with ingredients like soy sauce, ginger, garlic, sesame oil, and chili flakes to create delicious and satisfying meals.

6. Be Creative: Don't be afraid to get creative with how you use kelp in your cooking. Use it as a wrap for sushi, blend it into smoothies for a nutritional boost, or even bake it into savory snacks like crackers or chips.

7. Seek Inspiration: Look for recipes and cooking tutorials online or in cookbooks that feature kelp as a primary ingredient. There are countless inventive and delicious ways to incorporate kelp into your meals, so don't hesitate to get inspired and try new recipes.

8. Consider Convenience: If sourcing fresh kelp is challenging, consider using dried or powdered kelp as convenient alternatives. These forms are shelf-stable and can be easily stored in your pantry for whenever you want to add a dose of kelp to your meals.

9. Embrace the Health Benefits: Remind yourself of the numerous health benefits of consuming kelp, including its rich nutrient content, potential to support thyroid function, and role in promoting gut health. Keeping these benefits in mind can help motivate you to incorporate kelp into your diet regularly.

10. Be Patient and Persistent: Like any dietary change, transitioning to incorporating kelp into your diet may take time and patience. Be patient with yourself as you explore new recipes and flavors, and don't be discouraged if it takes some time to adjust to eating kelp regularly.

By following these tips and approaches, you can overcome any challenges associated with incorporating kelp into your diet and enjoy the myriad benefits that this nutrient-rich seaweed has to offer. Whether you're looking to expand your culinary horizons or boost your overall health and well-being, kelp can be a delicious and rewarding addition to your diet.

Conclusion:

Kelp, with its nutrient-rich composition and versatile uses, stands out as an oceanic superfood that offers a myriad of health benefits. From supporting thyroid function to promoting heart and bone health, kelp deserves a place on the plates of those seeking a nutritious and sustainable dietary choice. If you have specific health concerns, allergies, or conditions, it's advisable to consult with a healthcare professional or a registered dietitian before making significant changes to your diet.

Embrace the flavors and benefits of kelp, and dive into the world of this marine vegetable for a healthier and more vibrant lifestyle.

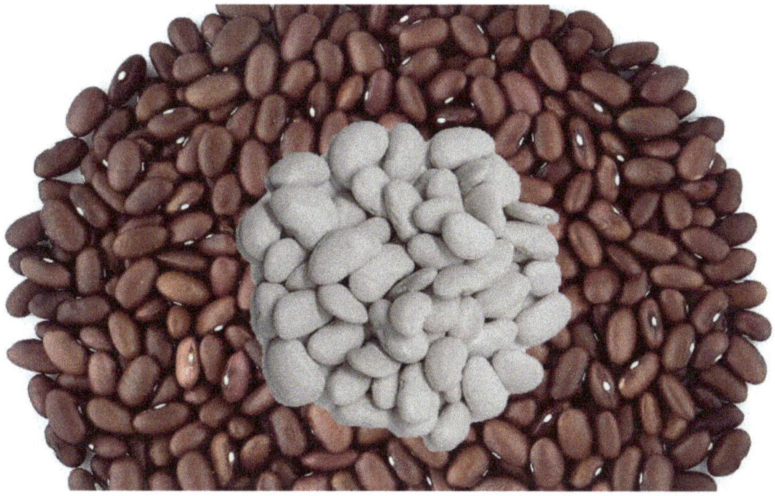

Kidney Beans

Nutrient-Rich Legumes Packed with Health Benefits and Culinary Versatility

Kidney beans, renowned for their kidney-shaped appearance, are not just a culinary delight but also a nutritional powerhouse. These legumes, scientifically known as Phaseolus vulgaris, have been a staple in various cuisines worldwide for centuries. In addition to their earthy flavor and creamy texture, kidney beans offer an impressive array of health benefits, making them a valuable inclusion in a balanced and wholesome diet. In this article, we'll explore the benefits and diverse uses of kidney beans, shedding light on why they are considered a nutritional gem.

Nutritional Powerhouse:

Kidney beans are a nutritional powerhouse, providing an abundance of essential nutrients that contribute to overall well-being. Key nutritional components of kidney beans include:

Protein:

- Kidney beans are an excellent source of plant-based protein, making them a valuable addition to vegetarian and vegan diets. Protein is essential for muscle repair, immune function, and overall growth and maintenance.

Dietary Fiber:

- Rich in both soluble and insoluble fiber, kidney beans support digestive health by promoting regular bowel movements, preventing constipation, and contributing to a healthy gut microbiota. Fiber also plays a role in heart health and blood sugar regulation.

Complex Carbohydrates:

- Kidney beans provide complex carbohydrates, offering a gradual release of energy. They have a low glycemic index, making them suitable for individuals aiming to manage blood sugar levels.

Vitamins and Minerals:

Kidney beans contain essential vitamins such as folate, vitamin B1 (thiamine), and minerals including iron, magnesium, phosphorus, and potassium. These nutrients play crucial roles in various bodily functions, including blood formation, energy metabolism, and bone health. **Essential Vitamins in Kidney Beans:**

Folate (Vitamin B9):

- **Benefits:** Folate is essential for DNA synthesis and repair. Adequate folate intake is crucial during periods of rapid cell division, such as pregnancy, and it helps prevent neural tube defects in developing fetuses.

Thiamine (Vitamin B1):

- **Benefits:** Thiamine is vital for energy metabolism, playing a key role in converting carbohydrates into energy. It also supports proper nerve function and is essential for the synthesis of neurotransmitters.

Vitamin B6:

- **Benefits:** Vitamin B6 is involved in over 100 enzymatic reactions in the body, including the metabolism of amino acids and the production of neurotransmitters. It plays a role in immune function, cognitive development, and the regulation of mood.

Niacin (Vitamin B3):

- **Benefits:** Niacin is crucial for energy metabolism, DNA repair, and the production of various enzymes. It contributes to maintaining healthy skin, nerves, and the digestive system.

Essential Minerals in Kidney Beans:

Iron:

- **Benefits:** Iron is essential for the formation of hemoglobin, the oxygen-carrying component of red blood cells. Adequate iron intake is crucial for preventing iron-deficiency anemia and supporting overall energy levels.

Magnesium:

- **Benefits:** Magnesium is involved in various physiological processes, including muscle and nerve function, bone health, and energy metabolism. It contributes to the regulation of blood pressure and supports the immune system.

Phosphorus:

- **Benefits:** Phosphorus is a structural component of DNA, RNA, and ATP (adenosine triphosphate), the primary energy carrier in cells. It is essential for bone health, kidney function, and the metabolism of macronutrients.

Potassium:

- **Benefits:** Potassium plays a crucial role in maintaining proper fluid balance, nerve impulses, and muscle contractions. It also supports heart health by helping to regulate blood pressure.

Health Benefits:

Heart Health:

- The high fiber content, potassium, and magnesium in kidney beans contribute to heart health. Fiber helps lower cholesterol levels, potassium regulates blood pressure, and magnesium supports overall cardiovascular function.

Blood Sugar Regulation:

- Kidney beans have a low glycemic index, providing a slow and steady release of glucose. This property makes them a suitable choice for individuals aiming to manage blood sugar levels and prevent insulin spikes.

Weight Management:

- The combination of protein and fiber in kidney beans promotes a feeling of fullness, aiding in weight management. Including kidney beans in meals can help control appetite and reduce overall calorie intake.

Antioxidant Properties:

- Kidney beans contain antioxidants, including flavonoids and polyphenols, which help neutralize free radicals in the body. Antioxidants play a role in reducing oxidative stress and inflammation.

Nutritional Content

Here's the approximate nutritional breakdown for 1 cup (about 177 grams) of cooked kidney beans, drained and without salt:

- Carbohydrates: Approximately 40 grams
- Protein: Roughly 15 grams
- Fiber: Around 11 grams
- Fat: Less than 1 gram
- Sugar: Approximately 0 grams

Kidney beans are a nutrient-dense food, rich in complex carbohydrates, protein, and dietary fiber. They're also low in fat and naturally free of cholesterol. The high fiber content in kidney beans can help promote digestive health, regulate blood sugar levels, and support weight management by promoting satiety. Additionally, kidney beans are a good source of plant-based protein, making them a valuable component of vegetarian and vegan diets.

Culinary Versatility:

Kidney beans are incredibly versatile in the kitchen, adapting well to various cooking methods and flavor profiles. Some common culinary uses include:

Chili Con Carne:

- A classic dish featuring kidney beans, ground meat, tomatoes, and chili spices. This hearty and flavorful dish is a comfort food favorite.

Red Beans and Rice:

- A popular dish in Caribbean and Creole cuisines, red beans and rice combine kidney beans with aromatic spices, rice, and sometimes sausage for a satisfying meal.

Kidney Bean Salad:

- A refreshing salad combining kidney beans with colorful vegetables, herbs, and a zesty dressing. This salad is both nutritious and visually appealing.

Vegetarian Kidney Bean Curry:

- A flavorful and protein-rich curry featuring kidney beans, vegetables, and aromatic spices. This vegetarian dish is a delightful option for those seeking plant-based meals.

Here are two delicious and nutritious recipes featuring kidney beans:

Vegetarian Three-Bean Chili:

Ingredients:

- 1 can (15 ounces) kidney beans, drained and rinsed
- 1 can (15 ounces) black beans, drained and rinsed
- 1 can (15 ounces) pinto beans, drained and rinsed
- 1 tablespoon olive oil
- 1 onion, diced
- 3 cloves garlic, minced
- 1 bell pepper, diced (any color)

- 1 zucchini, diced
- 1 can (28 ounces) crushed tomatoes
- 2 tablespoons tomato paste
- 2 teaspoons chili powder
- 1 teaspoon cumin
- 1 teaspoon smoked paprika
- Salt and pepper to taste
- Optional toppings: shredded cheese, sour cream, green onions, cilantro

Instructions:

1. In a large pot, heat olive oil over medium heat. Add diced onion and garlic, sautéing until softened.
2. Add diced bell pepper and zucchini to the pot, continuing to sauté for a few minutes until the vegetables are tender.
3. Stir in crushed tomatoes, tomato paste, chili powder, cumin, smoked paprika, salt, and pepper.
4. Add the drained and rinsed kidney beans, black beans, and pinto beans to the pot. Mix well.
5. Bring the chili to a simmer, then reduce the heat and let it simmer for at least 20-30 minutes to allow the flavors to meld.
6. Adjust the seasoning to taste and serve the vegetarian three-bean chili hot. Top with shredded cheese, sour cream, green onions, or cilantro if desired.

Mediterranean Kidney Bean Salad:

Ingredients:

- 2 cans (15 ounces each) kidney beans, drained and rinsed
- 1 cucumber, diced
- 1 cup cherry tomatoes, halved
- 1 red onion, finely chopped
- 1/2 cup Kalamata olives, sliced
- 1/2 cup feta cheese, crumbled
- Fresh parsley, chopped (for garnish)

For the Lemon Herb Dressing:

- 1/4 cup extra-virgin olive oil
- 2 tablespoons fresh lemon juice
- 1 teaspoon dried oregano
- 1 clove garlic, minced
- Salt and pepper to taste

Instructions:

1. In a large bowl, combine the drained and rinsed kidney beans, diced cucumber, cherry tomatoes, chopped red onion, Kalamata olives, and crumbled feta cheese.
2. In a small bowl, whisk together the ingredients for the lemon herb dressing: olive oil, fresh lemon juice, dried oregano, minced garlic, salt, and pepper.
3. Pour the dressing over the kidney bean salad and toss until all ingredients are well coated.
4. Garnish with fresh chopped parsley.
5. Chill the Mediterranean kidney bean salad in the refrigerator for at least 30 minutes before serving.
6. Serve the salad as a refreshing and protein-packed side dish or a light main course.

These recipes showcase the versatility of kidney beans, whether in a comforting chili or a vibrant salad. Kidney beans add both texture and nutritional value to dishes, making them a delicious and healthful choice for various meals.

Conclusion:

Incorporating kidney beans into your diet is a flavorful and health-conscious choice. Whether enjoyed in chili, salads, or as a side dish, kidney beans offer a nutrient-dense addition to meals. While kidney beans are generally safe and healthy to consume as part of a balanced diet. As with any food, moderation is key. If you have specific health concerns, allergies, or conditions, it's advisable to consult with a healthcare professional or a registered dietitian before making significant changes to your diet.

With their robust nutritional profile and culinary versatility, kidney beans stand as a testament to the idea that wholesome foods can be both delicious and beneficial for overall health and well-being.

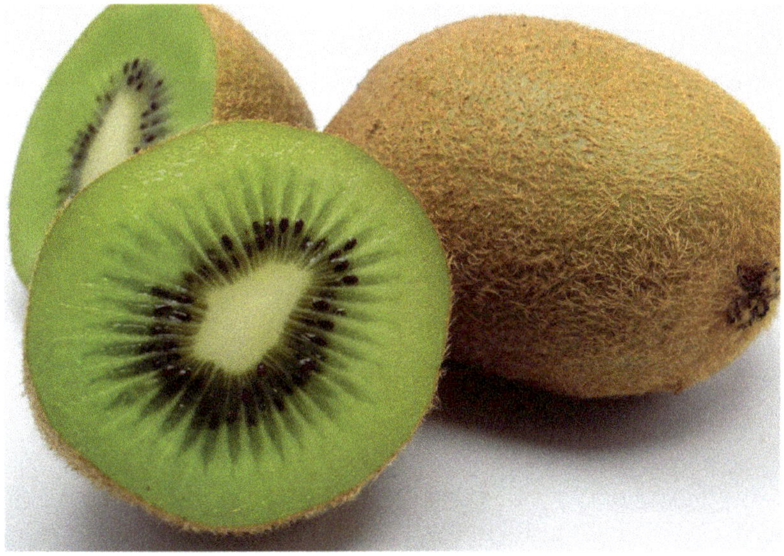

Kiwi

The Benefits and Culinary Versatility of this Nutrient-Packed Fruit

Kiwi, also known as the Chinese gooseberry, is a small but mighty fruit that has gained popularity for its unique taste and impressive nutritional profile. Packed with essential vitamins, minerals, and antioxidants, kiwi offers a plethora of health benefits. In this article, we'll delve into the various advantages of incorporating kiwi into your diet and explore its versatile uses in the culinary world.

Nutrient-Rich Goodness:

Kiwi is a nutritional powerhouse, boasting a range of essential nutrients that contribute to overall health. Here are some key nutritional components found in kiwi:

Vitamin C:

- **Benefits:** Boosts the immune system, supports skin health, acts as an antioxidant, aids in collagen production.

Dietary Fiber:

- **Benefits:** Promotes digestive health, helps regulate blood sugar levels, contributes to a feeling of fullness.

Vitamin K:

- **Benefits:** Essential for blood clotting, contributes to bone health, helps regulate calcium in the body.

Vitamin E:

- **Benefits:** Acts as an antioxidant, supports skin health, protects cells from damage.

Potassium:

- **Benefits:** Helps regulate blood pressure, supports heart and muscle function, aids in fluid balance.

Folate (Vitamin B9):

- **Benefits:** Important for DNA synthesis and repair, aids in red blood cell formation.

Vitamin A:

- **Benefits:** Essential for vision health, supports immune function, maintains healthy skin.

Copper:

- **Benefits:** Supports the formation of red blood cells, aids in iron absorption.

Phosphorus:

- **Benefits:** Essential for bone and teeth health, involved in energy metabolism.

Magnesium:

- **Benefits:** Important for muscle and nerve function, supports bone health.

Zinc:

- **Benefits:** Supports immune function, involved in wound healing, essential for DNA synthesis.

Iron:

- **Benefits:** Important for oxygen transport in the blood, supports energy metabolism.

Calcium:

- **Benefits:** Important for bone and teeth health, supports muscle and nerve function.

Vitamin B6 (Pyridoxine):

- **Benefits:** Important for brain development and function, helps the body convert food into energy, supports the nervous system.

Niacin (Vitamin B3):

- **Benefits:** Supports energy metabolism, helps maintain skin health.

Riboflavin (Vitamin B2):

- **Benefits:** Important for energy production, supports normal vision and skin health.

Thiamine (Vitamin B1):

- **Benefits:** Essential for energy metabolism, supports nerve function.

These vitamins and minerals make kiwi a nutritious and health-promoting fruit, contributing to various aspects of overall well-being. Including kiwi in your diet can be a flavorful and beneficial way to meet your nutritional needs.

Health Benefits:

Digestive Health:

- The dietary fiber in kiwi promotes healthy digestion, preventing constipation and supporting gut health.

Heart Health:

- Potassium in kiwi contributes to heart health by helping regulate blood pressure and supporting overall cardiovascular function.

Immune Support:

- The high Vitamin C content in kiwi strengthens the immune system, aiding the body in fighting off infections and illnesses.

Antioxidant Protection:

- Kiwi is rich in antioxidants that help neutralize free radicals, protecting cells from oxidative stress and reducing the risk of chronic diseases.

Nutritional Content

Here's the approximate nutritional breakdown for 1 cup (about 177 grams) of sliced kiwi fruit:

- Carbohydrates: Approximately 27 grams
- Protein: Roughly 2 grams
- Fiber: Around 5 grams
- Fat: Less than 1 gram
- Sugar: Approximately 16 grams

Kiwi fruit is low in calories and fat but rich in essential nutrients, particularly vitamin C, vitamin K, and dietary fiber. The high fiber content in kiwi can help support digestive health and promote feelings of fullness. Additionally, kiwi is a good source of antioxidants, such as vitamin C and vitamin E, which help protect cells from damage caused by free radicals.

Culinary Versatility:

Kiwi is not only a nutritious addition to your diet but also a versatile ingredient that can be enjoyed in various culinary creations. Here are some popular uses:

Fresh Snacking:

- Peel and slice kiwi for a refreshing and portable snack. Its sweet and tangy flavor makes it an excellent choice for satisfying your sweet tooth.

Smoothies and Juices:

- Blend kiwi into smoothies or juices for a burst of tropical flavor. Combine it with other fruits, yogurt, or a liquid of your choice for a nutritious and delicious beverage.

Fruit Salads:

- Add diced kiwi to fruit salads for a vibrant and flavorful twist. Kiwi pairs well with berries, melons, and citrus fruits.

Salsas and Relishes:

- Create salsas or relishes with kiwi to accompany grilled fish or chicken. The combination of sweetness and acidity adds complexity to savory dishes.

Here are two delightful recipes that highlight the unique flavor and nutritional benefits of kiwi:

Kiwi and Berry Parfait:

Ingredients:

- 2 cups Greek yogurt
- 4 kiwis, peeled and sliced
- 1 cup mixed berries (strawberries, blueberries, raspberries)
- 1/2 cup granola
- 2 tablespoons honey

Instructions:

1. In serving glasses or bowls, layer Greek yogurt at the bottom.
2. Add a layer of sliced kiwi on top of the yogurt.
3. Follow with a layer of mixed berries.
4. Sprinkle granola over the berries.
5. Repeat the layers until the glass or bowl is filled.
6. Drizzle honey over the top for a touch of sweetness.
7. Repeat for additional servings.

8. Serve immediately and enjoy this refreshing and nutritious Kiwi and Berry Parfait.

Kiwi Mint Smoothie:

Ingredients:

- 3 kiwis, peeled and sliced
- 1 banana, peeled
- 1 cup fresh spinach leaves
- 1/2 cup fresh mint leaves
- 1/2 cup plain yogurt
- 1 cup coconut water or water
- Ice cubes (optional)
- 1 tablespoon chia seeds (optional)

Instructions:

1. In a blender, combine kiwi slices, banana, fresh spinach leaves, fresh mint leaves, plain yogurt, and coconut water.
2. If desired, add ice cubes for a colder smoothie.
3. Blend until smooth and creamy.
4. Pour the smoothie into glasses.
5. Optionally, sprinkle chia seeds on top for added nutrition and texture.
6. Serve immediately and relish the invigorating taste of this Kiwi Mint Smoothie.

These recipes showcase the versatility of kiwi, whether layered in a parfait for a delightful treat or blended into a refreshing smoothie. Enjoy the vibrant flavors and nutritional benefits that kiwi brings to these creative and healthy dishes!

Conclusion:

Kiwi stands as a delicious and nutritious addition to a well-balanced diet. Whether enjoyed fresh, blended into beverages, or incorporated into various culinary creations, kiwi offers a unique combination of taste and health benefits. If you have specific health concerns, allergies, or conditions, it's advisable to consult with a healthcare professional or a registered dietitian before making significant changes to your diet.

Embrace the versatility and goodness of kiwi, and let this vibrant fruit become a staple in your journey towards a healthier and more flavorful lifestyle.

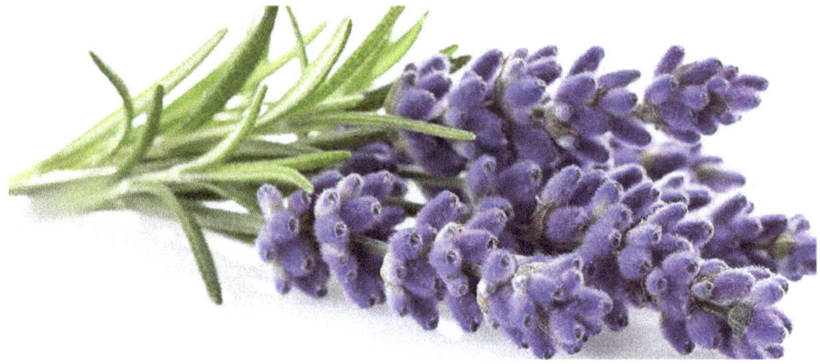

Lavender

A Guide to Its Benefits and Uses

Lavender, with its delightful fragrance and versatile properties, has been cherished for centuries for its numerous benefits and uses. This enchanting herb, known for its calming aroma and therapeutic qualities, has found its way into various aspects of our lives, from aromatherapy to culinary delights. In this article, we will explore the myriad benefits and diverse applications of lavender.

Aromatherapy and Stress Relief:

One of the most well-known benefits of lavender is its ability to induce relaxation and alleviate stress. The essential oil extracted from lavender contains compounds that interact with the nervous system, promoting a sense of calm and tranquility. A few drops of lavender oil in a diffuser or added to a warm bath can work wonders in reducing stress and promoting a restful sleep.

Skincare Marvel:

Lavender is a skincare powerhouse with its anti-inflammatory and antioxidant properties. It is often used in various skincare products such as creams, lotions, and oils. Lavender can help soothe irritated skin, reduce redness, and even promote wound healing. Its gentle nature makes it suitable for all skin types, including sensitive skin.

Lavender-infused Face Mask:

- Create a rejuvenating face mask by combining lavender essential oil with other skincare ingredients such as clay or honey. Lavender's anti-inflammatory and antioxidant properties can help soothe irritated skin, reduce redness, and promote a healthy complexion. Applying a lavender-infused face mask can be particularly beneficial for individuals with sensitive or acne-prone skin, as it may help calm inflammation and prevent breakouts.

Lavender-infused Body Scrub:

- Incorporate lavender into a homemade body scrub to exfoliate and nourish the skin. Mix lavender essential oil with ingredients like sugar, salt, or coffee grounds to create a fragrant scrub that not only buffs away dead skin cells but also provides aromatherapy benefits. Lavender's calming aroma can enhance the overall spa-like experience, while its antimicrobial properties contribute to maintaining healthy skin. Regular use of a lavender-infused body scrub can leave the skin feeling soft, smooth, and revitalized.

Lavender-infused Moisturizer or Oil:

- Enhance your skincare routine by incorporating lavender into your moisturizer or facial oil. Lavender's hydrating properties can help soothe dry or chapped skin, making it a valuable addition to your daily skincare regimen. Whether added to a store-bought product or mixed with a carrier oil like jojoba or almond oil, lavender contributes to maintaining skin elasticity and promoting a radiant complexion. Additionally, the calming scent of lavender can create a relaxing experience during your skincare routine, adding a touch of indulgence to self-care practices.

These lavender-infused skincare methods offer a natural and aromatic approach to promoting skin health and well-being. Whether you choose a face mask, body scrub, or moisturizer, incorporating lavender into your skincare routine can provide both tangible and sensory benefits for your skin.

Natural Sleep Aid:

Struggling with sleepless nights? Lavender might be the solution. The calming aroma of lavender can promote better sleep quality. Placing dried lavender sachets under your pillow or using a lavender-infused sleep spray can create a relaxing environment conducive to a good night's rest.

Culinary Delight:

Lavender is not just limited to aromatherapy and skincare; it has also found its way into the kitchen. Culinary lavender, known for its sweet and floral notes, can be used in various recipes. From lavender-infused desserts like ice cream and cookies to savory dishes like lavender-infused honey-glazed chicken, this herb adds a unique and delightful flavor to a wide range of culinary creations.

Lavender is a versatile herb that adds a unique floral flavor to both sweet and savory dishes.

Here are two recipes that feature lavender:

Lavender Honey Lemonade:

Ingredients:

- 4 cups water
- 1/2 cup honey
- 1/4 cup fresh lemon juice
- 2 tablespoons culinary lavender buds

- Ice cubes
- Lemon slices and fresh lavender sprigs for garnish (optional)

Instructions:

1. In a small saucepan, combine 2 cups of water and culinary lavender buds. Bring to a simmer over medium heat and let it simmer for about 5 minutes.
2. Remove the saucepan from heat and let the lavender-infused water cool for 10-15 minutes.
3. Strain the lavender buds from the water using a fine mesh strainer or cheesecloth, and discard the solids.
4. In a large pitcher, combine the lavender-infused water, honey, and fresh lemon juice. Stir until the honey is completely dissolved.
5. Add the remaining 2 cups of water to the pitcher and stir to combine.
6. Refrigerate the lavender honey lemonade for at least 1 hour to chill.
7. Serve the lavender honey lemonade over ice cubes, garnished with lemon slices and fresh lavender sprigs if desired. Enjoy this refreshing and aromatic beverage!

Lavender Lemon Shortbread Cookies:

Ingredients:

- 1 cup unsalted butter, softened
- 1/2 cup powdered sugar
- 2 cups all-purpose flour
- 1 tablespoon culinary lavender buds, finely chopped
- 1 tablespoon fresh lemon zest
- 1/4 teaspoon salt
- Additional powdered sugar for dusting (optional)

Instructions:

1. In a mixing bowl, cream together the softened butter and powdered sugar until light and fluffy.
2. Add the finely chopped culinary lavender buds, fresh lemon zest, and salt to the butter mixture. Mix until well combined.
3. Gradually add the all-purpose flour to the butter mixture, mixing until a dough forms.
4. Shape the dough into a ball, wrap it in plastic wrap, and refrigerate for at least 30 minutes to firm up.

5. Preheat the oven to 350°F (175°C). Line a baking sheet with parchment paper.
6. Roll out the chilled dough on a lightly floured surface to about 1/4 inch thickness.
7. Use cookie cutters to cut out desired shapes from the dough and place them onto the prepared baking sheet.
8. Bake the lavender lemon shortbread cookies in the preheated oven for 12-15 minutes, or until the edges are lightly golden.
9. Remove the cookies from the oven and let them cool on the baking sheet for a few minutes before transferring them to a wire rack to cool completely.
10. Once cooled, dust the lavender lemon shortbread cookies with powdered sugar if desired. Enjoy these fragrant and buttery cookies with a hint of lavender and lemon flavor!

These recipes showcase the delightful flavor of lavender and how it can be used to enhance both beverages and baked goods. Enjoy experimenting with these recipes in your kitchen!

Key Components in Lavender

However, Lavender does not typically serve as a significant dietary source of nutrients in the same way that fruits or vegetables do. However, lavender does contain certain compounds that contribute to its therapeutic properties. Here are some key components found in lavender and their associated benefits:

Linalool:

- **Benefit:** Linalool is a major component of lavender essential oil, and it contributes to lavender's calming and relaxing effects. It has been studied for its potential anti-anxiety and sedative properties, making it a valuable compound for stress relief and promoting a sense of tranquility.

Linalyl acetate:

- **Benefit:** Linalyl acetate is another important compound found in lavender oil. It is known for its anti-inflammatory and antispasmodic properties. This compound contributes to lavender's ability to soothe irritated skin and muscles, making it beneficial for skincare and relaxation.

Camphor:

- **Benefit:** Camphor is present in smaller amounts in lavender oil. It has been studied for its potential analgesic (pain-relieving) and anti-inflammatory effects. While lavender is not a primary source of camphor, its presence in the essential oil may contribute to the herb's ability to provide relief from headaches and muscle discomfort.

Caryophyllene:

- **Benefit:** Caryophyllene is a terpene found in lavender with anti-inflammatory properties. It has been studied for its potential in managing inflammatory conditions. While lavender contains caryophyllene in smaller amounts, it adds to the overall anti-inflammatory profile of the herb.

It's important to note that while lavender can provide therapeutic benefits through aromatherapy, skincare, and other applications, it is not commonly consumed in large quantities for its nutritional content. If you are considering using lavender for medicinal purposes, it's advisable to do so under the guidance of a healthcare professional, especially if you have any pre-existing conditions or are taking medications.

Natural Insect Repellent:

Lavender's pleasant fragrance serves as a natural deterrent for insects. Whether in the form of essential oil or dried lavender bundles, placing them around your living space can help keep mosquitoes and other unwanted pests at bay. Additionally, lavender-scented candles or sprays can be used outdoors to create a bug-free zone during gatherings.

Headache Relief:

Lavender's analgesic properties make it a natural remedy for headaches and migraines. Applying diluted lavender oil to the temples or inhaling its aroma can provide relief from tension headaches. The calming effect on the nervous system contributes to easing the discomfort associated with headaches.

Conclusion:

Lavender, with its enchanting aroma and versatile properties, has earned its place as a beloved herb in various aspects of our lives. Whether used for relaxation, skincare, culinary adventures, or as a natural insect repellent, lavender continues to prove its worth. Embrace the benefits of lavender and incorporate this fragrant herb into your daily routine for a touch of tranquility and well-being.

If you have specific health concerns, allergies, or conditions, it's advisable to consult with a healthcare professional or a registered dietitian before making significant changes to your diet.

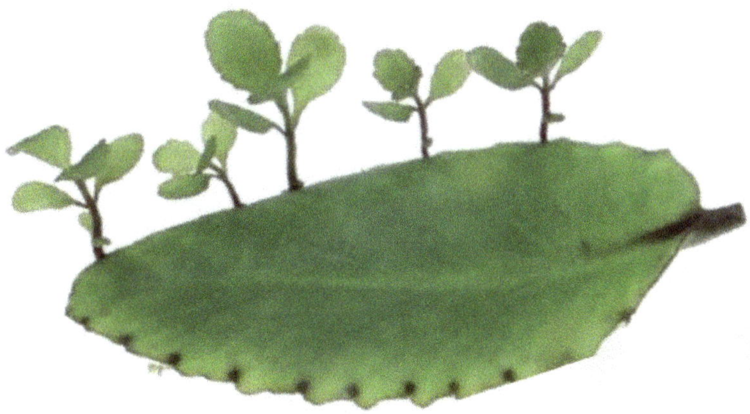

Leaf of Life

A Natural Wonder for Health and Healing

In the realm of natural remedies, there exists a plant revered for its myriad benefits and versatile applications—the Leaf of Life (Bryophyllum pinnatum). Known by various names such as "Air Plant," "Life Plant," or "Miracle Leaf," this succulent native to Madagascar has earned its reputation as a powerhouse of wellness in traditional medicine practices around the world.

Origins and Appearance

The Leaf of Life belongs to the Kalanchoe genus and is characterized by its thick, fleshy leaves arranged in a rosette pattern. Its botanical name, Bryophyllum pinnatum, stems from the Greek words "bryo" (to sprout) and "phyllon" (leaf), highlighting its propensity for proliferation through leaf propagation. This ability to reproduce new plants from its leaves contributes to its resilience and widespread distribution.

The leaves of the plant boast an impressive array of health-supporting activities, including neurosedative and muscle relaxant properties, along with antimicrobial, antiulcer, uterine contractility, antinociceptive, anti-inflammatory, antidiabetic, antihypertensive, and nephroprotective attributes. Antibacterial, antifungal, and antihistamine properties contribute to its efficacy in addressing insect bites, bruises, pain relief, and anxiety disorders.

Medicinal Properties

The Leaf of Life (Bryophyllum pinnatum) contains a variety of vitamins, minerals, and antioxidants, each contributing to its health-promoting properties. Here are some key nutrients found in the Leaf of Life along with their benefits:

Vitamins:

Vitamin C:

- *Benefits*: As a powerful antioxidant, Vitamin C helps protect cells from oxidative damage, supports immune function, aids in collagen production for skin health, and enhances iron absorption.

Minerals:

Calcium:

- *Benefits*: Essential for bone health, calcium also plays a role in muscle function, nerve transmission, and blood clotting.

Magnesium:

- *Benefits*: Magnesium is involved in hundreds of biochemical reactions in the body, including energy production, muscle and nerve function, blood sugar regulation, and bone health.

Potassium:

- *Benefits*: Potassium helps regulate fluid balance, muscle contractions, and nerve signals. It also plays a role in maintaining healthy blood pressure.

Phosphorus:

- *Benefits*: Phosphorus is essential for bone and teeth health, energy metabolism, cell membrane structure, and DNA synthesis.

Iron:

- *Benefits*: Iron is crucial for the production of hemoglobin, which carries oxygen in the blood. It also supports energy metabolism and immune function.

Antioxidants:

Flavonoids:

- *Benefits*: Flavonoids are potent antioxidants that help protect cells from oxidative damage caused by free radicals. They have anti-inflammatory, cardiovascular protective, and anticancer properties.

Phenols:

- *Benefits*: Phenolic compounds possess antioxidant properties, scavenging free radicals and reducing oxidative stress. They may help prevent chronic diseases such as cancer, cardiovascular diseases, and neurodegenerative disorders.

Triterpenes:

- *Benefits*: Triterpenes have been studied for their antioxidant activity, which helps combat oxidative stress and inflammation in the body. They may also contribute to skin health and wound healing.

Vitamin E:

- *Benefits*: Vitamin E is a fat-soluble antioxidant that protects cell membranes from damage. It supports immune function, skin health, and may reduce the risk of chronic diseases.

Beta-Carotene (Provitamin A):

- *Benefits*: Beta-carotene is converted into Vitamin A in the body, which is essential for vision, immune function, skin health, and normal growth and development.

These vitamins, minerals, and antioxidants found in the Leaf of Life contribute to its overall nutritional value and health benefits. Consuming the Leaf of Life or using it in various forms, such as teas, extracts, or topical applications, can help support overall health and well-being.

Bioactive Compounds

For centuries, the Leaf of Life has been treasured for its medicinal properties. Rich in bioactive compounds such as alkaloids, flavonoids, and phenols, this plant boasts an impressive array of therapeutic effects:

Alkaloids:

- *Benefits*: Alkaloids exhibit diverse pharmacological activities, including analgesic, anti-inflammatory, and antimicrobial properties. They can also have effects on the central nervous system, cardiovascular system, and digestive system.

Flavonoids:

- *Benefits*: Flavonoids are potent antioxidants, protecting cells from oxidative damage caused by free radicals. They also have anti-inflammatory, anti-allergic, anti-cancer, and cardiovascular protective effects.

Phenols:

- *Benefits*: Phenolic compounds possess antioxidant properties, scavenging free radicals and reducing oxidative stress. They may help prevent chronic diseases such as cancer, cardiovascular diseases, and neurodegenerative disorders.

Triterpenes:

- *Benefits*: Triterpenes have been studied for their anti-inflammatory, antimicrobial, and anticancer activities. They may also contribute to wound healing and skin regeneration.

Polysaccharides:

- *Benefits*: Polysaccharides have immunomodulatory effects, enhancing the activity of the immune system. They may also have antiviral, antioxidant, and anti-inflammatory properties.

Saponins:

- *Benefits*: Saponins have been investigated for their potential to lower cholesterol levels, boost immune function, and exhibit anticancer properties. They may also have anti-inflammatory and antimicrobial effects.

Organic Acids (e.g., malic acid, citric acid):

- *Benefits*: Organic acids play roles in metabolism and digestion. Malic acid, for example, is involved in the Krebs cycle and energy production, while citric acid is an antioxidant and may help prevent kidney stones.

These bioactive compounds work synergistically to provide the Leaf of Life with its wide range of therapeutic effects, including anti-inflammatory, antimicrobial, antioxidant, immunomodulatory, and wound-healing properties. It's important to note that the specific composition and concentrations of bioactive compounds may vary depending on factors such as plant maturity, growing conditions, and extraction methods.

Health Benefits

Anti-inflammatory: The Leaf of Life contains enzymes and compounds that help reduce inflammation, making it valuable in treating conditions like arthritis and rheumatism.

Wound Healing: Its antimicrobial properties aid in wound healing by preventing infections and promoting tissue regeneration. Applying crushed leaves or extracts topically can accelerate the healing process.

Respiratory Relief: Traditional medicine often employs Leaf of Life extracts to alleviate respiratory ailments such as asthma, bronchitis, and coughs. Its bronchodilator effects help to ease breathing and reduce symptoms.

Digestive Aid: Consuming Leaf of Life extracts or teas may soothe digestive issues like indigestion, bloating, and gastric ulcers. It is believed to stimulate the secretion of gastric juices, aiding in digestion.

Immune Support: With its rich antioxidant content, the Leaf of Life helps strengthen the immune system, protecting the body against oxidative stress and infections.

Skin Care: Its moisturizing and anti-inflammatory properties make it a popular ingredient in skincare products, renowned for its ability to soothe sunburns, rashes, and other skin irritations.

Antibacterial Properties:

Studies highlight the antimicrobial activity of "Leaf of Life" extracts against bacteria such as Escherichia coli (E. coli), Staphylococcus aureus (S. aureus), and Pseudomonas aeruginosa (P. aeruginosa), associated with various infections.

Antiviral Properties:

The plant exhibits antiviral activity against viruses including Herpes simplex virus (HSV), Human papillomavirus (HPV), Respiratory syncytial virus (RSV), and Hepatitis B virus (HBV). The presence of compounds like flavonoids, terpenoids, and phenolic compounds contributes to its antiviral efficacy.

How to Use Leaf of Life

The versatility of the Leaf of Life extends to its various applications:

- **Topical Use**: Crush fresh leaves to create poultices or extracts for topical application on wounds, burns, insect bites, and skin irritations.
- **Internal Consumption**: Brew dried Leaf of Life leaves into a tea for internal consumption, particularly to address digestive issues or respiratory ailments. However, it's essential to consult a healthcare professional before ingesting it, as excessive consumption may have adverse effects.
- **Supplements and Formulations**: Leaf of Life extracts are incorporated into various supplements and ointments available commercially for convenient use.

Methods of Juice Extraction:

- Blending the leaves and stems with a small amount of water, followed by straining.
- Beat the leaves and stems in a clean cloth or container, then separating the juice from the residue.
- Crushing the leaves and boiling, particularly suitable for making tea.

Culinary Uses

Here are two recipes that incorporate the Leaf of Life into delicious and nutritious dishes:

Leaf of Life Salad with Citrus Dressing

Ingredients:

- 2 cups fresh Leaf of Life leaves, washed and chopped
- 1 cup cherry tomatoes, halved
- 1 cucumber, thinly sliced
- 1 avocado, diced
- 1/4 cup red onion, thinly sliced
- 1/4 cup fresh parsley, chopped
- 1/4 cup olive oil
- 2 tablespoons freshly squeezed lemon juice

- 1 teaspoon honey
- Salt and pepper to taste

Instructions:

1. In a large salad bowl, combine the Leaf of Life leaves, cherry tomatoes, cucumber, avocado, red onion, and parsley.
2. In a small bowl, whisk together the olive oil, lemon juice, honey, salt, and pepper to make the dressing.
3. Pour the dressing over the salad and toss gently to coat all the ingredients evenly.
4. Serve immediately as a refreshing side dish or light meal.

Leaf of Life Infused Tea

Ingredients:

- 2 cups water
- 5-7 fresh Leaf of Life leaves (Depending on their size)
- Honey or sweetener of choice (optional)
- Lemon slices (optional)

Instructions:

1. Bring the water to a boil in a small saucepan.
2. Meanwhile, wash the Leaf of Life leaves thoroughly and chop them into smaller pieces.
3. Once the water is boiling, add the chopped leaves to the saucepan.
4. Reduce the heat to low and let the leaves simmer in the water for about 5-7 minutes, allowing their beneficial compounds to infuse into the water.
5. Remove the saucepan from the heat and let the tea steep for an additional 2-3 minutes.
6. Strain the tea to remove the leaves, then pour it into cups.
7. Add honey or sweetener to taste, if desired, and garnish with lemon slices for extra flavor.
8. Enjoy your soothing and nutritious Leaf of Life infused tea as a calming beverage.

These recipes offer creative ways to incorporate the Leaf of Life into your diet, allowing you to experience its health benefits while enjoying delicious and satisfying dishes.

Various Historical Medicinal Applications:

Consumption of fresh leaves for medicinal remedy in asthma, bronchitis, and intestinal problems.

Utilization of leaf extract on an empty stomach for treating urinary bladder stones and fever in children.

Application of heated leaves for treating swellings and abscesses.

Soaking leaves in cold water overnight, boiling, squeezing, or roasting for diverse medicinal extracts.

The "Leaf of Life" finds diverse applications, serving as a blood purifier, liver protector, diuretic, and remedy for ailments ranging from high blood pressure to leucorrhoea. Its antioxidant properties contribute to its inclusion in herbal green tea mixtures, and its potential benefits for hair nourishment, gray hair treatment, piles, stomachache, and jaundice underscore its holistic medicinal significance.

Historical Uses

The leaf of life plant has been utilized for various purposes throughout history. Here are two historical uses:

Traditional Medicine: The leaf of life plant has a long history of use in traditional medicine systems, particularly in regions where it is native, such as parts of Africa, Asia, and the Americas. In these cultures, the plant has been used to treat various ailments such as wounds, burns, infections, gastrointestinal disorders, respiratory issues, and inflammatory conditions. The leaves of the plant are often crushed or made into poultices and applied directly to the affected area or ingested in the form of teas or extracts.

Folklore and Rituals: In addition to its medicinal uses, the leaf of life plant has also held significance in folklore and cultural rituals in some communities. For example, in certain cultures, the plant is believed to possess protective qualities and is placed in homes to ward off negative energies or evil spirits. It has also been used in rituals associated with healing ceremonies or spiritual practices, where it may be burned, carried, or used as an offering to deities or spirits as a symbol of healing and vitality.

Precautions and Considerations

While the Leaf of Life offers numerous health benefits, it's crucial to exercise caution:

- **Allergic Reactions**: Some individuals may be allergic to the sap or compounds present in the Leaf of Life. Perform a patch test before using it topically and start with small doses when consuming internally.
- **Pregnancy and Lactation**: Pregnant and breastfeeding women should avoid using Leaf of Life products due to limited safety data.
- **Medical Interactions**: Individuals on medication, allergic or with pre-existing medical conditions should consult healthcare professionals before incorporating Leaf of Life supplements into their regimen, as it may interact with certain drugs.

Conclusion:

The Leaf of Life stands as a testament to the wonders of nature, offering a wealth of health benefits and therapeutic applications. From its anti-inflammatory and antimicrobial properties to its digestive and respiratory support, this remarkable plant continues to captivate the attention of herbalists and modern researchers alike. As with any herbal remedy, it's essential to approach its usage with knowledge, caution, and respect for its potent capabilities. Whether brewed into a healing tea, applied topically to soothe the skin, or incorporated into supplements for holistic wellness, the Leaf of Life remains a cherished ally in the pursuit of health and healing.

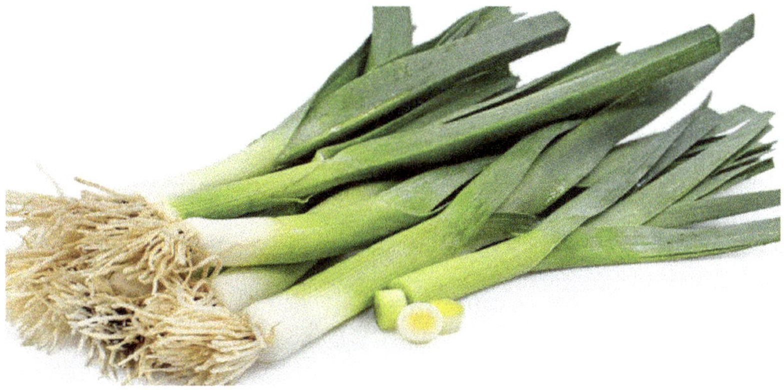

Leeks

Unlocking the Potential of Leeks: A Nutritious Addition to Your Diet

Leeks, with their mild yet distinctive flavor, have been cherished in culinary traditions across the globe for centuries. These versatile vegetables not only add depth and aroma to dishes but also offer an array of health benefits. From supporting heart health to boosting immunity, leeks are a nutritious addition to any diet. Let's delve into the benefits and uses of this underappreciated member of the allium family.

Nutritional Profile:

Leeks are low in calories and fat but pack a powerful punch of essential nutrients. They are an excellent source of dietary fiber, vitamins, and minerals, including:

Vitamins:

Vitamin A: Essential for vision, immune function, and skin health.

Vitamin C: An antioxidant that supports immune function, collagen synthesis, and iron absorption.

Vitamin K: Crucial for blood clotting and bone health.

Vitamin B6 (Pyridoxine): Involved in energy metabolism and neurotransmitter synthesis.

Folate (Vitamin B9): Important for cell division, DNA synthesis, and red blood cell formation.

Niacin (Vitamin B3): Supports energy metabolism and nervous system function.

Riboflavin (Vitamin B2): Essential for energy production and antioxidant activity.

Thiamine (Vitamin B1): Necessary for energy metabolism and nerve function.

Vitamin E: An antioxidant that protects cells from oxidative damage.

Minerals:

Potassium: Important for nerve function, muscle contraction, and blood pressure regulation.

Manganese: Essential for bone formation, metabolism, and antioxidant defense.

Iron: Necessary for oxygen transport in the blood and energy production.

Calcium: Crucial for bone health, muscle function, and nerve transmission.

Magnesium: Involved in hundreds of enzymatic reactions in the body, including energy metabolism and muscle function.

Phosphorus: Essential for bone and teeth formation, DNA synthesis, and energy metabolism.

Copper: Important for iron absorption, enzyme function, and antioxidant activity.

Zinc: Necessary for immune function, wound healing, and DNA synthesis.

Antioxidants and Phytonutrients:

Polyphenols: Including flavonoids, such as kaempferol and quercetin, which have antioxidant and anti-inflammatory properties.

Sulfur Compounds: Including allyl sulfides, which may have antioxidant and anti-cancer effects.

Carotenoids: Including beta-carotene, lutein, and zeaxanthin, which have antioxidant properties and contribute to eye health.

These vitamins, minerals, and antioxidants contribute to the overall health benefits of leeks, including supporting immune function, promoting bone health, and reducing inflammation. Incorporating leeks into your diet can be a delicious way to boost your nutrient intake and enhance your overall well-being.

Health Benefits:

Heart Health: Leeks are rich in antioxidants and flavonoids, which help lower the risk of cardiovascular diseases by reducing inflammation and preventing the oxidation of LDL cholesterol. The folate content in leeks also supports heart health by regulating homocysteine levels in the blood.

Digestive Health: Being a good source of dietary fiber, leeks promote digestive health by supporting regular bowel movements, preventing constipation, and maintaining a healthy gut microbiome. The prebiotic fibers in leeks nourish beneficial gut bacteria, contributing to overall digestive wellness.

Immune Support: The high vitamin C content in leeks strengthens the immune system, helping the body fend off infections and illnesses. Additionally, the antioxidant properties of leeks combat oxidative stress and inflammation, further supporting immune function.

Bone Health: Vitamin K, present abundantly in leeks, is essential for bone health as it helps in calcium absorption and regulates bone metabolism. Including leeks in your diet can contribute to maintaining strong and healthy bones, reducing the risk of osteoporosis and fractures.

Detoxification: The sulfur compounds in leeks, particularly allyl sulfides, support liver health and aid in detoxification processes. They help the liver in breaking down toxins and promoting their elimination from the body, supporting overall detoxification.

Nutritional Content

The nutritional content in 1 cup (89 grams) of raw leeks typically includes:

- Carbohydrates: Around 12.6 grams
- Protein: Roughly 1.5 grams
- Fiber: About 1.6 grams
- Fat: Less than 0.3 grams

It's important to note that nutritional values may vary slightly depending on factors such as the specific variety of leeks and growing conditions. Additionally, cooking methods can also influence the nutritional content of leeks.

Culinary Uses:

Leeks are incredibly versatile and can be used in a variety of culinary applications:

- **Soups and Stews:** Leeks add a rich, savory flavor to soups and stews, such as potato leek soup or chicken and leek stew.
- **Sautéed or Grilled:** Sautéed or grilled leeks make a delicious side dish or topping for salads, pizzas, and sandwiches.
- **Quiches and Frittatas:** Leeks can be incorporated into quiches, frittatas, or savory tarts for added flavor and texture.
- **Roasted or Braised:** Roasted or braised leeks make an elegant and flavorful side dish, perfect for special occasions or holiday dinners.
- **Incorporated into Casseroles:** Leeks can be added to casseroles, gratins, and pasta dishes for a subtle onion-like flavor.

Here are two delicious recipes that make excellent use of leeks:

Creamy Potato Leek Soup

Ingredients:

- 3 large leeks, white and light green parts only, thinly sliced
- 3 medium potatoes, peeled and diced
- 4 cups vegetable broth

- 1 cup milk (or dairy-free alternative)
- 2 tablespoons butter (or olive oil for vegan option)
- Salt and pepper to taste
- Chopped fresh chives or parsley for garnish (optional)

Instructions:

1. In a large pot, melt the butter over medium heat. Add the sliced leeks and sauté until softened, about 5-7 minutes.
2. Add the diced potatoes and vegetable broth to the pot. Bring to a boil, then reduce heat to low and simmer until the potatoes are tender, about 15-20 minutes.
3. Use an immersion blender to blend the soup until smooth. Alternatively, transfer the soup to a blender and blend in batches until smooth.
4. Stir in the milk and season with salt and pepper to taste. Simmer for an additional 5 minutes.
5. Serve hot, garnished with chopped fresh chives or parsley if desired. Enjoy this comforting and creamy potato leek soup!

Leek and Mushroom Quiche

Ingredients:

- 1 pre-made pie crust (homemade or store-bought)
- 2 large leeks, white and light green parts only, thinly sliced
- 2 cups sliced mushrooms (such as button or cremini)
- 4 eggs
- 1 cup milk (or half-and-half for a richer quiche)
- 1 cup shredded cheese (such as Gruyere or Swiss)
- Salt and pepper to taste
- Olive oil for sautéing

Instructions:

1. Preheat the oven to 375°F (190°C). Place the pie crust in a pie dish and set aside.
2. In a skillet, heat a drizzle of olive oil over medium heat. Add the sliced leeks and mushrooms, and sauté until softened, about 8-10 minutes. Season with salt and pepper to taste.
3. In a mixing bowl, whisk together the eggs and milk until well combined. Stir in the shredded cheese.

4. Spread the sautéed leeks and mushrooms evenly over the bottom of the pie crust. Pour the egg mixture over the vegetables.
5. Bake the quiche in the preheated oven for 35-40 minutes, or until the center is set and the top is golden brown.
6. Allow the quiche to cool for a few minutes before slicing and serving. Enjoy warm or at room temperature as a satisfying meal or appetizer!

These recipes highlight the versatility and delicious flavor of leeks, whether they're used in a comforting soup or a savory quiche. Feel free to customize the recipes with your favorite ingredients and seasonings for a personalized touch.

Tips for Selection and Storage:

When selecting leeks, look for ones with firm, straight, white stalks and bright green leaves. Avoid leeks with wilted or yellowing leaves or those that feel soft to the touch. Store unwashed leeks in the refrigerator, wrapped in a damp paper towel or cloth, for up to one week.

Tips on Growing Leeks (3 to 6 months)

The time it takes for leeks to grow from seed to harvest depends on several factors, including the variety of leeks, environmental conditions, and cultivation practices. Here is a detailed breakdown of the typical growth stages of leeks:

1. **Seed Germination (7-14 days)**:
    - Leek seeds are typically sown indoors or in a seedbed outdoors.
    - Germination usually occurs within 7 to 14 days after planting, depending on temperature and moisture levels.
2. **Seedling Stage (6-8 weeks)**:
    - After germination, leek seedlings begin to grow.
    - During this stage, seedlings require adequate moisture and light to develop healthy roots and foliage.
    - Seedlings are often transplanted into the garden or larger containers once they have reached a suitable size, usually around 6 to 8 weeks after germination.
3. **Vegetative Growth (10-12 weeks)**:
    - Once transplanted, leeks enter a period of vegetative growth.
    - During this stage, leeks develop their characteristic long, slender leaves and gradually increase in size.
    - Leeks require consistent watering and regular fertilization to support healthy growth.

4. **Bulb Formation (variable)**:
   - Leeks do not form bulbs in the same way as onions, but they do develop a thickened stem base known as the "shank."
   - The time it takes for leeks to reach harvestable size varies depending on the desired size and growing conditions.
   - Typically, leeks are ready for harvest when they reach a diameter of about 1 to 2 inches (2.5 to 5 centimeters) and have a length of 6 to 12 inches (15 to 30 centimeters).
   - Depending on the variety and growing conditions, leeks may take anywhere from 3 to 6 months from sowing to reach maturity.
5. **Harvest (variable)**:
   - Leeks can be harvested once they have reached the desired size.
   - To harvest, carefully loosen the soil around the base of the leek and gently pull it from the ground.
   - Leeks can typically be harvested over an extended period, allowing for successive harvests as needed.

It's essential to monitor the growth of leeks throughout their development and provide appropriate care to ensure optimal growth and yield. Additionally, factors such as temperature, soil quality, and pest management can impact the growth and maturity of leeks.

Conclusion:

Leeks are not only a delicious addition to culinary creations but also offer an array of health benefits, from supporting heart health to boosting immunity and promoting digestive wellness. If you have specific health concerns, allergies, or conditions, it's advisable to consult with a healthcare professional or a registered dietitian before making significant changes to your diet.

Incorporating leeks into your diet can be a flavorful and nutritious way to enhance your overall health and well-being. So, next time you're at the market, don't overlook these humble yet mighty vegetables—your taste buds and your body will thank you for it!

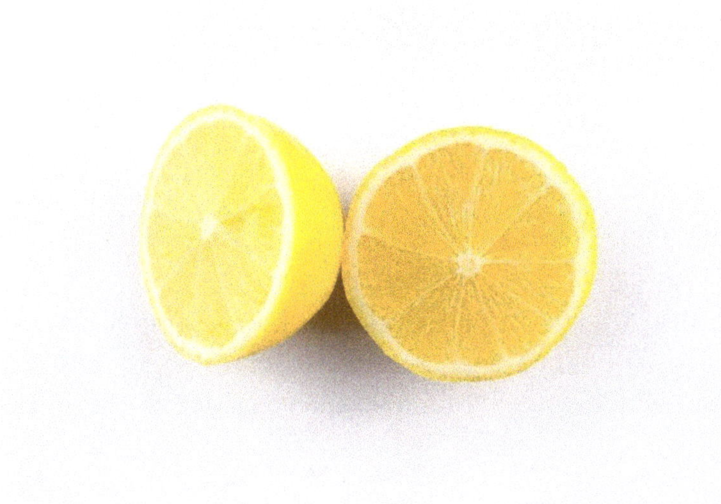

Lemon

The Zesty Elixir: Exploring the Health Benefits and Culinary Marvels of Lemon

Lemons, with their vibrant yellow hue and unmistakable citrus aroma, stand as a symbol of freshness and vitality. Beyond being a popular kitchen staple, lemons boast a myriad of health benefits and culinary uses. In this article, we will delve into the rich nutritional profile, medicinal properties, and diverse applications of lemons that make them a versatile and indispensable addition to our daily lives.

Nutritional Profile:

Lemons (Citrus limon) are a nutritional powerhouse, packed with essential vitamins and minerals. Here are some key components of their nutritional profile:

Vitamin C:

- Lemons are renowned for their high vitamin C content. This antioxidant vitamin plays a crucial role in the production of white blood cells, which are essential for fighting off infections, supporting the immune system, promoting skin health, and aiding in the absorption of iron. Additionally, vitamin C supports skin health and collagen synthesis.

Vitamin B6 (Pyridoxine):

- *Benefits:*

  Metabolism and Nervous System: Vitamin B6 is involved in numerous metabolic processes, including the breakdown of carbohydrates and the synthesis of neurotransmitters. It contributes to the proper functioning of the nervous system and helps convert food into energy.

Folate (Vitamin B9):

- *Benefits:*

Cell Division and DNA Synthesis: Folate is crucial for cell division and DNA synthesis. It plays a vital role in the formation of red blood cells and supports overall cellular health. Folate is particularly important during periods of rapid growth, such as pregnancy.

Vitamin A:

- *Benefits:*

  Eye Health: Vitamin A is essential for maintaining healthy vision. It supports the function of the retina and contributes to low-light and color vision. Adequate vitamin A intake is crucial for overall eye health.

Citric Acid:

- Citric acid, abundant in lemons, contributes to their tart flavor. This compound is known for its alkalizing effect on the body and may help prevent the formation of kidney stones.

Fiber:

- Lemons contain dietary fiber, which supports digestive health. Fiber aids in maintaining bowel regularity and can contribute to a feeling of fullness.

While lemons are not particularly high in minerals, they do contain trace amounts of some essential minerals that contribute to overall health. Here are four minerals found in lemons and their associated benefits:

Potassium:

- *Benefits:*

  Heart Health: Potassium is crucial for maintaining proper fluid balance in the body and supporting heart health. It helps regulate blood pressure, promoting cardiovascular well-being.

Calcium:

- *Benefits:*

  Bone Health: Calcium is essential for the development and maintenance of strong and healthy bones. While lemons contain only small amounts of calcium, every bit contributes to overall bone health.

Magnesium:

- *Benefits:*

  Nerve and Muscle Function: Magnesium is vital for nerve function and muscle contraction. It supports the proper functioning of the nervous and muscular systems, contributing to overall neuromuscular health.

Phosphorus:

- *Benefits:*

  Bone Health and Energy Metabolism: Phosphorus is involved in bone health, working in conjunction with calcium. It also plays a role in energy metabolism and various cellular processes in the body.

Health Benefits:

Immune System Support:

- The vitamin C in lemons is a potent antioxidant that helps protect cells from damage and supports the immune system. Regular consumption of lemons may contribute to overall immune health.

Digestive Health:

- The combination of citric acid and fiber in lemons promotes digestive health. Lemon water, a popular beverage, is often consumed in the morning to kickstart digestion and hydration.

Hydration and Detoxification:

- Lemon water serves as a refreshing and hydrating beverage. Additionally, lemons are believed to have detoxifying properties, supporting the liver in its natural cleansing processes.

Culinary Uses:

Flavorful Enhancements:

- Lemons add a burst of citrusy flavor to both sweet and savory dishes. Their juice and zest are widely used in salads, marinades, dressings, and desserts, elevating the taste of various culinary creations.

Beverages:

- Lemonade is a classic and refreshing beverage enjoyed worldwide. Additionally, lemon slices or wedges are commonly added to water, teas, and cocktails for a zesty twist.

Preservation:

- The acidity of lemons makes them a natural preservative. Lemon juice can be used to prevent fruits like apples and avocados from browning and to add a tangy kick to homemade preserves.

Recipes

Here are two recipes that incorporate lemon as a key ingredient:

Lemon Garlic Butter Shrimp:

- Ingredients:
    - 1 pound (450g) shrimp, peeled and deveined
    - 4 tablespoons butter
    - 4 cloves garlic, minced
    - 1 lemon, juiced and zested
    - Salt and pepper, to taste
    - Fresh parsley, chopped (for garnish)
- ***Instructions:***

1. In a large skillet, melt the butter over medium heat. Add minced garlic and cook until fragrant, about 1-2 minutes.
2. Add the shrimp to the skillet and cook until pink and opaque, about 2-3 minutes per side.
3. Squeeze lemon juice over the shrimp and sprinkle with lemon zest, salt, and pepper. Stir to combine.
4. Remove from heat and garnish with chopped parsley.
5. Serve the lemon garlic butter shrimp hot, with your choice of sides such as rice, pasta, or crusty bread.

Lemon Blueberry Yogurt Cake:

- ***Ingredients:***
    - 1 1/2 cups all-purpose flour
    - 1 teaspoon baking powder
    - 1/4 teaspoon baking soda
    - 1/4 teaspoon salt
    - 1/2 cup unsalted butter, softened
    - 1 cup granulated sugar
    - 2 large eggs
    - 1/2 cup Greek yogurt
    - Zest of 1 lemon

- 2 tablespoons lemon juice
- 1 teaspoon vanilla extract
- 1 cup fresh blueberries
- For the glaze:
    - 1 cup powdered sugar
    - 2-3 tablespoons lemon juice

- ***Instructions:***

1. Preheat your oven to 350°F (175°C). Grease and flour a 9x5-inch loaf pan.
2. In a medium bowl, whisk together flour, baking powder, baking soda, and salt. Set aside.
3. In a large mixing bowl, cream together softened butter and granulated sugar until light and fluffy.
4. Beat in eggs, one at a time, until well combined. Mix in Greek yogurt, lemon zest, lemon juice, and vanilla extract.
5. Gradually add the dry ingredients to the wet ingredients, mixing until just combined. Gently fold in the fresh blueberries.
6. Pour the batter into the prepared loaf pan and smooth the top.
7. Bake in the preheated oven for 50-60 minutes, or until a toothpick inserted into the center comes out clean.
8. Allow the cake to cool in the pan for 10 minutes before transferring to a wire rack to cool completely.
9. To make the glaze, whisk together powdered sugar and lemon juice until smooth. Drizzle the glaze over the cooled cake.
10. Slice and serve the lemon blueberry yogurt cake as a delightful dessert or snack. Enjoy!

Aromatherapy:

The aromatic essential oil extracted from lemon peels is used in aromatherapy for its uplifting and invigorating scent. Lemon-scented candles and essential oil diffusers can create a fresh and energizing atmosphere.

Historical Uses:

Ancient Mediterranean Civilizations:

- ***Benefit:*** In ancient Mediterranean civilizations, including Greek and Roman cultures, lemons were not specifically known, but their precursor, citron, was cultivated. Citron had religious significance and was used in religious ceremonies. It was also valued for its pleasant aroma. The use of citron laid the foundation for the later development and cultivation of lemon varieties.

Maritime Medicine:

- ***Benefit:*** During the Age of Sail in the 18th century, British sailors carried lemons on long sea voyages to prevent scurvy—a disease caused by vitamin C deficiency. The high vitamin C content in lemons helped combat scurvy, and sailors consuming lemon juice experienced improved health. This historical use highlighted the importance of lemons in preventing nutritional deficiencies.

Middle Ages in Europe:

- ***Benefit:*** In the Middle Ages, lemons were introduced to Europe via trade routes, and their rarity made them a symbol of wealth and prestige. During this time, lemons were used not only in culinary pursuits but also for their aromatic properties. Lemon peels were often used to add fragrance to homes and clothing.

Traditional Ayurvedic Medicine:

- ***Benefit:*** In traditional Ayurvedic medicine in India, lemons were valued for their health benefits. Lemon water was commonly consumed to aid digestion and detoxify the body. The sour taste of lemons was believed to stimulate digestive enzymes and promote a healthy metabolism.

These historical uses of lemons underscore their multifaceted significance, from religious ceremonies in ancient civilizations to practical applications in maritime medicine. As lemons gained prominence and accessibility, their diverse benefits became more widely recognized, contributing to their cultural and culinary importance across different regions and time periods.

Conclusion:

Lemons, with their invigorating flavor and impressive nutritional profile, are a true kitchen essential. From supporting immune health to enhancing the flavor of dishes, lemons offer a delightful combination of health benefits and culinary versatility. Embrace the zest of lemons in your daily routine and savor the multifaceted joys they bring to both your well-being and your plate.

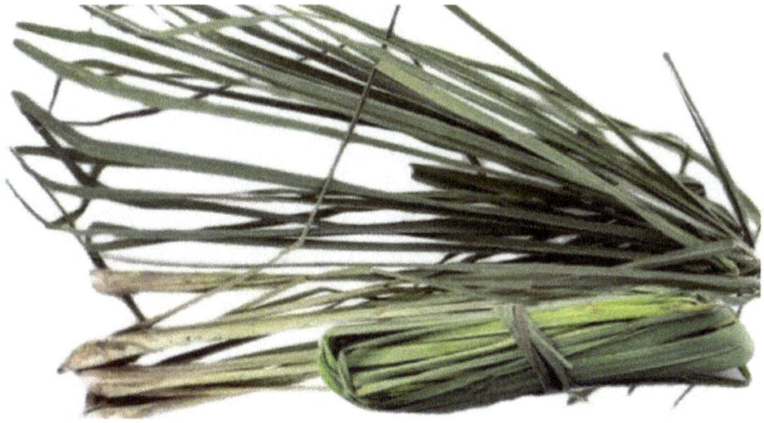

Lemongrass / Fever Grass

A Citrus Infusion of Health and Culinary Delight

Lemongrass, with its refreshing aroma and zesty flavor, has earned its place as a versatile herb in both culinary and medicinal realms. Native to tropical regions, this tall, slender plant is celebrated for its myriad benefits, ranging from digestive support to aromatic enhancements in various dishes. In this article, we will explore the rich history, nutritional components, and diverse uses of lemongrass that make it a cherished herb around the globe.

History and Origin:

Lemongrass (Cymbopogon citratus) has its roots in Southeast Asia, where it has been used for centuries in traditional medicine and culinary practices. Known for its ability to alleviate fevers, the herb earned the moniker "fever grass" in some cultures, reflecting its historical association with promoting health during times of illness.

From Thai cuisine to Indian Ayurveda, lemongrass has spread its influence across cultures, appreciated not only for its unique flavor but also for its potential health benefits.

Nutritional Profile:

Lemongrass is rich in essential oils, including citronella, which gives it its distinct citrusy fragrance. It also contains vitamins such as vitamin A, vitamin C, and various B-vitamins. Additionally, lemongrass is a source of minerals like potassium, magnesium, and calcium.

Vitamin A:

Benefits:

- ***Eye Health:*** Vitamin A is essential for maintaining healthy vision. It supports the function of the retina and helps prevent conditions such as night blindness. Consuming lemongrass, which contains vitamin A, contributes to eye health.

Vitamin C:

Benefits:

- ***Immune Support:*** Lemongrass is a good source of vitamin C, an antioxidant that supports the immune system. Vitamin C helps protect cells from damage, aids in the absorption of iron, and contributes to overall immune health.

Vitamin B6 (Pyridoxine):

Benefits:

- ***Brain Health:*** Vitamin B6 plays a crucial role in brain development and function. It is involved in the synthesis of neurotransmitters, including serotonin and dopamine, contributing to mood regulation and cognitive function.

Folate (Vitamin B9):

Benefits:

- ***Cell Division and DNA Synthesis:*** Folate is essential for cell division and DNA synthesis. It is particularly important during periods of rapid cell growth, such as pregnancy. Consuming lemongrass can contribute to folate intake, supporting overall cellular health.

Lemongrass (Fever Grass) contains several minerals that contribute to its nutritional profile and potential health benefits. Here are some key minerals found in lemongrass and their associated benefits:

Potassium:

Benefits:

- ***Heart Health**:* Potassium is essential for maintaining proper fluid balance in the body and plays a crucial role in heart health. It helps regulate blood pressure, supporting cardiovascular function.

Magnesium:

Benefits:

- ***Nerve and Muscle Function:*** Magnesium is crucial for nerve function and muscle contraction. It contributes to the proper functioning of the nervous and muscular systems, promoting overall neuromuscular health.

Phosphorus:

Benefits:

- ***Bone Health:*** Phosphorus is a key mineral for bone health, working in conjunction with calcium to maintain strong and healthy bones. It also plays a role in energy metabolism and various cellular processes.

Copper:

Benefits:

- ***Iron Absorption and Connective Tissue Formation:*** Copper is involved in the absorption of iron and the formation of connective tissues. It plays a role in maintaining healthy bones, blood vessels, and skin.

Incorporating lemongrass into your diet, whether through teas, culinary dishes, or infusions, provides not only a refreshing flavor but also essential minerals that contribute to overall health and well-being.

Health Benefits:

Digestive Health:

- Lemongrass is known for its digestive properties. It may help alleviate indigestion, bloating, and abdominal discomfort. Consuming lemongrass tea or incorporating lemongrass into meals can contribute to digestive well-being.

Antioxidant and Anti-Inflammatory Properties:

- The citral in lemongrass contributes to its antioxidant and anti-inflammatory effects. These properties may help combat oxidative stress, reduce inflammation, and support overall immune health.

Immune Support:

- The citronella and other compounds in fever grass contribute to its immune-boosting properties. Regular consumption may help support the immune system, providing a natural defense against infections.

Aromatherapy and Relaxation:

- The essential oils in lemongrass are often used in aromatherapy to promote relaxation and reduce stress. Diffusing lemongrass oil or adding it to bath products can create a soothing and invigorating atmosphere.

Culinary Uses:

Lemongrass adds a burst of citrusy freshness to a variety of dishes. Whether used in soups, curries, marinades, or teas, lemongrass imparts a unique flavor that enhances the overall culinary experience. Lemongrass pairs well with ingredients like ginger, garlic, and coconut milk.

Lemongrass Tea:

- Prepare a refreshing lemongrass tea by steeping fresh or dried lemongrass leaves in hot water. Add honey or a slice of ginger for added flavor.

Lemongrass Marinade:

- Create a flavorful marinade by blending lemongrass with garlic, ginger, soy sauce, and a touch of honey. Use it to marinate poultry, fish, or tofu before grilling or roasting.

Lemongrass Infused Coconut Milk:

- Infuse coconut milk with lemongrass to elevate the flavor of curries, soups, or rice dishes. Simmer coconut milk with lemongrass and other aromatic spices for a fragrant and delicious base.

Lemongrass Infused Oil:

- Infuse cooking oils with fever grass to impart its citrusy flavor to stir-fries, sautés, or salad dressings. Simply heat the oil with chopped lemongrass and strain before using.

Historical uses:

Traditional Medicine in Southeast Asia:

- ***Benefit:*** Lemongrass has a rich history in traditional medicine in Southeast Asia, where it has been used to address various health concerns. Its aromatic leaves and stems were often brewed into teas or infusions believed to aid digestion, relieve stomach discomfort, and promote overall well-being. Additionally, lemongrass was valued for its potential to reduce fevers, leading to its nickname "fever grass" in some cultures.

Ayurvedic Medicine in India:

- ***Benefit:*** In Ayurvedic medicine, lemongrass is recognized for its digestive properties and its ability to balance doshas. It has been traditionally used to alleviate digestive issues, including bloating and indigestion. The citrusy herb was also employed to promote mental clarity and uplift the spirits.

Ancient Egyptian and Roman Culinary Practices:

- ***Benefit:*** Lemongrass found its way into ancient Egyptian and Roman culinary practices, where it was used to enhance the flavor of various dishes. The aromatic herb was valued for its culinary versatility, adding a refreshing and citrusy note to soups, stews, and sauces.

Traditional Brazilian Folk Medicine:

- ***Benefit:*** In traditional Brazilian folk medicine, lemongrass has been utilized for its potential diuretic properties. It was believed to support kidney health and help alleviate water retention. Lemongrass teas and infusions were often consumed for their purported detoxifying effects.

These historical uses of lemongrass highlight its diverse applications in traditional medicine and culinary practices across different cultures. From addressing digestive discomfort to providing a burst of flavor in culinary creations, lemongrass has been valued for its aromatic properties and potential health benefits throughout history.

Tips on Growing Lemongrass / Fever Grass (3 – 6 months)

Lemongrass is a tropical grass that is widely cultivated for its culinary and medicinal uses. The time it takes for lemongrass to grow from planting to harvest varies depending on various factors such as climate, soil conditions, and cultivation methods. Here's a detailed breakdown of the typical growth stages of lemongrass:

1. **Planting (0-2 weeks)**:
    - Lemongrass can be propagated from seeds, divisions, or transplants.
    - If grown from seeds, germination usually takes about 1-2 weeks. Seedlings will emerge from the soil during this time.
2. **Establishment (4-8 weeks)**:
    - During the first few weeks after planting or transplanting, lemongrass focuses on establishing its root system.
    - Adequate moisture and warm temperatures are essential for root development.
    - Lemongrass plants may not show significant above-ground growth during this stage.
3. **Vegetative Growth (8-16 weeks)**:
    - Once established, lemongrass begins to grow vigorously.
    - The grass blades elongate, and new shoots may emerge from the base of the plant.
    - Lemongrass requires regular watering and fertilization to support healthy growth.
    - Under optimal conditions, lemongrass can grow several inches in height per week during this stage.
4. **Maturation (3-6 months)**:
    - Lemongrass typically reaches maturity and is ready for harvest within 3 to 6 months after planting, depending on growing conditions.

- Mature lemongrass plants typically have thick, robust stems and abundant foliage.
- The timing of maturity can vary based on factors such as temperature, sunlight, and soil fertility.

5. **Harvest**:
    - Lemongrass can be harvested once the stalks reach a suitable size, usually around 12-24 inches (30-60 cm) tall.
    - To harvest lemongrass, cut the stalks close to the ground using sharp pruning shears or a knife.
    - Regular harvesting encourages new growth and helps maintain the vigor of the plant.
6. **Continued Growth and Maintenance**:
    - After harvesting, lemongrass will continue to grow and produce new shoots.
    - Provide ongoing care such as watering, fertilizing, and occasional pruning to promote healthy growth and productivity.

It's important to note that the growth timeline provided is approximate and can vary based on factors such as cultivar, growing conditions, and local climate. Additionally, lemongrass is a perennial plant in tropical regions but may be grown as an annual or overwintered indoors in colder climates.

Adverse Effects:

While lemongrass is generally considered safe for consumption and has been used traditionally for various health benefits, it's essential to be aware that some individuals may be allergic or experience side effects. It's advisable to exercise caution and consult with a healthcare professional, especially if you have pre-existing health conditions or are taking medications.

Conclusion:

Lemongrass stands as a testament to the harmonious fusion of culinary delight and wellness. From its origins in traditional medicine to its widespread use in global cuisines, lemongrass continues to captivate with its refreshing aroma and versatile applications. Whether sipped as a soothing tea or savored in savory dishes, lemongrass adds a citrusy zest to life, enhancing both health and culinary experiences. Embrace the invigorating essence of lemongrass and let its benefits infuse vitality into your daily routine.

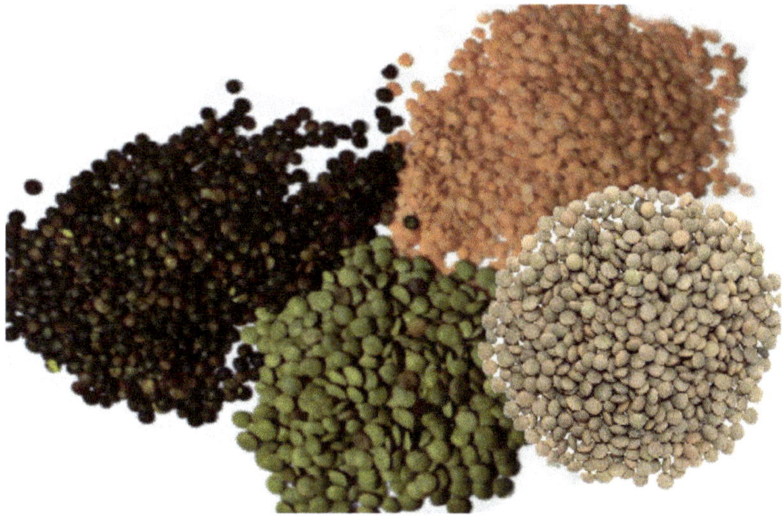

Lentils

Nutrient-Rich Legumes Packed with Health Benefits and Culinary Versatility

Lentils, a staple in many cuisines around the world, are small but mighty legumes that have been cultivated for thousands of years. These versatile seeds come in various colors, including brown, green, red, and black, each with its unique flavor and texture. Beyond their delightful taste and ease of preparation, lentils are celebrated for their impressive nutritional profile and numerous health benefits. In this article, we will explore the benefits and diverse uses of lentils, highlighting why they deserve a prominent place in a balanced and wholesome diet.

Nutritional Powerhouse:

Lentils are a nutritional powerhouse, offering an array of essential nutrients that contribute to overall health and well-being. Key nutritional components of lentils include:

Protein:

- Lentils are an excellent source of plant-based protein, making them an essential food for vegetarians and vegans. Protein is crucial for muscle repair, growth, and the overall functioning of the body.

Dietary Fiber:

- Lentils are rich in dietary fiber, both soluble and insoluble. Fiber supports digestive health by promoting regular bowel movements, preventing constipation, and aiding in the maintenance of a healthy gut microbiota.

Complex Carbohydrates:

- Lentils provide complex carbohydrates, offering a steady release of energy. They have a low glycemic index, making them a suitable choice for individuals looking to manage blood sugar levels.

Vitamins and Minerals:

Lentils contain essential vitamins such as folate, vitamin B6, thiamine, and minerals including iron, phosphorus, potassium, and magnesium. These nutrients play vital roles in various bodily functions, including blood formation, energy metabolism, and bone health.

Essential Vitamins in Lentils:

Folate (Vitamin B9):

- **Benefits:** Folate is crucial for DNA synthesis and repair, making it essential during periods of rapid cell division and growth. Adequate folate intake is particularly important for pregnant women to prevent neural tube defects in developing fetuses.

Thiamine (Vitamin B1):

- **Benefits:** Thiamine is essential for energy metabolism, aiding in the conversion of carbohydrates into energy. It also supports proper nerve function and is crucial for the synthesis of neurotransmitters.

Vitamin B6:

- **Benefits:** Vitamin B6 is involved in over 100 enzymatic reactions in the body, including the metabolism of amino acids and the production of neurotransmitters. It plays a role in immune function, cognitive development, and the regulation of mood.

Niacin (Vitamin B3):

- **Benefits:** Niacin plays a key role in energy metabolism, DNA repair, and the production of various enzymes. It contributes to maintaining healthy skin, nerves, and digestive system.

Essential Minerals in Lentils:

Iron:

- **Benefits:** Iron is vital for the formation of hemoglobin, the oxygen-carrying component of red blood cells. Adequate iron intake is essential for preventing iron-deficiency anemia and supporting overall energy levels.

Phosphorus:

- **Benefits:** Phosphorus is a structural component of DNA, RNA, and ATP (adenosine triphosphate), the primary energy carrier in cells. It is essential for bone health, kidney function, and the metabolism of macronutrients.

Potassium:

- **Benefits:** Potassium plays a crucial role in maintaining proper fluid balance, nerve impulses, and muscle contractions. It also supports heart health by helping to regulate blood pressure.

Magnesium:

- **Benefits:** Magnesium is involved in various physiological processes, including muscle and nerve function, bone health, and energy metabolism. It contributes to the regulation of blood pressure and supports the immune system.

Health Benefits:

Heart Health:

- The high fiber content in lentils contributes to heart health by helping to lower cholesterol levels. Lentils are also a good source of potassium, which supports healthy blood pressure levels.

Blood Sugar Regulation:

- Lentils have a low glycemic index and are rich in soluble fiber. These characteristics contribute to stable blood sugar levels, making lentils a valuable addition to diets aimed at managing diabetes or preventing insulin resistance.

Weight Management:

- The combination of protein and fiber in lentils promotes a feeling of fullness, aiding in weight management. Including lentils in meals can help control appetite and reduce overall calorie intake.

Nutrient Absorption:

- Lentils contain folate, a B-vitamin that plays a role in DNA synthesis and repair. Folate is essential for pregnant women to prevent neural tube defects in developing fetuses.

Nutritional Content

Here's the approximate nutritional content in 1 cup (198 grams) of cooked lentils:

- Calories: Around 230 kcal
- Carbohydrates: Approximately 39.9 grams
- Protein: Roughly 17.9 grams
- Fiber: About 15.6 grams
- Fat: Less than 1 gram

Please note that these values are approximate and can vary depending on factors such as the specific type of lentils, cooking method, and any additional ingredients added during cooking. Lentils are a nutritious food source rich in protein, fiber, and various vitamins and minerals.

Culinary Versatility:

Lentils are incredibly versatile in the kitchen, adapting well to various cooking methods and flavor profiles. Some common culinary uses include:

Lentil Soups and Stews:

- Lentils add texture, protein, and nutritional value to hearty soups and stews. Popular examples include lentil soup, dal, and lentil curry.

Lentil Salads:

- Cold lentil salads, combined with fresh vegetables, herbs, and a flavorful dressing, make for refreshing and nutrient-packed meals.

Lentil Casseroles:

- Lentils can be used in casseroles and bakes, providing a wholesome and satisfying base for a variety of ingredients.

Lentil Burgers and Patties:

- Lentils make an excellent base for vegetarian burgers and patties, offering a protein-rich alternative to meat.

Here are two delicious and nutritious recipes featuring lentils:

Spiced Lentil Soup:

Ingredients:

- 1 cup dried lentils (any color), rinsed and drained
- 1 onion, finely chopped
- 2 carrots, diced
- 2 celery stalks, diced
- 3 cloves garlic, minced
- 1 teaspoon ground cumin
- 1 teaspoon ground coriander
- 1/2 teaspoon turmeric
- 1/2 teaspoon paprika
- 1 can (14 ounces) diced tomatoes

- 6 cups vegetable or chicken broth
- Salt and pepper to taste
- Fresh lemon wedges (for serving)
- Fresh cilantro or parsley, chopped (for garnish)

Instructions:

1. In a large pot, sauté the chopped onion, carrots, celery, and garlic in a bit of olive oil until the vegetables are softened.
2. Add the ground cumin, ground coriander, turmeric, and paprika. Stir well to coat the vegetables in the spices.
3. Pour in the rinsed lentils, diced tomatoes, and broth. Bring the mixture to a boil.
4. Reduce the heat, cover the pot, and simmer for about 25-30 minutes or until the lentils are tender.
5. Season with salt and pepper to taste.
6. Serve the spiced lentil soup hot, garnished with fresh lemon wedges and chopped cilantro or parsley.

Mediterranean Lentil Salad:

Ingredients:

- 1 cup dried green or brown lentils, rinsed and drained
- 1 cucumber, diced
- 1 cup cherry tomatoes, halved
- 1 red bell pepper, diced
- 1/2 red onion, finely chopped
- 1/3 cup Kalamata olives, sliced
- 1/2 cup crumbled feta cheese
- 1/4 cup fresh parsley, chopped

For the Dressing:

- 3 tablespoons extra-virgin olive oil
- 2 tablespoons red wine vinegar
- 1 teaspoon Dijon mustard

- 1 clove garlic, minced
- Salt and pepper to taste

Instructions:

1. Cook the lentils according to package instructions. Drain and let them cool to room temperature.
2. In a large bowl, combine the cooked lentils, cucumber, cherry tomatoes, red bell pepper, red onion, Kalamata olives, feta cheese, and fresh parsley.
3. In a small bowl, whisk together the dressing ingredients: olive oil, red wine vinegar, Dijon mustard, minced garlic, salt, and pepper.
4. Pour the dressing over the lentil salad and toss to coat the ingredients evenly.
5. Chill the Mediterranean lentil salad in the refrigerator for at least 30 minutes before serving.
6. Enjoy the refreshing and flavorful lentil salad as a side dish or a light main course.

These recipes showcase the versatility of lentils, whether in a comforting soup or a vibrant salad. Lentils not only provide a rich source of protein and fiber but also add depth and heartiness to a variety of dishes.

Conclusion:

Incorporating lentils into your diet can be a delicious and healthful choice. Their versatility, combined with a nutritional profile that supports heart health, weight management, and overall well-being, makes lentils a valuable addition to a diverse and balanced diet. While lentils are generally safe and healthy to consume as part of a balanced diet. As with any food, moderation is key. If you have specific health concerns, allergies, or conditions, it's advisable to consult with a healthcare professional or a registered dietitian before making significant changes to your diet.

Whether enjoyed in comforting soups, vibrant salads, or savory main dishes, lentils stand as a testament to the fact that good health and great taste can go hand in hand.

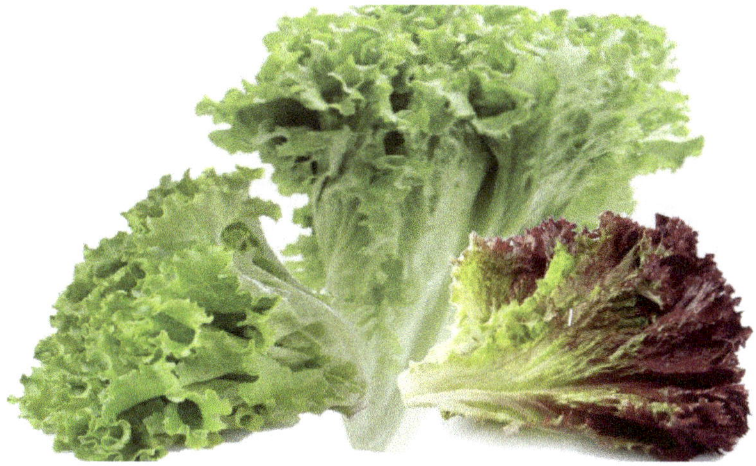

Lettuce

The Green Powerhouse: Unveiling the Health Benefits and Culinary Versatility of lettuce.

Lettuce, a crisp and vibrant leafy green, is a staple in salads and a versatile ingredient that adds freshness to a myriad of dishes. Beyond its delightful crunch, lettuce offers a range of health benefits that make it a valuable addition to a balanced diet. In this article, we will explore the nutritional value, health advantages, and diverse culinary uses of lettuce.

Nutritional Value of Lettuce:

Low-Calorie, High-Nutrient Content:

- Lettuce is a low-calorie food, making it an excellent choice for those aiming to maintain or lose weight.
- Despite its low caloric density, lettuce is rich in essential nutrients such as vitamins A, C, and K, as well as folate and iron.

Rich in Antioxidants:

- The presence of antioxidants, particularly vitamin C and beta-carotene, in lettuce helps combat oxidative stress.
- Antioxidants protect cells from damage caused by free radicals, contributing to overall health and potentially reducing the risk of chronic diseases.

Good Source of Fiber:

- Lettuce contains dietary fiber, promoting digestive health by aiding in regular bowel movements and preventing constipation.
- The fiber content in lettuce contributes to a feeling of fullness, which can be beneficial for weight management and maintaining a healthy digestive system.

Health Benefits of Lettuce:

Heart Health Support:

- The high fiber and potassium content in lettuce contribute to cardiovascular health.
- Fiber helps lower cholesterol levels, while potassium assists in maintaining healthy blood pressure, reducing the risk of heart disease.

Vision Protection:

- Lettuce is rich in vitamin A and beta-carotene, essential for eye health.
- These nutrients contribute to maintaining good vision and may help prevent age-related macular degeneration.

Bone Health Enhancement:

- Vitamin K, present in lettuce, plays a crucial role in bone health by aiding in calcium absorption and bone mineralization.
- Regular consumption of lettuce can contribute to maintaining strong and healthy bones.

Nutritional Content

The nutritional content in 1 cup (or approximately 56 grams) of raw lettuce can vary slightly depending on the specific type of lettuce, but here are the approximate values:

- Calories: Around 5 kcal
- Carbohydrates: Approximately 1 gram
- Protein: Roughly 0.5 grams
- Fiber: About 0.5 grams
- Fat: Less than 0.1 gram

Lettuce is low in calories and carbohydrates but contains small amounts of fiber and protein. It is also a good source of various vitamins and minerals, including vitamin A, vitamin K, folate, and potassium.

Culinary Uses of Lettuce:

Classic Salads:

- Lettuce is a staple ingredient in various salads, from the classic Caesar salad to mixed greens with vinaigrette.
- Its crisp texture and mild flavor provide a refreshing base for a wide range of salad combinations.

Wraps and Sandwiches:

- Large lettuce leaves, such as those from iceberg or romaine varieties, make excellent substitutes for traditional wraps.
- Lettuce leaves can also be used as a crunchy layer in sandwiches or burgers, adding both texture and nutritional value.

Stir-Fries and Soups:

- Certain lettuce varieties, like butterhead or iceberg, can be added to stir-fries and soups.
- The addition of lettuce enhances the texture of cooked dishes while preserving its nutritional benefits.

Ancient Medicinal Uses:

Historical records indicate that ancient Egyptians used lettuce for its medicinal properties.

Benefits: Lettuce was believed to have calming effects and was used to induce sleep. The milky substance (latex) in certain lettuce varieties was considered to have sedative properties, making it a natural remedy for insomnia and anxiety.

Roman Culinary and Therapeutic Applications:

Romans not only consumed lettuce as a culinary ingredient but also recognized its therapeutic qualities.

Benefits: Lettuce was thought to have cooling effects on the body, and it was often consumed to alleviate symptoms of fever. Additionally, it was believed to aid digestion and was included in meals for its potential digestive benefits.

Traditional Chinese Medicine:

Lettuce has been utilized in Traditional Chinese Medicine (TCM) for centuries.

Benefits: Lettuce was considered to have cooling properties and was used to balance the body's internal heat. It was often recommended for individuals experiencing symptoms related to excessive internal heat, such as irritability and inflammation. Additionally, lettuce was believed to support liver health.

Tips on Growing Lettuce (3 to 8 weeks)

The time it takes for lettuce to grow from seed to harvest varies depending on several factors, including the variety of lettuce, growing conditions, and desired size at harvest. Here's a detailed breakdown of the typical growth stages of lettuce:

1. **Germination (7-14 days)**:
    - Lettuce seeds typically germinate within 7 to 14 days when soil temperatures are around 50-80°F (10-27°C).
    - During germination, the seeds absorb water and begin to sprout, sending out roots and a shoot.
2. **Seedling Stage (2-4 weeks)**:
    - After germination, lettuce seedlings emerge from the soil.
    - During this stage, seedlings require adequate moisture, sunlight, and nutrients to develop healthy leaves and roots.
    - Seedlings may be thinned to ensure proper spacing, which helps prevent overcrowding and competition for resources.
3. **Vegetative Growth (3-6 weeks)**:
    - As lettuce plants continue to grow, they enter a phase of vegetative growth where they focus on producing leaves.
    - Lettuce requires consistent watering and fertilization to support rapid leaf growth.
    - Depending on the variety, environmental conditions, and desired size at harvest, lettuce may take 3 to 6 weeks to reach maturity from the time of planting.
4. **Head Formation (varies by type)**:
    - Some lettuce varieties form tight heads, while others produce loose leaf rosettes.
    - Head-forming lettuce varieties typically require longer growing periods to develop fully formed heads, which may take an additional 1-2 weeks or more beyond the vegetative growth stage.
    - Loose-leaf lettuce varieties can be harvested continuously as individual leaves mature, allowing for multiple harvests over time without waiting for a single head to form.
5. **Harvest**:
    - Lettuce leaves can be harvested at any stage of growth, depending on personal preference and culinary needs.
    - Loose-leaf lettuce can be harvested by cutting individual leaves as needed, leaving the plant to continue growing and producing more leaves.
    - Head-forming lettuce varieties are typically harvested by cutting the entire head at the base when it reaches the desired size and maturity.
    - Lettuce leaves are best harvested in the morning when they are crisp and hydrated.

6. **Continued Growth and Successive Plantings**:

    - After harvesting, lettuce plants may regrow new leaves if the growing conditions are favorable, allowing for multiple harvests from the same plant.
    - Successive plantings of lettuce can be made throughout the growing season to ensure a continuous supply of fresh greens.

Overall, lettuce is a relatively fast-growing crop that can be ready for harvest within a few weeks to a couple of months, depending on the variety and growing conditions.

Conclusion:

Lettuce stands out not only for its crisp and refreshing taste but also for its numerous health benefits. Whether enjoyed in salads, wraps, or cooked dishes, lettuce proves to be a versatile and nutritious addition to a well-rounded diet. As we embrace the green goodness of lettuce, we invite not only a burst of flavor but also a wealth of nutrients that contribute to our overall well-being.

If you have specific health concerns, allergies, or conditions, it's advisable to consult with a healthcare professional or a registered dietitian before making significant changes to your diet.

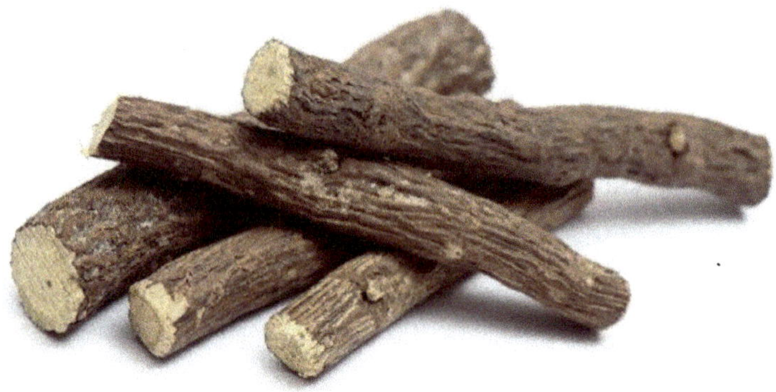

Licorice

Unveiling the Sweetness of Licorice

Licorice, scientifically known as Glycyrrhiza glabra, is a perennial herb native to the Mediterranean region and parts of Asia. Renowned for its distinct sweet flavor and medicinal properties, licorice has been used for thousands of years in traditional medicine and culinary practices across various cultures. Let's delve into the myriad benefits and versatile uses of this remarkable herb.

A Sweet History:

Licorice has a rich and storied history dating back to ancient times. It was prized by the ancient Egyptians, Greeks, Romans, and Chinese for its medicinal properties and unique flavor. In traditional Chinese medicine (TCM), licorice root, known as "gan cao," is considered one of the 50 fundamental herbs and is valued for its harmonizing and tonifying effects on the body.

Licorice root contains various vitamins, minerals, and antioxidants that contribute to its numerous health benefits. Here's a list of some of the key nutrients found in licorice and their associated benefits:

Vitamins:

Vitamin B1 (Thiamine):

- Benefits: Essential for energy metabolism, nerve function, and carbohydrate metabolism.

Vitamin B2 (Riboflavin):

- Benefits: Supports energy production, helps maintain healthy skin and eyes, and aids in the metabolism of carbohydrates, fats, and proteins.

Vitamin B3 (Niacin):

- Benefits: Plays a crucial role in energy metabolism, supports cardiovascular health, and helps maintain healthy skin and nerves.

Vitamin B5 (Pantothenic Acid):

- Benefits: Essential for synthesizing and metabolizing fats, proteins, and carbohydrates, and supports adrenal gland function.

Vitamin B6 (Pyridoxine):

- Benefits: Supports brain health, neurotransmitter synthesis, and hormone regulation, and may help reduce symptoms of PMS and morning sickness.

Minerals:

Magnesium:

- Benefits: Supports muscle and nerve function, regulates blood sugar levels, aids in energy production, and promotes bone health.

Potassium:

- Benefits: Regulates fluid balance, supports proper muscle function, helps maintain healthy blood pressure levels, and plays a role in nerve transmission.

Calcium:

- Benefits: Essential for building and maintaining strong bones and teeth, supports muscle function, and aids in nerve transmission.

Manganese:

- Benefits: Necessary for bone formation, wound healing, metabolism of carbohydrates and cholesterol, and antioxidant defense.

Antioxidants:

Glycyrrhizin:

- Benefits: Acts as an anti-inflammatory and immune-modulating agent, may help protect against liver damage, and exhibits antiviral properties.

Flavonoids:

- Benefits: Possess antioxidant and anti-inflammatory properties, support cardiovascular health, and may help reduce the risk of chronic diseases such as heart disease and cancer.

Coumarins:

- Benefits: Exhibit antioxidant and anti-inflammatory effects, may help improve blood circulation, and have potential anticancer properties.

Phenolic Acids:

- Benefits: Act as antioxidants, scavenging free radicals and reducing oxidative stress, which may help protect against chronic diseases and support overall health.

Saponins:

- Benefits: Exhibit anti-inflammatory and immune-modulating properties, may help reduce cholesterol levels, and have potential anticancer effects.

These vitamins, minerals, and antioxidants found in licorice contribute to its numerous health benefits, including supporting digestive health, promoting respiratory health, reducing inflammation, and boosting immune function. Incorporating licorice root into your diet or using it as a herbal supplement can be a flavorful and nutritious way to reap these benefits and support overall well-being.

Health Benefits:

Soothes Digestive Discomfort:

- Licorice root contains compounds that help soothe gastrointestinal irritation and promote digestive health. It is commonly used to alleviate symptoms of acid reflux, indigestion, and heartburn.

Supports Respiratory Health:

- Licorice has expectorant and demulcent properties, making it beneficial for respiratory conditions such as coughs, colds, and bronchitis. It helps to loosen and expel mucus from the respiratory tract, providing relief from congestion and coughing.

Anti-inflammatory Effects:

- Glycyrrhizin, a compound found in licorice root, exhibits potent anti-inflammatory properties that can help reduce inflammation and alleviate symptoms associated with inflammatory conditions such as arthritis and allergies.

Hormonal Balance:

- Licorice root contains phytoestrogens that may help balance hormone levels in the body, making it beneficial for women experiencing menopausal symptoms such as hot flashes and mood swings.

Immune Support:

- Licorice root has been traditionally used to support immune function and enhance the body's natural defenses against infections and illnesses. Its antiviral and antimicrobial properties may help fend off pathogens and boost overall immunity.

Culinary and Herbal Uses:

Herbal Teas:

- Licorice root is commonly used as an ingredient in herbal teas and infusions for its sweet flavor and medicinal properties. It blends well with other herbs such as peppermint, ginger, and chamomile.

While licorice is commonly used in herbal remedies and candies, it's not typically used in culinary recipes due to its intense flavor and potential side effects when consumed in large quantities. However, licorice-flavored products, such as licorice tea, can be enjoyed as beverages.

Here are two recipes featuring licorice:

Licorice Infusion Tea:

Ingredients:

- 1 tablespoon dried licorice root
- 1 cup water
- Optional: honey or sweetener of choice

Instructions:

1. Bring 1 cup of water to a boil in a small saucepan.
2. Add the dried licorice root to the boiling water.
3. Reduce the heat to low and let the licorice root simmer in the water for about 5 minutes.
4. Remove the saucepan from the heat and let the licorice root steep in the hot water for an additional 5-10 minutes, depending on desired strength.
5. Strain the licorice infusion into a cup using a fine mesh strainer or tea infuser.
6. Sweeten the tea with honey or your preferred sweetener, if desired.
7. Serve the licorice infusion tea hot and enjoy its soothing flavor.

Licorice Root and Peppermint Herbal Blend:

Ingredients:

- 1 tablespoon dried licorice root
- 1 tablespoon dried peppermint leaves
- 1 cup water
- Optional: honey or sweetener of choice

Instructions:

1. Bring 1 cup of water to a boil in a small saucepan.
2. Add the dried licorice root and dried peppermint leaves to the boiling water.
3. Reduce the heat to low and let the herbs simmer in the water for about 5 minutes.
4. Remove the saucepan from the heat and let the herbal blend steep in the hot water for an additional 5-10 minutes, depending on desired strength.
5. Strain the herbal blend into a cup using a fine mesh strainer or tea infuser.
6. Sweeten the tea with honey or your preferred sweetener, if desired.
7. Serve the licorice root and peppermint herbal blend hot or chilled, depending on preference.

These recipes showcase licorice's potential as a flavorful herbal infusion. It's important to enjoy licorice in moderation and consult with a healthcare professional before consuming large quantities, especially if you have any underlying health conditions or are pregnant or breastfeeding.

Traditional Medicine:

- Licorice root is a key ingredient in traditional herbal medicine systems such as Ayurveda and traditional Chinese medicine (TCM). It is used in various formulations to treat a wide range of ailments, including digestive disorders, respiratory conditions, and hormonal imbalances.

Confectionery and Flavoring:

- Licorice extract is used as a flavoring agent in confectionery products such as candies, chewing gums, and soft drinks. Its sweet and distinctive flavor adds depth and complexity to various culinary creations.

Skincare:

- Licorice extract is prized in skincare products for its anti-inflammatory and skin-soothing properties. It is used in creams, lotions, and serums to calm irritation, reduce redness, and even out skin tone.

Historical uses:

Licorice has a long history of use in various cultures around the world, dating back thousands of years. Here are two historical uses of licorice:

Traditional Medicine in Ancient Civilizations:

Ancient Egypt:

- Licorice root was highly valued in ancient Egypt for its medicinal properties. It was used as a remedy for various ailments, including sore throat, cough, and digestive issues.

- Licorice root was also used topically as a treatment for skin conditions and to promote wound healing.

Traditional Chinese Medicine (TCM):

- In traditional Chinese medicine, licorice root, known as "gan cao," has been used for thousands of years as a harmonizing and tonifying herb.
- Licorice root is considered one of the 50 fundamental herbs in TCM and is often prescribed in herbal formulations to enhance the effects of other herbs, balance the body's energy (Qi), and support various organ systems.
- Licorice root is commonly used in TCM to treat conditions such as cough, sore throat, fatigue, digestive disorders, and hormonal imbalances.

Ancient Greece and Rome:

Hippocrates and Theophrastus:

- Licorice was known to ancient Greek and Roman physicians, including Hippocrates and Theophrastus, who wrote about its medicinal properties and uses.
- Hippocrates, often referred to as the "father of medicine," recommended licorice root as a treatment for coughs, respiratory ailments, and gastrointestinal issues.

Culinary and Cultural Uses:

- Licorice was also enjoyed in ancient Greece and Rome as a flavorful ingredient in confections and beverages.
- Licorice-flavored candies, drinks, and desserts were popular among the ancient Greeks and Romans, who valued licorice for its sweet taste and aromatic qualities.

These historical uses of licorice highlight its longstanding reputation as a valuable medicinal herb and culinary ingredient. Licorice continues to be cherished today for its diverse applications in traditional medicine, herbal remedies, and culinary creations.

Tips on Growing Licorice

Growing licorice (Glycyrrhiza glabra) is a process that requires patience and specific conditions to ensure successful cultivation. Here's a detailed breakdown of the typical timeline for growing licorice:

1. Seed Germination (3-4 weeks):

- Licorice seeds have a hard outer coat that needs to be scarified (scratched or nicked) before planting to aid in germination.

- After scarification, licorice seeds are sown in well-draining soil in early spring, either directly in the ground or in pots if started indoors.
- Germination typically occurs within 3 to 4 weeks under optimal conditions, including warmth and moisture.

2. Seedling Stage (6-8 weeks):

- Once the seeds have germinated, they will develop into seedlings with small, true leaves.
- Licorice seedlings require consistent moisture and adequate sunlight to support healthy growth during this stage.
- Seedlings are typically ready for transplanting when they have developed several sets of true leaves and are sturdy enough to handle.

3. Transplanting (8-12 weeks):

- Licorice seedlings can be transplanted into their permanent growing location after 8 to 12 weeks, once the risk of frost has passed and the weather is consistently warm.
- Choose a sunny location with well-draining soil for transplanting. Space the seedlings at least 18 to 24 inches apart to allow for proper root development.
- Water the transplanted seedlings thoroughly to help them establish in their new environment.

4. Vegetative Growth (1-2 years):

- Licorice plants undergo a period of vegetative growth, during which they develop a deep taproot and lush foliage.
- Regular watering and occasional fertilization with a balanced fertilizer can support healthy growth and development.
- Licorice plants may not produce significant harvestable roots until they have been growing for at least 1 to 2 years.

5. Harvesting (2-3 years):

- Licorice roots are typically harvested in the fall of the plant's second or third year of growth, once they have reached a sufficient size and maturity.
- To harvest licorice roots, carefully dig around the base of the plant to expose the roots without damaging them.
- Harvest only a portion of the roots, leaving some behind to allow the plant to regrow and continue producing.

6. Maintenance (ongoing):

- Licorice plants require minimal maintenance once established. Regular weeding and occasional watering during dry periods can help keep the plants healthy.
- In colder climates, licorice plants may benefit from mulching in the winter to protect the roots from freezing temperatures.

By following these guidelines and providing proper care and attention, you can expect to grow licorice successfully and enjoy a bountiful harvest of its sweet, flavorful roots.

Precautions:

While licorice offers numerous health benefits, it's essential to use it judiciously and under the guidance of a healthcare professional, especially for individuals with certain medical conditions, allergic or those taking medications. Excessive consumption of licorice or prolonged use of high-dose licorice supplements may lead to side effects such as elevated blood pressure, potassium depletion, and hormonal imbalances.

Conclusion:

Licorice stands as a testament to the power of nature's remedies and the enduring legacy of traditional herbal medicine. Whether enjoyed as a soothing tea, a flavorful culinary ingredient, or a therapeutic herbal remedy, licorice continues to captivate with its sweet charm and multifaceted benefits for health and well-being. Embrace the sweetness of licorice and discover the wonders it holds for mind, body, and spirit.

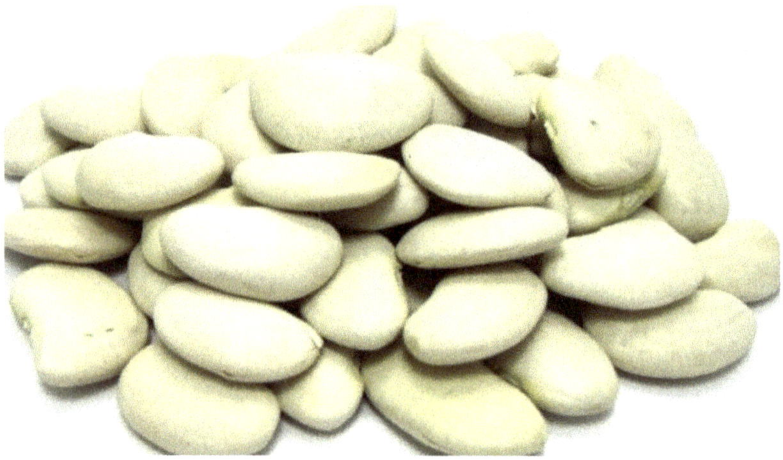

Lima Beans / Butter Beans

Unlocking the Nutritional Treasure Trove: Lima Beans

Lima beans, also known as butter beans, are a versatile legume celebrated for their rich flavor, creamy texture, and impressive nutritional profile. These beans have been cultivated for thousands of years and are cherished in cuisines around the world for their versatility and health benefits. Let's explore the wonders of lima beans, uncovering their remarkable benefits and diverse culinary uses.

Nutritional Profile of Lima Beans:

Lima beans are a nutritional powerhouse, offering an abundance of essential nutrients that promote overall health and well-being. Here's a glimpse into the impressive nutritional profile of lima beans:

Protein: Lima beans are a rich source of plant-based protein, making them an excellent option for vegetarians, vegans, and individuals looking to reduce their meat consumption. Protein is essential for muscle repair, growth, and overall body function.

Dietary Fiber: Lima beans are high in dietary fiber, both soluble and insoluble, which supports digestive health, regulates bowel movements, and promotes feelings of fullness and satiety. Fiber also helps lower cholesterol levels and stabilize blood sugar levels.

Complex Carbohydrates: Lima beans provide complex carbohydrates, which are digested slowly, providing a steady source of energy and helping to maintain stable blood sugar levels. This makes lima beans an excellent choice for individuals with diabetes or those looking to manage their weight.

Vitamins and Minerals:

Lima beans are packed with essential vitamins and minerals, including folate, potassium, magnesium, iron, zinc, and manganese. These nutrients are crucial for immune function, energy metabolism, bone health, and various biochemical processes in the body.

Folate (Vitamin B9): Folate is important for DNA synthesis, cell division, and the production of red blood cells. Adequate folate intake is crucial during pregnancy to prevent neural tube defects in the developing fetus. Folate also supports cardiovascular health and may reduce the risk of certain cancers.

Potassium: Potassium is an electrolyte that helps regulate fluid balance, nerve function, and muscle contractions. It also supports heart health by helping to lower blood pressure and reduce the risk of stroke.

Magnesium: Magnesium is involved in over 300 biochemical reactions in the body, including energy production, muscle function, and nerve transmission. Magnesium also supports bone health, heart health, and blood sugar regulation.

Iron: Iron is essential for oxygen transport, energy metabolism, and the synthesis of hemoglobin and myoglobin. Adequate iron intake helps prevent iron deficiency anemia and supports immune function and cognitive health.

Zinc: Zinc is important for immune function, wound healing, and DNA synthesis. It also supports growth and development, reproductive health, and the maintenance of healthy skin, hair, and nails.

Copper: Copper is necessary for the formation of red blood cells, collagen synthesis, and the absorption of iron. Copper also acts as an antioxidant and supports immune function, bone health, and connective tissue health.

Manganese: Manganese is involved in bone formation, cartilage formation, and the metabolism of carbohydrates, proteins, and cholesterol. Manganese also acts as an antioxidant and supports immune function and blood sugar regulation.

Phosphorus: Phosphorus is important for bone and teeth health, energy metabolism, and cell membrane structure. Phosphorus also supports kidney function, nerve function, and muscle contractions.

Incorporating butter beans into your diet can help you meet your daily requirements for these essential vitamins and minerals, promoting overall health and well-being. Whether enjoyed in soups, salads, stews, or main dishes, butter beans offer a delicious and nutritious addition to any meal.

Antioxidants:

Lima beans contain antioxidants such as flavonoids and phenolic compounds, which help protect cells from oxidative damage caused by free radicals. Antioxidants play a key role in reducing inflammation, preventing chronic diseases, and promoting longevity.

Flavonoids: Lima beans contain flavonoids such as quercetin, kaempferol, and myricetin. These flavonoids have potent antioxidant properties that help neutralize free radicals, reduce inflammation, and lower the risk of chronic diseases such as heart disease, cancer, and neurodegenerative disorders like Alzheimer's disease.

Phenolic Compounds: Lima beans are rich in phenolic compounds, including phenolic acids and tannins. These compounds have antioxidant and anti-inflammatory properties, which help protect cells from damage, reduce inflammation, and support overall health.

Anthocyanins: Anthocyanins are pigments responsible for the red, purple, or blue colors in fruits and vegetables. While lima beans may not be as rich in anthocyanins as some other foods, they still contain small amounts of these antioxidants, which contribute to their overall antioxidant activity.

Vitamin C: Lima beans are a good source of vitamin C, a powerful antioxidant that helps boost the immune system, protect against oxidative stress, and promote skin health. Vitamin C also supports collagen production, wound healing, and the absorption of iron.

Vitamin E: Lima beans contain vitamin E, including tocopherols and tocotrienols, which have antioxidant properties and help protect cell membranes from oxidative damage. Vitamin E may also support immune function, cardiovascular health, and skin health.

Saponins: Lima beans contain saponins, plant compounds with antioxidant and anti-inflammatory properties. Saponins may help lower cholesterol levels, regulate blood sugar levels, and support immune function. They also have potential anticancer effects and may protect against certain infections.

These antioxidants found in lima beans work synergistically to combat oxidative stress, reduce inflammation, and promote overall health and well-being. Incorporating lima beans into your diet can help increase your intake of these beneficial antioxidants, supporting optimal health and disease prevention.

Health Benefits of Lima Beans:

Heart Health: The combination of fiber, potassium, and antioxidants in lima beans supports heart health by lowering cholesterol levels, regulating blood pressure, and reducing the risk of cardiovascular disease. Consuming lima beans as part of a balanced diet may help prevent heart attacks, strokes, and other cardiovascular complications.

Digestive Health: The high fiber content of lima beans promotes digestive health by preventing constipation, regulating bowel movements, and nourishing beneficial gut bacteria. Fiber also helps reduce the risk of digestive disorders such as diverticulitis and irritable bowel syndrome (IBS).

Blood Sugar Control: The complex carbohydrates and soluble fiber in lima beans help stabilize blood sugar levels and improve insulin sensitivity. Including lima beans in meals can help prevent spikes and crashes in blood glucose levels, making them a valuable food for individuals with diabetes or those at risk of developing the condition.

Bone Health: Lima beans are a good source of calcium, magnesium, and manganese, which are essential minerals for bone health and density. Regular consumption of lima beans may help prevent osteoporosis and reduce the risk of fractures and bone-related disorders.

Weight Management: The high protein and fiber content of lima beans promote feelings of fullness and satiety, reducing overall calorie intake and aiding in weight loss or weight management efforts. Including lima beans in meals can help control appetite and prevent overeating.

Nutritional Content

The nutritional content in 1 cup (approximately 188 grams) of cooked lima beans typically includes:

- Calories: Around 216 kcal
- Carbohydrates: Approximately 39.2 grams
- Protein: Roughly 12.9 grams
- Fiber: About 9.2 grams
- Fat: Approximately 0.7 grams

Please note that these values are approximate and can vary depending on factors such as the specific variety of lima beans, cooking method, and any additional ingredients added during preparation. Lima beans are a nutritious source of carbohydrates, protein, fiber, and various vitamins and minerals.

Culinary Uses of Lima Beans:

Lima beans are incredibly versatile and can be used in a variety of culinary applications, including:

Soups and Stews: Lima beans add texture, flavor, and nutritional value to soups, stews, and chili recipes. They pair well with vegetables, herbs, and spices, creating hearty and satisfying dishes.

Salads: Lima beans can be tossed into salads for added protein, fiber, and creaminess. They complement leafy greens, tomatoes, cucumbers, and avocados, as well as tangy dressings or vinaigrettes.

Dips and Spreads: Lima beans can be blended into creamy dips and spreads, such as hummus or bean dip, for a nutritious and delicious snack or appetizer.

Side Dishes: Lima beans can be served as a standalone side dish, seasoned with herbs, spices, and a drizzle of olive oil. They pair well with rice, quinoa, or other grains, as well as roasted or steamed vegetables.

Vegetarian Entrees: Lima beans can be the star ingredient in vegetarian or vegan entrees, such as bean burgers, bean casseroles, or bean-based curries. They provide protein, fiber, and flavor, making them a satisfying meat alternative.

Here are two delicious recipes featuring lima beans:

Lima Bean Salad with Herbs and Lemon Dressing:

Ingredients:

- 2 cups cooked lima beans (or canned, drained, and rinsed)
- 1 cup cherry tomatoes, halved
- 1/2 red onion, thinly sliced
- 1/4 cup fresh parsley, chopped
- 1/4 cup fresh cilantro, chopped
- 1/4 cup fresh mint leaves, chopped
- 2 tablespoons extra virgin olive oil
- 2 tablespoons lemon juice
- 1 garlic clove, minced
- Salt and pepper to taste

Instructions:

1. In a large bowl, combine the cooked lima beans, cherry tomatoes, red onion, parsley, cilantro, and mint.
2. In a small bowl, whisk together the olive oil, lemon juice, minced garlic, salt, and pepper to make the dressing.
3. Pour the dressing over the salad ingredients and toss until everything is evenly coated.
4. Taste and adjust seasoning if needed.
5. Let the salad marinate in the refrigerator for at least 30 minutes before serving to allow the flavors to meld together.
6. Serve chilled as a refreshing side dish or light lunch.

Jamaican Oxtail with Butter Beans:

Ingredients:

- 3 lbs oxtail, cut into pieces
- 2 tablespoons vegetable oil
- 1 onion, chopped
- 4 garlic cloves, minced

- 2 carrots, chopped
- 2 celery stalks, chopped
- 2 tablespoons tomato paste
- 1 teaspoon dried thyme
- 1 teaspoon ground allspice
- 1 teaspoon smoked paprika
- 1 bay leaf
- 4 cups beef broth
- 2 cans (15 oz each) butter beans, drained and rinsed
- Salt and pepper to taste
- Fresh parsley for garnish

Instructions:

1. Heat the vegetable oil in a large pot or Dutch oven over medium heat. Add the oxtail pieces and brown them on all sides, working in batches if necessary. Remove the oxtail and set aside.
2. In the same pot, add the chopped onion, minced garlic, carrots, and celery. Cook until softened, about 5 minutes.
3. Stir in the tomato paste, dried thyme, ground allspice, smoked paprika, and bay leaf. Cook for another 2 minutes, stirring constantly.
4. Return the browned oxtail pieces to the pot. Pour in the beef broth and bring to a simmer.
5. Cover and cook over low heat for 2-3 hours, or until the oxtail is tender and falls off the bone.
6. Stir in the drained and rinsed butter beans. Cook for an additional 15-20 minutes until the beans are heated through.
7. Season with salt and pepper to taste.
8. Garnish with fresh parsley before serving.
9. Serve the Jamaican oxtail with butter beans hot over rice or with your favorite side dishes.

These recipes highlight the versatility of lima beans, whether used in a refreshing salad or as a hearty addition to a flavorful stew. Enjoy these dishes bursting with flavor and nutritional goodness!

Conclusion:

Lima beans are a versatile and nutrient-dense legume that offers a wide range of health benefits and culinary possibilities. Whether enjoyed in soups, salads, dips, or main dishes, lima beans are a valuable addition to any diet, providing protein, fiber, vitamins, minerals, and antioxidants to support overall health and well-being. Embrace the goodness of lima beans and explore the endless ways to incorporate them into your favorite recipes for a nutritious and flavorful dining experience.

If you have specific health concerns, allergies, or conditions, it's advisable to consult with a healthcare professional or a registered dietitian before making significant changes to your diet.

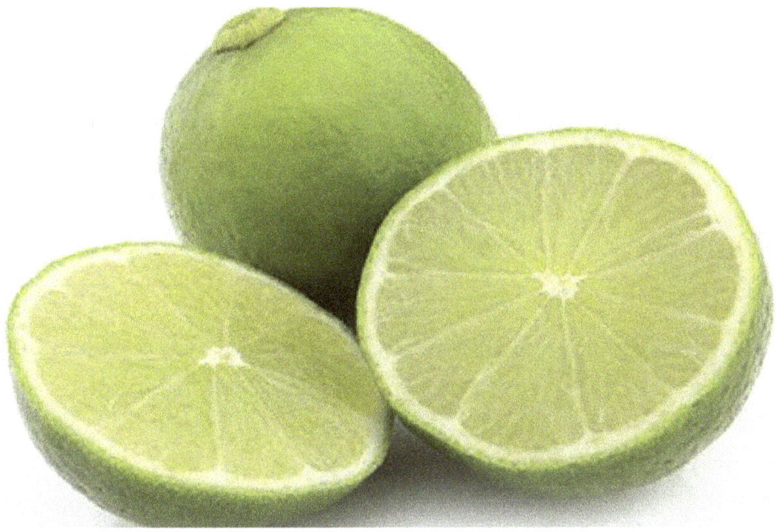

Lime

The Versatility and Health Benefits of Lime: A Citrus Gem

Lime, with its vibrant green hue and tangy flavor, has long been celebrated as a versatile fruit in culinary, medicinal, and household applications. Beyond its refreshing taste, lime boasts an array of health benefits and practical uses that make it a staple in kitchens and beyond. Let's delve into the wonders of lime, exploring its diverse applications and the numerous ways it can enhance our lives.

Nutritional Value

Limes are packed with essential nutrients, including vitamin C, vitamin A, potassium, and antioxidants. Just one lime can provide a significant portion of your daily recommended intake of vitamin C, which plays a crucial role in immune function, collagen production, and skin health. Additionally, limes contain flavonoids and other compounds that contribute to their antioxidant properties, helping to combat oxidative stress and inflammation in the body.

Vitamins:

Vitamin C: Limes are particularly rich in vitamin C, also known as ascorbic acid. This vitamin is essential for immune function, collagen synthesis, wound healing, and antioxidant defense against free radicals. Consuming limes can help boost your immune system and promote healthy skin.

Minerals:

Potassium: Limes contain potassium, an essential mineral that plays a vital role in maintaining proper heart function, muscle contraction, and fluid balance within the body. Adequate potassium intake can help regulate blood pressure and support overall cardiovascular health.

Antioxidants:

The presence of antioxidants in limes has demonstrated effectiveness in reducing inflammation and preventing specific chronic illnesses. Notably, the substantial vitamin C content in limes serves as a protective measure against infections while expediting the body's healing processes. Scientific evidence also supports the role of citrus fruits, including limes, in deterring the formation of kidney stones. The antioxidants found in limes may reduce the risk of chronic diseases, such as heart disease and certain types of cancer.

Flavonoids (including flavonol glycosides and flavanones): These antioxidants found in limes help neutralize harmful free radicals in the body, reducing oxidative stress and inflammation. Flavonoids have been associated with various health benefits, including improved heart health and reduced risk of chronic diseases.

Limonoids: Limonoids are a group of phytochemicals found in citrus fruits like limes. They have antioxidant and anti-inflammatory properties and have been studied for their potential anticancer effects.

Beta-Carotene: Limes contain beta-carotene, a precursor to vitamin A. Beta-carotene acts as an antioxidant and is essential for maintaining healthy vision, skin, and immune function.

Beyond their tangy flavor, limes house a multitude of benefits encompassing citric acid, ascorbic acid (vitamin C), flavonoids, and various minerals. A singular lime can supply 22% of the recommended daily intake of vitamin C, establishing it as a noteworthy source of vitamin B6, folate, potassium, calcium, and magnesium.

Limes and lime leaf extract have a rich history in traditional medicine, particularly in Southeast Asia. Presently, scientists are delving into the mechanisms through which the plant contributes to the healing process.

Health Benefits

The consumption of lime has been associated with several health benefits. Lime juice is also known to aid digestion, stimulate the liver, and promote healthy skin due to its cleansing properties.

- **Immune Support**: The high vitamin C content in limes helps strengthen the immune system, making them useful in preventing and fighting off colds, flu, and other infections.
- **Skin Health**: Vitamin C and antioxidants in limes contribute to healthy skin by promoting collagen production, reducing signs of aging, and protecting against damage from UV radiation and environmental pollutants.
- **Heart Health**: Potassium and antioxidants found in limes support cardiovascular health by helping regulate blood pressure, reducing cholesterol levels, and protecting against oxidative stress and inflammation.

- **Digestive Health**: Limes contain soluble fiber and compounds like limonoids, which may help support digestive health by promoting regularity, preventing constipation, and supporting a healthy gut microbiota.
- **Weight Management**: Limes are low in calories and rich in fiber, making them a good choice for weight management and promoting feelings of fullness and satiety.
- **Blood Sugar Regulation:** Limes, being low in carbohydrates, offer an advantageous choice for individuals seeking to regulate blood sugar levels. Their consumption is particularly beneficial for those managing diabetes, as the low carbohydrate content reduces the likelihood of causing spikes in blood sugar.

Incorporating limes into your diet can provide a wide range of health benefits, but it's essential to consume them as part of a balanced diet that includes a variety of fruits, vegetables, whole grains, and lean proteins.

Are Limes Effective Against Inflammation?

In a 2020 study, researchers from Brazil discovered that the flavonoids present in Tahitian limes exhibited comparable efficacy to the anti-inflammatory drug meloxicam in alleviating the pain and heavy bleeding associated with menstrual periods.

During the COVID-19 pandemic in 2020, a family in the USA reported positive outcomes, attributing the elimination of COVID-19 in one family member to the regular consumption of natural lime juice. The rest of the family, by incorporating natural lime juice into their daily routine, successfully prevented any further instances of contracting the disease. They also experience eliminating stomach viruses with natural lime consumption.

Culinary Uses

Lime adds a burst of flavor to countless culinary creations, from savory dishes to sweet treats. Its acidic tang can enhance the taste of salads, seafood, and marinades, while its zest can lend a refreshing aroma to baked goods and desserts. Lime juice is a popular ingredient in cocktails and beverages, adding a refreshing twist to classics like margaritas and mojitos. Moreover, lime is a versatile condiment, as its juice can be used to create tangy sauces, dressings, and salsas.

Here are two recipes featuring lime as a key ingredient:

Cilantro Lime Chicken:

Ingredients:

- 4 boneless, skinless chicken breasts
- 2 limes (juiced and zested)
- 3 cloves garlic, minced
- 2 tablespoons olive oil

- 1/4 cup chopped fresh cilantro
- Salt and pepper to taste

Instructions:

1. In a small bowl, mix together the lime juice, lime zest, minced garlic, olive oil, chopped cilantro, salt, and pepper to create the marinade.
2. Place the chicken breasts in a resealable plastic bag or shallow dish and pour the marinade over them, ensuring they are well coated. Marinate in the refrigerator for at least 30 minutes (or up to 4 hours for maximum flavor).
3. Preheat the grill to medium-high heat. Remove the chicken from the marinade and discard any excess marinade.
4. Grill the chicken breasts for about 6-7 minutes per side, or until they are cooked through and reach an internal temperature of 165°F (75°C).
5. Serve the grilled cilantro lime chicken with your favorite sides, such as rice, grilled vegetables, or a fresh salad.

Key Lime Pie:

Ingredients:

1. 1 1/2 cups graham cracker crumbs
2. 1/3 cup granulated sugar
3. 6 tablespoons unsalted butter, melted
4. 3 large egg yolks
5. 14 ounces sweetened condensed milk
6. 1/2 cup key lime juice (regular lime juice can be used as well)
7. 1 tablespoon lime zest
8. Whipped cream for topping (optional)

Instructions:

1. Preheat the oven to 350°F (175°C).
2. In a medium bowl, mix together the graham cracker crumbs, granulated sugar, and melted butter until well combined. Press the mixture into the bottom and up the sides of a 9-inch pie dish to form the crust.
3. Bake the crust in the preheated oven for 10 minutes, then remove and let it cool slightly.

4. In another bowl, whisk together the egg yolks, sweetened condensed milk, lime juice, and lime zest until smooth and well combined.
5. Pour the lime filling into the cooled crust and spread it out evenly.
6. Bake the pie in the oven for 15 minutes, or until the filling is set but still slightly jiggly in the center.
7. Remove the pie from the oven and let it cool to room temperature, then refrigerate for at least 2 hours (or overnight) to chill and set.
8. Serve slices of key lime pie chilled, topped with whipped cream if desired.

Enjoy these delicious recipes featuring the refreshing flavor of lime!

Healthy Sugar Alternative:

Lime water serves as a commendable substitute for sugary sodas. Enjoying the refreshing citrus flavor of lime water allows individuals to steer clear of the potential blood sugar spikes associated with sugary beverages. Furthermore, opting for lime water contributes to hydration, facilitating the body's ability to regulate blood glucose levels effectively.

Household Applications:

Beyond the kitchen, lime has practical uses in household cleaning and aromatherapy. The acidic properties of lime juice make it an effective natural cleaner for surfaces, removing stains, grease, and odors. Additionally, the fresh scent of lime can uplift and invigorate your surroundings when used in homemade air fresheners or diffused in essential oil blends.

Beauty and Skincare:

Lime is not only beneficial when consumed but also when applied topically to the skin. The vitamin C and antioxidants in lime juice can help brighten the complexion, fade dark spots, and promote collagen production, resulting in smoother, more youthful-looking skin. Lime juice can also be used as a natural astringent to tone and tighten pores, making it a popular ingredient in DIY skincare treatments.

Conclusion:

From its nutritional value and health benefits to its culinary versatility and household applications, lime truly deserves its status as a citrus gem. Whether you're squeezing it over a dish to add flavor, using it to clean your home naturally, or incorporating it into your skincare routine, lime proves to be a valuable addition to any lifestyle. Embrace the zestiness of lime and discover the myriad ways it can enrich your life, both inside and out.

If you have specific health concerns, allergies, or conditions, it's advisable to consult with a healthcare professional or a registered dietitian before making significant changes to your diet.

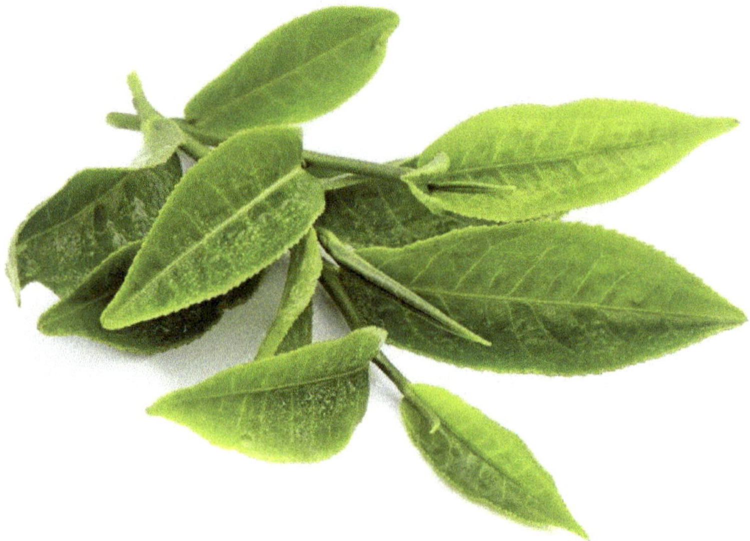

L-Theanine

Health Benefits and Nutritional Content

What is L-Theanine?

L-theanine is a unique amino acid primarily found in tea leaves, especially **green tea (Camellia sinensis)** and black tea, as well as in certain mushrooms. It is known for its calming effects on the brain and body, making it a popular supplement for stress relief, cognitive enhancement, and relaxation. Unlike other amino acids, L-theanine is not used to build proteins but instead interacts with neurotransmitters in the brain to promote a state of mental clarity and relaxation.

Health Benefits of L-Theanine

1. Promotes Relaxation and Reduces Stress

L-theanine is best known for its ability to reduce stress and anxiety without causing drowsiness. It increases the production of calming neurotransmitters such as gamma-aminobutyric acid (GABA), serotonin, and dopamine. These chemicals help regulate mood, relaxation, and overall mental well-being.

2. Enhances Cognitive Function

Research suggests that L-theanine can improve focus, attention, and mental clarity. It works synergistically with caffeine to boost cognitive performance without the jittery side effects often associated with caffeine consumption. This is why green tea, which naturally contains both L-theanine and caffeine, is known for providing a balanced energy boost.

3. Improves Sleep Quality

Although L-theanine does not act as a sedative, it helps promote relaxation, which can lead to better sleep quality. Studies show that individuals who take L-theanine before bed experience improved sleep duration and quality, making it a useful supplement for those struggling with insomnia or restless nights.

4. Supports Heart Health

L-theanine has been linked to cardiovascular health benefits, including reduced blood pressure and improved circulation. By lowering stress-related blood pressure spikes and promoting relaxation, L-theanine may contribute to overall heart health.

5. Boosts Immune Function

Some studies suggest that L-theanine may enhance the immune system by increasing the production of certain infection-fighting cells. This makes it a potential ally in protecting against colds and other illnesses.

6. Helps with Weight Management

L-theanine, when combined with caffeine (as found in tea), may aid in weight management by increasing metabolism and promoting fat oxidation. Additionally, its stress-reducing properties can help prevent stress-related overeating.

L-Theanine is primarily found in tea leaves, especially **green tea (Camellia sinensis)**. While it is not commonly present in most plant-based foods, here are some sources where you may find L-Theanine or related compounds:

1. **Green Tea** – The richest source of L-Theanine
2. **Black Tea** – Contains lower amounts than green tea
3. **White Tea** – Less processed, but still contains L-Theanine
4. **Oolong Tea** – Moderate amounts of L-Theanine
5. **Matcha Green Tea** – High concentration due to whole-leaf consumption
6. **Gyokuro Tea** – A Japanese green tea with high L-Theanine content
7. **Shiitake Mushrooms** – While not a major source, some mushrooms contain similar amino acids
8. **Bay Bolete Mushrooms** – A wild mushroom containing small amounts of L-Theanine

Nutritional Content of L-Theanine

L-theanine is not a nutrient in the traditional sense, as it is an amino acid rather than a vitamin or mineral. However, it is naturally found in:

- **Green Tea** (20–60 mg per cup)

- **Black Tea** (20–40 mg per cup)
- **Certain Mushrooms** (small amounts)
- **L-Theanine Supplements** (100–400 mg per dose)

How to Take L-Theanine

L-theanine can be consumed through tea or taken as a supplement in capsule or powder form. The recommended dosage typically ranges from **100 to 400 mg per day**, depending on the intended use.

Safety and Side Effects

L-theanine is generally considered safe with few reported side effects. Some individuals may experience mild symptoms such as dizziness, headaches, or nausea. However, it is advisable to consult a healthcare professional before taking L-theanine supplements, especially if you are pregnant, nursing, or taking medication.

Conclusion

L-theanine is a powerful amino acid known for its calming and cognitive-enhancing effects. Whether consumed through tea or supplements, it offers a range of health benefits, including stress reduction, improved focus, better sleep, and heart health support. For those seeking a natural way to enhance mental clarity and relaxation, L-theanine is a safe and effective option.

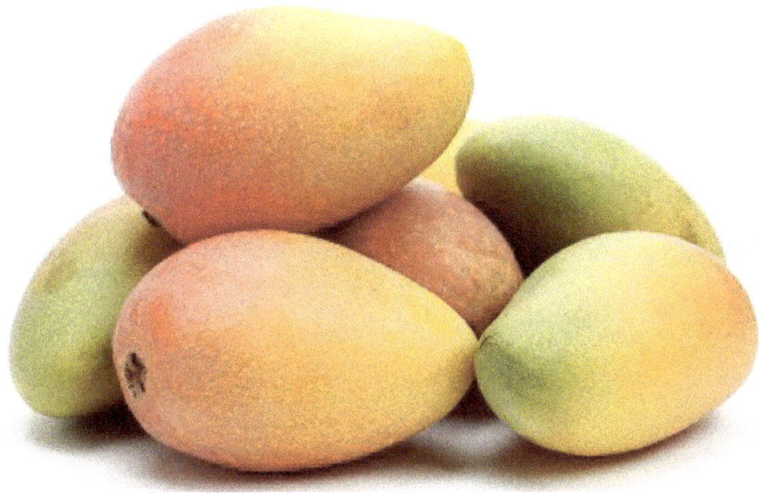

Mango

The King of Fruits - A Sweet and Nutrient-Packed Delight

Mango, often hailed as the "King of Fruits," is not only celebrated for its rich, sweet flavor but also revered for its myriad health benefits. Originating from the tropical regions of South Asia, this luscious fruit has become a global favorite, finding its way into a wide array of culinary creations. In this article, we delve into the nutritional benefits and versatile uses of mango.

Nutritional Benefits:

Rich in Vitamins:

Mangoes are a powerhouse of vitamins, particularly vitamin C, which supports immune function and promotes healthy skin. They also contain vitamin A, contributing to vision health and immune support.

Here are four vitamins found in mangoes and their benefits:

Vitamin C:

- **Benefits:**
    - Boosts the immune system by supporting the production of white blood cells.
    - Acts as an antioxidant, protecting cells from oxidative stress.
    - Promotes healthy skin by aiding in collagen synthesis.
    - Enhances the absorption of non-heme iron from plant-based foods.

Vitamin A:

- **Benefits:**
    - Essential for maintaining healthy vision and preventing night blindness.
    - Supports immune function, helping the body fight infections.
    - Contributes to the health of the skin and mucous membranes.
    - Plays a role in cell differentiation and gene expression.

Vitamin E:

- **Benefits:**
    - Acts as an antioxidant, protecting cells from oxidative damage.
    - Supports immune function.
    - Contributes to skin health and may help with skin conditions.

Vitamin K:

- **Benefits:**
    - Essential for blood clotting and proper wound healing.
    - Contributes to bone health by regulating calcium.
    - Plays a role in cardiovascular health.

High in Dietary Fiber:

- With a significant fiber content, mangoes aid digestion, promote bowel regularity, and help maintain a healthy weight by providing a feeling of fullness.

Packed with Antioxidants:

Mangoes are loaded with antioxidants, including quercetin, beta-carotene, and astragalin. These compounds help combat oxidative stress, reducing the risk of chronic diseases.

Beta-Carotene:

- **Benefits:**
    - Acts as a precursor to vitamin A, essential for maintaining healthy vision.
    - Functions as an antioxidant, protecting cells from oxidative stress.
    - Supports immune function and skin health.

Quercetin:

- **Benefits:**
    - Exhibits anti-inflammatory properties, helping reduce inflammation in the body.
    - Acts as an antioxidant, neutralizing free radicals and reducing oxidative damage.
    - May have potential cardiovascular benefits by promoting heart health.

Source of Minerals:

Mangoes contain essential minerals such as potassium, magnesium, and copper. These minerals contribute to heart health, regulate blood pressure, and support overall physiological functions.

Here are some minerals found in mangoes and their benefits:

Potassium:

- **Benefits:**
    - Supports heart health by helping regulate blood pressure.
    - Facilitates proper muscle and nerve function.
    - Contributes to fluid balance in the body.

Magnesium:

- **Benefits:**
    - Aids in muscle and nerve function.
    - Supports bone health by working in conjunction with calcium.
    - Contributes to energy metabolism.

Copper:

- **Benefits:**
    - Essential for the formation of red blood cells and hemoglobin.
    - Supports the immune system.
    - Plays a role in the maintenance of healthy connective tissues.

Manganese:

- **Benefits:**
    - Supports bone formation and maintenance.

- Contributes to collagen production, promoting skin health.
- Participates in antioxidant enzyme function, helping combat oxidative stress.

Health Benefits:

Immune System Support:

- The high vitamin C content in mangoes boosts the immune system, aiding the body in defending against infections and illnesses.

Eye Health:

- Vitamin A, present in mangoes, is crucial for maintaining healthy vision and preventing conditions like night blindness.

Digestive Health:

- The fiber content in mangoes supports digestive health by preventing constipation and promoting a healthy gut microbiome.

Skin Health:

- Antioxidants in mangoes contribute to skin health by neutralizing free radicals and reducing oxidative stress. Mangoes are also used in some skincare products for their nourishing properties.

Nutritional Content

The nutritional content in 1 cup (approximately 165 grams) of diced mango typically includes:

- Calories: Around 99 kcal
- Carbohydrates: Approximately 25.7 grams
- Protein: Roughly 1.4 grams
- Fiber: About 2.8 grams
- Fat: Approximately 0.6 grams
- Sugar: Around 22 grams

Please note that these values are approximate and can vary slightly depending on factors such as the ripeness and variety of the mango. Mangos are delicious and nutritious fruit rich in vitamins, minerals, and antioxidants.

Culinary Versatility:

Fresh Mango Salsa:

- Dice ripe mangoes and combine them with tomatoes, red onion, cilantro, lime juice, and a hint of chili for a refreshing salsa. Perfect as a topping for grilled chicken or fish.

Mango Smoothie:

- Blend mango chunks with yogurt, banana, and a splash of orange juice for a delicious and nutritious smoothie.

Mango Sticky Rice:

- A popular dessert in Southeast Asia, mango sticky rice features sweet sticky rice topped with ripe mango slices and drizzled with coconut milk.

Mango Chutney:

- Cook diced mangoes with spices, vinegar, and sugar to create a flavorful mango chutney. Perfect as a condiment for grilled meats or as a dip.

Mangoes' sweet and tropical flavor makes them a delightful addition to various recipes, both sweet and savory.

Here are two delicious recipes featuring mango:

Mango Salsa:

Ingredients:

- 2 ripe mangoes, peeled, pitted, and diced
- 1 red bell pepper, diced
- 1/2 red onion, finely chopped
- 1 jalapeño, seeded and finely chopped
- 1/4 cup fresh cilantro, chopped
- Juice of 2 limes
- Salt and pepper to taste

Instructions:

1. In a large bowl, combine diced mangoes, red bell pepper, red onion, jalapeño, and cilantro.
2. Squeeze lime juice over the mixture and toss gently to combine.
3. Season with salt and pepper to taste.

4. Refrigerate for at least 30 minutes to allow the flavors to meld.
5. Serve the mango salsa with tortilla chips, grilled chicken, fish, or as a refreshing topping for tacos.

Mango Coconut Smoothie:

Ingredients:

- 1 ripe mango, peeled, pitted, and diced
- 1/2 cup coconut milk
- 1/2 cup plain Greek yogurt
- 1 tablespoon honey (optional, depending on sweetness preference)
- Ice cubes

Instructions:

1. In a blender, combine diced mango, coconut milk, Greek yogurt, and honey (if using).
2. Add ice cubes to achieve the desired consistency and blend until smooth.
3. Pour the mango coconut smoothie into glasses.
4. Garnish with additional mango slices or a sprinkle of shredded coconut if desired.
5. Enjoy this tropical and creamy smoothie as a refreshing breakfast or snack.

These recipes showcase the versatility of mangoes, whether used in a vibrant salsa or blended into a tropical smoothie. Enjoy the burst of flavor and nutritional benefits that mangoes bring to your table!

Conclusion:

Mangoes not only tantalize the taste buds with their sweetness but also contribute to overall health and well-being. If you have specific health concerns or conditions, it's advisable to consult with a healthcare professional or a registered dietitian for personalized advice. Whether enjoyed fresh, blended into smoothies, or incorporated into savory dishes, the versatility of mango makes it a delightful addition to a diverse range of culinary creations. So, savor the season's bounty and relish the benefits of the King of Fruits.

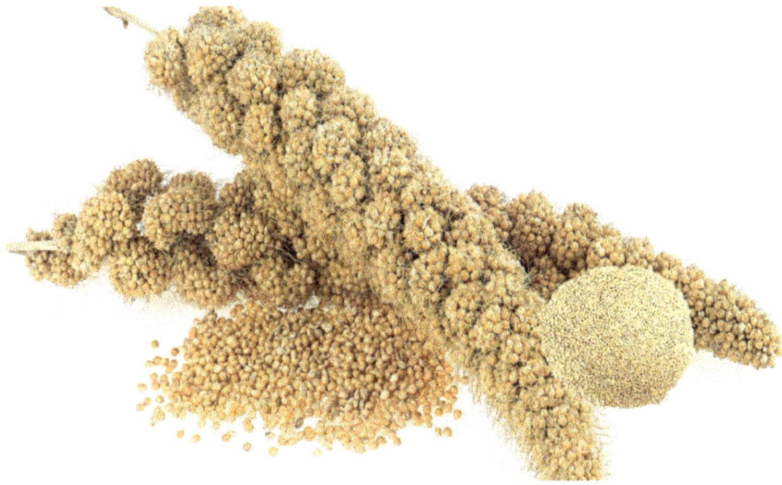

Millet

The Ancient Grain with Modern Appeal

Millet, often referred to as the "forgotten grain," has been a staple in diets across the world for thousands of years. While it may have faded from the spotlight in recent times, this ancient grain is making a comeback as a popular choice for those seeking nutritious and versatile alternatives to traditional grains. From its impressive health benefits to its wide range of culinary uses, millet is reclaiming its well-deserved place on the table.

Nutritional Powerhouse:

Millet boasts an impressive nutritional profile, packed with essential vitamins, minerals, fiber, and antioxidants. Here's a closer look at the key nutrients found in millet:

- **Protein:** Millet is a rich source of plant-based protein, making it an excellent option for vegetarians and vegans looking to meet their protein needs.
- **Dietary Fiber:** High in dietary fiber, millet supports digestive health, promotes satiety, and helps regulate blood sugar levels.

Vitamins:

Millet contains various vitamins, including B vitamins like niacin, thiamine, and folate, which are important for energy metabolism and overall health.

Vitamin B1 (Thiamine): Important for energy metabolism, nerve function, and maintaining a healthy appetite.

Vitamin B2 (Riboflavin): Necessary for energy production, cell growth, and antioxidant activity.

Vitamin B3 (Niacin): Supports energy metabolism, DNA repair, and skin health.

Vitamin B5 (Pantothenic Acid): Involved in energy metabolism, hormone synthesis, and nerve function.

Vitamin B6 (Pyridoxine): Essential for amino acid metabolism, neurotransmitter synthesis, and immune function.

Vitamin B9 (Folate): Important for cell division, DNA synthesis, and fetal development during pregnancy.

Vitamin E: An antioxidant that protects cells from oxidative damage and supports immune function.

Vitamin K: Crucial for blood clotting, bone health, and heart health.

These vitamins play various roles in the body, including supporting energy metabolism, promoting healthy cell growth and repair, aiding in immune function, and contributing to overall health and vitality. Incorporating millet into your diet can be a nutritious way to ensure you're getting these important vitamins.

Minerals:

Millet is rich in minerals such as magnesium, phosphorus, manganese, and iron, which are essential for bone health, energy production, and immune function.

1. **Magnesium:** Important for nerve function, muscle contraction, bone health, and energy metabolism.
2. **Phosphorus:** Essential for bone and teeth formation, DNA synthesis, and energy production.
3. **Potassium:** Crucial for nerve function, muscle contraction, and maintaining fluid balance in the body.
4. **Calcium:** Necessary for bone and teeth health, muscle function, and nerve transmission.
5. **Iron:** Vital for oxygen transport in the blood, energy production, and immune function.
6. **Zinc:** Essential for immune function, wound healing, and DNA synthesis.
7. **Copper:** Important for iron metabolism, antioxidant defense, and connective tissue formation.
8. **Manganese:** Necessary for bone formation, metabolism, and antioxidant activity.
9. **Selenium:** Acts as an antioxidant, supports thyroid function, and may have anti-inflammatory properties.
10. **Phytosterols:** Plant compounds that may help lower cholesterol levels and reduce the risk of heart disease.
11. **Phytic Acid (Phytate):** While considered an anti-nutrient due to its ability to bind to minerals and inhibit their absorption, phytic acid may also have antioxidant and anti-cancer properties.

12. **Fiber:** While not a mineral, fiber is abundant in millet and contributes to digestive health, blood sugar control, and satiety.

13. **Sulfur:** Found in various organic compounds, including amino acids, and plays a role in protein synthesis and overall cellular function.

These minerals play various critical roles in the body, including maintaining bone health, supporting energy production, aiding in immune function, and protecting against oxidative stress. Incorporating millet into your diet can be a nutritious way to ensure you're getting these important minerals.

Antioxidants:

Millet contains antioxidants like phenolic compounds, which help protect cells from oxidative damage and reduce the risk of chronic diseases.

Phenolic Compounds: Millet contains phenolic compounds such as ferulic acid, caffeic acid, and coumaric acid, which have antioxidant properties and contribute to its health benefits.

Lignans: Millet contains lignans, which are phytoestrogens with antioxidant properties that may help reduce the risk of chronic diseases such as heart disease and cancer.

Flavonoids: Flavonoids are a group of polyphenolic compounds found in plants, including millet. Examples of flavonoids found in millet include quercetin, kaempferol, and luteolin, which have antioxidant and anti-inflammatory properties.

Tocotrienols: Millet contains tocotrienols, a form of vitamin E, which have antioxidant properties and help protect cells from oxidative damage.

Carotenoids: Millet contains carotenoids such as lutein and zeaxanthin, which have antioxidant properties and contribute to eye health.

These antioxidants work together to scavenge free radicals, reduce oxidative stress, and support overall health. Incorporating millet into your diet as part of a balanced and varied plant-based diet can help provide a wide range of antioxidants to support your health and well-being.

Health Benefits:

Heart Health: The fiber, magnesium, and potassium in millet may help lower cholesterol levels, reduce blood pressure, and promote overall cardiovascular health.

Digestive Health: The high fiber content of millet supports digestive health by promoting regular bowel movements and preventing constipation.

Blood Sugar Control: Millet has a low glycemic index, meaning it causes a slower rise in blood sugar levels compared to refined grains. This can help stabilize blood sugar levels and reduce the risk of type 2 diabetes.

Weight Management: The fiber and protein in millet help promote feelings of fullness and satiety, which can aid in weight management and prevent overeating.

Bone Health: Millet is rich in minerals like calcium, phosphorus, and magnesium, which are important for bone health and may help reduce the risk of osteoporosis.

Nutritional Content

The nutritional content in 1 cup (approximately 174 grams) of cooked millet typically includes:

- Calories: Around 207 kcal
- Carbohydrates: Approximately 41 grams
- Protein: Roughly 6 grams
- Fiber: About 2.3 grams
- Fat: Approximately 1.7 grams
- Sugar: Less than 1 gram

Please note that these values are approximate and can vary slightly depending on factors such as the specific variety of millet and the cooking method. Millet is a nutritious whole grain that is gluten-free and rich in various vitamins, minerals, and antioxidants.

Culinary Uses:

Millet is incredibly versatile and can be used in a variety of culinary applications:

- **Grains:** Millet can be cooked and served as a nutritious and flavorful side dish, similar to rice or quinoa.
- **Porridge:** Millet can be cooked into a creamy porridge, sweetened with honey or maple syrup, and topped with fruits, nuts, or seeds for a hearty breakfast.
- **Baking:** Millet flour can be used in baking to make bread, muffins, pancakes, and other baked goods.
- **Salads:** Cooked millet can be added to salads for added texture and nutrition or used as a base for grain salads.
- **Stir-fries:** Millet can be added to stir-fries or fried rice for a nutritious and filling meal.

Here are two delicious recipes featuring millet:

Millet Veggie Stir-Fry

Ingredients:

- 1 cup millet, rinsed and drained
- 2 cups vegetable broth or water
- 2 tablespoons olive oil

- 2 cloves garlic, minced
- 1 onion, diced
- 2 carrots, diced
- 1 bell pepper, diced
- 1 cup broccoli florets
- 1 cup snow peas, trimmed
- 1/4 cup soy sauce or tamari
- 1 tablespoon rice vinegar
- 1 tablespoon sesame oil
- Salt and pepper to taste
- Optional garnish: sliced green onions, sesame seeds

Instructions:

1. In a medium saucepan, combine the rinsed millet and vegetable broth or water. Bring to a boil, then reduce heat to low, cover, and simmer for about 20-25 minutes, or until the millet is tender and the liquid is absorbed. Remove from heat and let it sit, covered, for 5 minutes. Fluff with a fork.
2. In a large skillet or wok, heat the olive oil over medium-high heat. Add the minced garlic and diced onion, and cook for 2-3 minutes, until softened and fragrant.
3. Add the diced carrots, bell pepper, broccoli florets, and snow peas to the skillet. Cook, stirring frequently, for 5-7 minutes, or until the vegetables are tender-crisp.
4. Add the cooked millet to the skillet with the vegetables, along with the soy sauce or tamari, rice vinegar, and sesame oil. Stir well to combine and coat everything evenly. Cook for an additional 2-3 minutes to heat through.
5. Season with salt and pepper to taste. Garnish with sliced green onions and sesame seeds, if desired.
6. Serve the millet veggie stir-fry hot as a flavorful and nutritious main dish.

Millet Breakfast Porridge

Ingredients:

- 1 cup millet, rinsed and drained
- 2 cups unsweetened almond milk or other plant-based milk
- 1 ripe banana, mashed

- 1 teaspoon ground cinnamon
- 1/2 teaspoon vanilla extract
- 1 tablespoon maple syrup or honey (optional)
- Fresh fruit, nuts, and seeds for topping (e.g., berries, sliced banana, chopped nuts, chia seeds)

Instructions:

1. In a medium saucepan, combine the rinsed millet and almond milk. Bring to a boil, then reduce heat to low, cover, and simmer for about 15-20 minutes, or until the millet is tender and the liquid is absorbed. Stir occasionally to prevent sticking.
2. Once the millet is cooked, remove from heat and stir in the mashed banana, ground cinnamon, vanilla extract, and maple syrup or honey (if using). Mix well to combine.
3. Serve the millet porridge hot, topped with your favorite fresh fruit, nuts, and seeds. Enjoy this comforting and nutritious breakfast to start your day on a delicious note.

These recipes showcase the versatility of millet and its ability to be incorporated into a variety of dishes, from savory stir-fries to sweet breakfast porridge. Feel free to customize the recipes with your favorite vegetables, spices, and toppings for a personalized touch!

Historical uses:

Millet has been cultivated and consumed by various cultures around the world for thousands of years. Here are two historical uses of millet:

Ancient Grain in China and East Asia:

Millet has a long history of cultivation in China and other parts of East Asia, dating back thousands of years. It was one of the earliest domesticated grains in the region and played a crucial role in the diet of ancient Chinese civilizations. Millet was grown in diverse climates and soil conditions, making it a resilient and adaptable crop for farmers. It was commonly used to make various staple foods, including porridge, flatbreads, noodles, and fermented beverages like millet wine. Millet also held cultural significance and was often featured in rituals, ceremonies, and religious offerings.

Traditional Grain in Africa:

Millet has been a staple food in many parts of Africa for centuries, particularly in regions with arid or semi-arid climates where other grains may not thrive. In sub-Saharan Africa, millet is commonly grown and consumed by various ethnic groups as a primary source of sustenance. It is used to make traditional dishes such as millet porridge, couscous, flatbreads, and fermented beverages like millet beer. Millet's drought-resistant nature and nutritional value make it an important crop for food security in regions prone to erratic rainfall and climate extremes.

These historical uses of millet highlight its importance as a staple food crop in diverse cultures and regions throughout history. Its resilience, nutritional value, and versatility have ensured its enduring popularity as a dietary staple for millions of people worldwide.

Conclusion:

Millet may have been overshadowed by other grains in recent times, but its nutritional benefits and culinary versatility make it a grain worth rediscovering. Whether you're looking to improve your health, diversify your diet, or experiment with new recipes, millet offers a delicious and nutritious alternative to traditional grains. So, the next time you're planning your meals, consider adding millet to your shopping list—you won't be disappointed!

If you have specific health concerns, allergies, or conditions, it's advisable to consult with a healthcare professional or a registered dietitian before making significant changes to your diet.

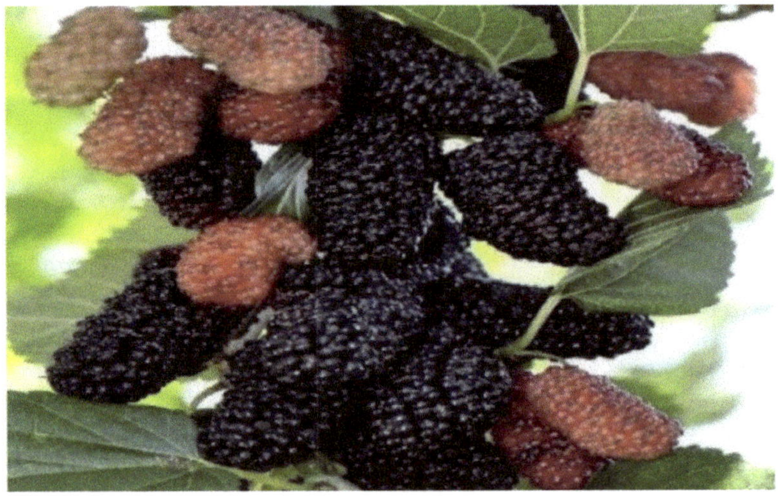

Mulberries

Unveiling the Nutritional Wonders of Mulberries: Benefits and Uses

Mulberries, the sweet and succulent fruits derived from the Morus genus of trees, have been cherished for centuries for both their delightful taste and impressive nutritional content. From boosting overall health to serving as a versatile ingredient in various culinary creations, mulberries have carved a niche as a wholesome and beneficial addition to diverse diets around the world.

Nutrient-Rich Powerhouse:

Mulberries are a nutritional powerhouse, offering a rich array of essential vitamins and minerals. Among the key nutrients found in mulberries are vitamin C, vitamin K, vitamin A, iron, potassium, and dietary fiber. Let's delve into the benefits associated with these essential elements:

Vitamin C:

- **Benefits:** Boosts the immune system, supports skin health, acts as an antioxidant, and aids in collagen production.

Vitamin K:

- **Benefits:** Essential for blood clotting, contributes to bone health, and helps regulate calcium in the body.

Vitamin A:

- **Benefits:** Supports vision health, immune function, and skin health; acts as an antioxidant.

Iron:

- **Benefits:** Important for oxygen transport in the blood, supports energy metabolism.

Potassium:

- **Benefits:** Helps regulate blood pressure, supports heart and muscle function, aids in fluid balance.

Dietary Fiber:

- **Benefits:** Promotes digestive health, helps regulate blood sugar levels, contributes to a feeling of fullness.

Vitamin E:

- **Benefits:** Acts as an antioxidant, supports skin health, protects cells from damage.

Vitamin B Complex (B1, B2, B3, B5, B6, B9):

- **Benefits:** Important for energy metabolism, supports nervous system function, aids in red blood cell formation.

Copper:

- **Benefits:** Important for iron absorption, supports the formation of red blood cells.

Manganese:

- **Benefits:** Contributes to bone formation, supports metabolism, acts as an antioxidant.

Zinc:

- **Benefits:** Supports immune function, involved in wound healing, essential for DNA synthesis.

Magnesium:

- **Benefits:** Important for muscle and nerve function, supports bone health, regulates blood sugar levels.

Antioxidant Rich:

Mulberries are known for their high levels of anthocyanins, a type of antioxidant responsible for the fruit's vibrant color. Antioxidants play a crucial role in neutralizing free radicals in the body, helping to protect cells from oxidative stress and reduce the risk of chronic diseases.

Heart Health:

Regular consumption of mulberries has been associated with heart health benefits. The potassium content helps maintain healthy blood pressure levels, while the antioxidants contribute to overall cardiovascular well-being. The dietary fiber in mulberries also aids in managing cholesterol levels.

Weight Management:

The high fiber content in mulberries makes them a satisfying and low-calorie snack, supporting weight management goals. The fiber contributes to a feeling of fullness, reducing the likelihood of overeating.

Nutritional Content

The nutritional content in 1 cup (approximately 140 grams) of fresh mulberries typically includes:

- Calories: Around 60 kcal
- Carbohydrates: Approximately 14 grams
- Protein: Roughly 2 grams
- Fiber: About 2.5 grams
- Fat: Approximately 0.4 grams
- Sugar: Around 10 grams

Please note that these values are approximate and can vary slightly depending on factors such as the variety of mulberries and their ripeness. Mulberries are a nutritious fruit rich in vitamins, minerals, and antioxidants.

Culinary Versatility:

Mulberries can be enjoyed in various culinary forms, adding a burst of flavor and nutrition to meals and snacks. Here are some popular uses:

Fresh Snacking: Enjoy mulberries on their own as a sweet and nutritious snack.

Smoothies and Yogurt Bowls: Add fresh or dried mulberries to smoothies or yogurt bowls for a tasty and nutrient-rich boost.

Baking: Incorporate mulberries into muffins, pancakes, or desserts for a natural sweetness and added nutritional value.

Jam and Preserves: Make homemade mulberry jam or preserves to spread on toast or use as a topping for desserts.

Here are two delicious recipes that incorporate the sweet and nutritious flavor of mulberries:

Mulberry Smoothie Bowl:

Ingredients:

- 1 cup frozen mixed berries (including mulberries)
- 1 ripe banana

- 1/2 cup Greek yogurt
- 1/2 cup almond milk (or any preferred milk)
- 1 tablespoon chia seeds
- Toppings: Fresh mulberries, sliced banana, granola, and a drizzle of honey

Instructions:

1. In a blender, combine frozen mixed berries, banana, Greek yogurt, almond milk, and chia seeds.
2. Blend until smooth and creamy, adjusting the consistency with more milk if needed.
3. Pour the smoothie into a bowl.
4. Top with fresh mulberries, sliced banana, granola, and a drizzle of honey.
5. Enjoy this vibrant and nutrient-packed mulberry smoothie bowl for a delicious and satisfying breakfast or snack.

Mulberry and Almond Oat Bars:

Ingredients:

- 1 cup rollcd oats
- 1/2 cup almond butter
- 1/3 cup honey or maple syrup
- 1/2 cup chopped almonds
- 1/2 cup dried mulberries
- 1/4 cup shredded coconut
- 1 teaspoon vanilla extract
- A pinch of salt

Instructions:

1. Preheat the oven to 350°F (180°C) and line a baking dish with parchment paper.
2. In a mixing bowl, combine rolled oats, almond butter, honey or maple syrup, chopped almonds, dried mulberries, shredded coconut, vanilla extract, and a pinch of salt.
3. Mix until all ingredients are well combined.
4. Press the mixture into the prepared baking dish, creating an even layer.
5. Bake for 15-20 minutes or until the edges are golden brown.

6. Allow the bars to cool completely before cutting them into squares or bars.
7. Store in an airtight container for a delicious and wholesome snack.

These recipes showcase the versatility of mulberries, whether blended into a refreshing smoothie bowl or incorporated into nutritious oat bars. Enjoy the unique and delightful taste of mulberries in these creative and health-conscious recipes!

Conclusion:

Mulberries stand out not only for their delectable taste but also for the multitude of health benefits they offer. From supporting immune function to promoting heart health and aiding in weight management, mulberries are a versatile and nutritious addition to a well-balanced diet. If you have specific health concerns, allergies, or conditions, it's advisable to consult with a healthcare professional or a registered dietitian before making significant changes to your diet.

Whether enjoyed fresh, dried, or incorporated into various culinary creations, mulberries are a delightful way to embrace the goodness of nature and enhance overall well-being.

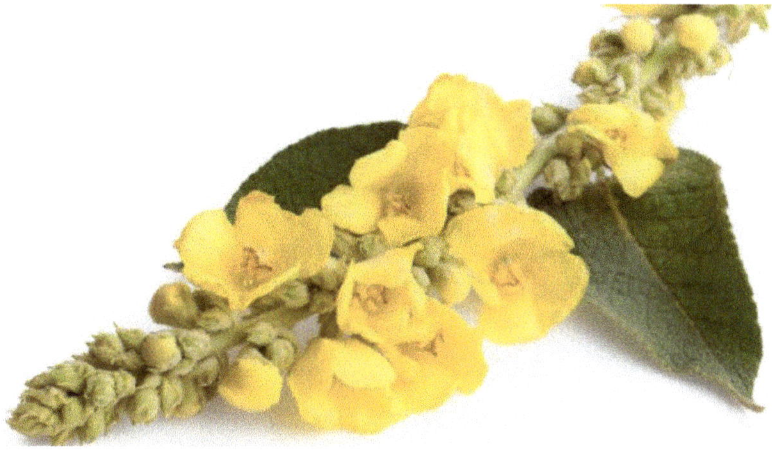

Mullein

Unveiling the Versatility of Mullein: Benefits and Uses

Mullein, scientifically known as Verbascum thapsus, is a biennial herb native to Europe, Asia, and North Africa, but it has since naturalized in various regions around the world. Revered for its striking appearance and myriad medicinal properties, mullein has been used for centuries in traditional herbal medicine and cultural practices. Let's explore the numerous benefits and versatile uses of this remarkable herb.

A Botanical Profile:

Mullein is characterized by its tall, erect stem adorned with soft, fuzzy leaves and vibrant yellow flowers. The leaves and flowers of the mullein plant are the primary parts used for medicinal and therapeutic purposes. Historically, mullein leaves were used as torches or candlewicks due to their flammability and absorbent qualities, earning the plant the nickname "torch plant" or "candlewick plant."

Mullein, scientifically known as Verbascum thapsus, is a flowering plant native to Europe, Asia, and North Africa, but it has since been naturalized to various regions around the world. Revered for its numerous medicinal properties, mullein has a long history of use in traditional herbal medicine. While mullein is not particularly rich in vitamins, minerals, or antioxidants compared to some other plants, it does contain certain beneficial compounds. Here are some of the components found in mullein and their potential benefits:

Components of Mullein:

Flavonoids:

- Flavonoids are antioxidants found in mullein that help protect cells from oxidative damage caused by free radicals. They may contribute to reducing inflammation and supporting overall health.

Saponins:

- Saponins are natural compounds with expectorant properties, which means they help loosen mucus and facilitate its expulsion from the respiratory tract. This makes mullein beneficial for respiratory conditions such as coughs and bronchitis.

Mucilage:

- Mullein contains mucilage, a gel-like substance that has demulcent properties. Mucilage forms a soothing coating when ingested, which can help alleviate irritation and inflammation in the throat and digestive tract.

Tannins:

- Tannins are astringent compounds found in mullein that may have antimicrobial and anti-inflammatory properties. They help tighten and tone mucous membranes, making them useful for treating diarrhea and other gastrointestinal issues.

Minerals:

- While mullein is not particularly high in specific minerals, it does contain small amounts of potassium, calcium, magnesium, and iron. These minerals play essential roles in various bodily functions, including nerve function, muscle contraction, and blood oxygenation.

Health Benefits:

Respiratory Support:

- Mullein has long been prized for its respiratory benefits, particularly for addressing coughs, bronchitis, and congestion. It acts as an expectorant, helping to expel mucus from the respiratory tract and soothe irritated airways.

Anti-inflammatory Properties:

- The anti-inflammatory compounds found in mullein make it effective for reducing inflammation and discomfort associated with conditions such as sore throat, earaches, and swollen glands.

Pain Relief:

- Mullein is known for its mild analgesic properties, which can help alleviate pain and discomfort caused by various ailments, including arthritis, headaches, and minor injuries.

Ear Health:

- Mullein oil or ear drops made from mullein flowers infused in oil have been traditionally used to address ear infections, earaches, and excess ear wax buildup. The oil helps soften ear wax and soothe inflammation in the ear canal.

Skin Care:

- Mullein possesses emollient properties that can benefit the skin. Mullein-infused oils or salves are used topically to soothe dry, irritated skin, relieve minor burns, and promote wound healing.

Digestive Support:

- Mucilage and tannins found in mullein can help soothe digestive discomfort, alleviate diarrhea, and support overall gastrointestinal health.

Culinary and Cultural Uses:

Herbal Teas and Infusions:

- Mullein leaves and flowers are commonly used to prepare herbal teas and infusions. The mild, slightly sweet flavor of mullein makes it a pleasant addition to herbal blends designed to support respiratory health and overall well-being.

Mullein, with its subtle flavor and medicinal properties, is not commonly used in culinary recipes due to its primarily medicinal role. However, it can be incorporated into herbal preparations such as teas or infused oils.

Here are two simple recipes featuring mullein:

Mullein Tea:

Ingredients:

- 1-2 teaspoons dried mullein leaves and/or flowers
- 1 cup water
- Optional: honey, lemon, or other flavorings

Instructions:

1. Bring 1 cup of water to a boil in a small saucepan.
2. Add 1-2 teaspoons of dried mullein leaves and/or flowers to the boiling water.
3. Reduce the heat to low and let the mullein steep in the water for 10-15 minutes.
4. Strain the tea into a cup using a fine mesh strainer or tea infuser.
5. Sweeten the tea with honey and add lemon or other flavorings to taste, if desired.
6. Enjoy the soothing and medicinal benefits of mullein tea.

Mullein Infused Oil:

Ingredients:

- Fresh mullein flowers and/or leaves
- Carrier oil (such as olive oil or coconut oil)

Instructions:

1. Harvest fresh mullein flowers and/or leaves from the plant.
2. Wash and dry the mullein thoroughly to remove any dirt or debris.
3. Chop or crush the mullein flowers and leaves to release their aromatic oils.
4. Place the chopped mullein into a clean, dry glass jar.
5. Pour enough carrier oil over the mullein to completely cover it, ensuring that there are no air bubbles.
6. Seal the jar tightly with a lid and place it in a warm, sunny location to infuse for 4-6 weeks, shaking the jar gently every few days.
7. After the infusion period, strain the oil through a fine mesh strainer or cheesecloth to remove the mullein plant material.

8. Transfer the infused oil to a clean, dry glass bottle or jar for storage.
9. Use the mullein infused oil topically as a soothing massage oil or herbal remedy for various skin conditions.

These recipes demonstrate simple ways to incorporate mullein into herbal preparations for both internal and external use. As always, it's essential to harvest mullein ethically and ensure that you have correctly identified the plant before use. If you are unsure, consult with a knowledgeable herbalist or botanist.

Smoking and Vaporization:

Historically, mullein leaves were smoked or vaporized for their potential respiratory benefits. While smoking is generally discouraged due to its health risks, some individuals use mullein leaves in smoking blends as a tobacco alternative.

Harvesting and Preparation:

Mullein leaves are typically harvested in the summer months when the plant is in full bloom. The leaves can be dried and stored for later use in teas, tinctures, or herbal preparations. Mullein flowers can also be harvested and infused in oil to create mullein oil, which is used topically for various purposes.

Tips on Growing Mullein

Mullein (Verbascum thapsus) is a biennial plant, meaning it completes its life cycle over two growing seasons. Here's a detailed breakdown of the growth timeline for mullein:

Year 1:

1. **Spring**: Mullein seeds germinate in early spring when temperatures begin to warm, typically within 1 to 3 weeks after sowing.
2. **Seedling Stage**: After germination, mullein plants develop into rosettes of large, fuzzy leaves during the first growing season. These basal leaves remain close to the ground and do not produce a flowering stalk in the first year.
3. **Vegetative Growth**: Throughout the spring and summer, mullein plants focus on establishing a strong root system and accumulating energy through photosynthesis. They continue to grow and develop more leaves but do not flower.
4. **Winter Dormancy**: In colder climates, mullein plants may enter a period of dormancy or semi-dormancy during the winter months. The rosettes of leaves persist through the winter, ready to resume growth in the following spring.

Year 2:

1. **Spring**: As temperatures warm in the second year, mullein plants begin to send up a tall flowering stalk from the center of the leaf rosette. This usually occurs in late spring or early summer.
2. **Flowering Stage**: The flowering stalk of mullein can grow rapidly, reaching heights of 3 to 8 feet (1 to 2.5 meters) or more. The stalk produces numerous small, yellow flowers arranged in dense spikes along its length. Mullein flowers are pollinated by insects.
3. **Seed Production**: After flowering, mullein plants produce seed capsules containing many tiny seeds. These capsules mature and dry on the plant over the summer months.

4. **Seed Dispersal**: By late summer or early fall, the seed capsules of mullein mature and split open, releasing the seeds. Mullein seeds are small and lightweight, allowing them to be dispersed by wind, animals, or human activity.
5. **End of Life Cycle**: After completing the flowering and seed production stages, mullein plants typically die back and senesce. By the end of the second growing season, the plants have completed their life cycle, and new seedlings may emerge from the dispersed seeds to start the process anew.

Overall Duration:

- From germination to the end of the plant's life cycle, mullein typically takes about 1.5 to 2 years to grow and complete its reproductive cycle. The exact timing may vary depending on factors such as climate, soil conditions, and growing conditions.

Precautions and Considerations:

While mullein is generally considered safe for most people when used appropriately, it's essential to exercise caution and consult with a healthcare professional before using mullein, especially if you are pregnant, breastfeeding, or taking medications. Some individuals may experience allergic reactions or adverse effects when using mullein.

Conclusion:

Mullein stands as a testament to the power of nature's remedies and the enduring legacy of traditional herbal medicine. Whether enjoyed as a soothing herbal tea, a natural remedy for respiratory ailments, or a topical treatment for skin conditions, mullein continues to captivate with its diverse benefits and versatile uses. Embrace the healing properties of mullein and discover the wonders it holds for mind, body, and spirit.

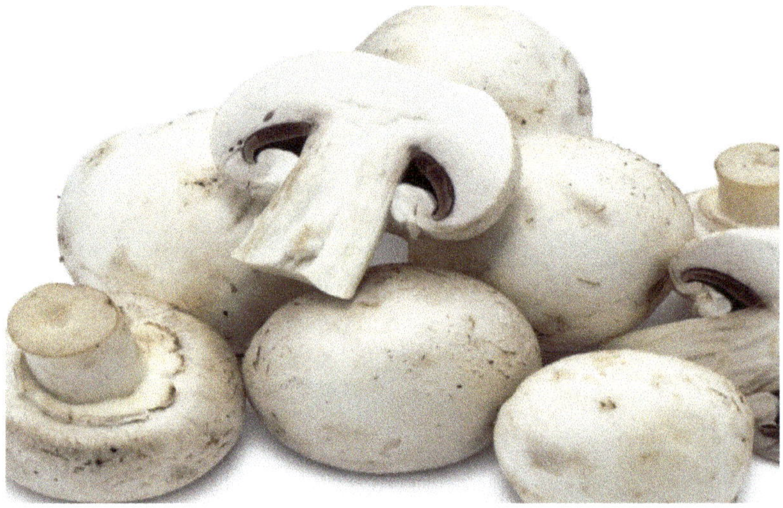

Mushrooms

The Magic of Mushrooms: A Nutrient-Rich Fungi with Health Benefits and Culinary Versatility

Mushrooms, the earthy wonders that emerge from the forest floor, have captivated the human palate for centuries. Beyond their unique taste and texture, mushrooms boast an impressive nutritional profile and a multitude of health benefits. In this article, we will explore the advantages of incorporating mushrooms into your diet, as well as the diverse culinary uses that make them a beloved ingredient across various cuisines.

Nutritional Powerhouse:

Mushrooms are a nutritional powerhouse, offering an array of vitamins, minerals, antioxidants, and other bioactive compounds. While the nutritional content can vary between mushroom varieties, a typical serving provides:

B Vitamins:

Mushrooms are a rich source of various B vitamins, including riboflavin (B2), niacin (B3), pantothenic acid (B5), and biotin (B7). These vitamins play crucial roles in energy metabolism, red blood cell formation, and overall cellular function.

B1 (Thiamine):

- **Benefits:** Thiamine is essential for energy metabolism. It helps convert carbohydrates into usable energy for the body. Thiamine also plays a role in nerve function and overall cellular health.

B2 (Riboflavin):

- **Benefits:** Riboflavin is involved in energy production and metabolism. It contributes to the conversion of food into usable energy and supports the health of the skin, eyes, and nerve functions.

B3 (Niacin):

- **Benefits:** Niacin is important for energy production, DNA repair, and skin health. It also helps regulate cholesterol levels and supports overall cardiovascular health.

B5 (Pantothenic Acid):

- **Benefits:** Pantothenic acid is involved in the synthesis of fatty acids and is essential for the metabolism of carbohydrates, proteins, and fats. It also plays a role in supporting adrenal function.

B6 (Pyridoxine):

- **Benefits:** Vitamin B6 is involved in various metabolic processes, including amino acid metabolism and neurotransmitter synthesis. It contributes to the formation of red blood cells and supports the immune system.

B7 (Biotin):

- **Benefits:** Biotin plays a role in energy metabolism, supporting the conversion of food into usable energy. It is also involved in the synthesis of fatty acids and the maintenance of healthy skin, hair, and nails.

B9 (Folate):

- **Benefits:** Folate is crucial for DNA synthesis and cell division. Adequate folate intake is particularly important during pregnancy as it helps prevent neural tube defects in the developing fetus. Folate also supports overall cellular function.

B12 (Cobalamin):

- **Benefits:** While mushrooms naturally contain minimal amounts of B12, some varieties may be exposed to B12 during processing. B12 is essential for nerve function, the formation of red blood cells, and DNA synthesis.

Vitamin D:

- Some mushrooms, when exposed to sunlight or ultraviolet (UV) light during growth, can produce vitamin D. This nutrient is essential for bone health, immune function, and overall well-being.

Minerals:

Mushrooms provide minerals such as selenium, copper, potassium, and phosphorus, which contribute to various physiological functions, including antioxidant defense and bone health.

Copper:

- **Benefits:** Copper is essential for the formation of red blood cells, collagen production, and the proper functioning of the nervous and immune systems. It also acts as an antioxidant, helping to protect cells from oxidative damage.

Selenium:

- **Benefits:** Selenium is an important antioxidant that helps protect cells from oxidative stress. It also supports the immune system and thyroid function. Selenium in mushrooms may vary based on the selenium content of the soil in which they are grown.

Potassium:

- **Benefits:** Potassium is crucial for maintaining proper fluid balance, nerve transmission, and muscle contraction. It also helps regulate blood pressure and support heart health.

Phosphorus:

- **Benefits:** Phosphorus is essential for bone and teeth formation, energy metabolism, and the synthesis of DNA and RNA. It also plays a role in maintaining the pH balance of body fluids.

Zinc:

- **Benefits:** Zinc is involved in immune function, wound healing, and the synthesis of DNA. It also plays a role in taste and smell perception. Zinc content in mushrooms may vary depending on the growing conditions.

Iron:

- **Benefits:** Iron is essential for the formation of hemoglobin, the protein in red blood cells that carries oxygen. Adequate iron intake helps prevent anemia and supports overall energy metabolism.

Magnesium:

- **Benefits:** Magnesium is involved in over 300 enzymatic reactions in the body, including energy metabolism, muscle and nerve function, and bone health. It also contributes to the regulation of blood pressure.

Calcium:

- **Benefits:** While mushrooms contain smaller amounts of calcium compared to dairy products, calcium is essential for bone and teeth formation, blood clotting, and muscle function.

Antioxidants:

Rich in antioxidants like ergothioneine and glutathione, mushrooms help combat oxidative stress and inflammation in the body. These compounds may contribute to a reduced risk of chronic diseases.

Ergothioneine:

- **Benefits:** Ergothioneine is a powerful antioxidant that helps protect cells from oxidative stress. It has been linked to anti-inflammatory properties and may contribute to overall cellular health.

Glutathione:

- **Benefits:** Glutathione is a potent antioxidant that plays a crucial role in the detoxification of harmful substances in the body. It also supports the immune system and helps neutralize free radicals.

Vitamin C:

- **Benefits:** Ascorbic acid, or vitamin C, is a well-known antioxidant that protects cells from oxidative stress. It supports the immune system, aids in the absorption of non-heme iron, and contributes to collagen synthesis for skin health.

Vitamin E:

- **Benefits:** Tocopherols, collectively known as vitamin E, are antioxidants that protect cell membranes from oxidative damage. They contribute to skin health and support the immune system.

Polyphenols:

- **Benefits:** Polyphenols are a group of antioxidants found in various plant foods, including mushrooms. They have anti-inflammatory and antioxidant properties, potentially reducing the risk of chronic diseases.

Beta-Glucans:

- **Benefits:** Beta-glucans are compounds found in the cell walls of mushrooms. They have immune-modulating properties and act as antioxidants, contributing to overall health and well-being.

Health Benefits:

Immune Support:

- The beta-glucans present in mushrooms have been linked to immune system modulation, enhancing the body's ability to fight infections and diseases.

Heart Health:

- Mushrooms can help maintain heart health by contributing to the regulation of cholesterol levels. Beta-glucans and fiber in mushrooms play a role in managing blood lipid profiles.

Weight Management:

- With their low calorie and high fiber content, mushrooms can be a valuable addition to a weight management plan. They provide satiety without contributing excess calories.

Anti-Inflammatory Properties:

- Bioactive compounds in mushrooms, such as ergothioneine, possess anti-inflammatory properties that may contribute to reducing the risk of chronic inflammatory conditions.

Nutritional Content

The nutritional content in 1 cup (approximately 70 grams) of sliced mushrooms typically includes:

- Calories: Around 15 kcal
- Carbohydrates: Approximately 2.3 grams
- Protein: Roughly 2.2 grams
- Fiber: About 0.7 grams
- Fat: Approximately 0.2 grams
- Sugar: Less than 1 gram

Please note that these values are approximate and can vary slightly depending on factors such as the specific type of mushrooms and whether they are cooked or raw. Mushrooms are low in calories and fat but rich in various vitamins, minerals, and antioxidants.

Culinary Uses:

Sautéed Mushrooms:

- Sautéing mushrooms in olive oil with garlic and herbs creates a versatile and flavorful side dish. Enjoy them on their own or use them as a topping for steaks, pasta, or omelets.

Mushroom Risotto:

- Incorporate mushrooms into a creamy risotto for a comforting and satisfying meal. The earthy flavor of mushrooms pairs well with the richness of Arborio rice and Parmesan cheese.

Grilled Portobello Mushrooms:

- Marinate large Portobello mushrooms and grill them for a delicious meaty texture. Serve them as a burger substitute or as a flavorful topping for salads.

Mushroom Soup:

- A classic mushroom soup, whether creamy or broth-based, showcases the depth of flavor mushrooms can bring to a dish. Add herbs and spices for an extra layer of complexity.

Creamy Mushroom Risotto:

Ingredients:

- 1 cup Arborio rice
- 8 oz (about 225g) mushrooms, sliced (button, cremini, or shiitake)
- 1 small onion, finely chopped
- 2 cloves garlic, minced
- 1/2 cup dry white wine
- 4 cups vegetable or chicken broth, kept warm
- 2 tablespoons olive oil
- 1/2 cup Parmesan cheese, grated
- Salt and pepper to taste
- Fresh parsley, chopped (for garnish)

Instructions:

1. In a large pan, heat olive oil over medium heat. Add chopped onions and garlic, sauté until softened.
2. Add sliced mushrooms and cook until they release their moisture and become golden brown.
3. Stir in Arborio rice and cook for 1-2 minutes until the rice is lightly toasted.
4. Pour in the white wine and cook until it's mostly absorbed by the rice.
5. Begin adding warm broth one ladle at a time, stirring frequently. Allow each ladle of broth to be absorbed before adding the next.
6. Continue this process until the rice is creamy and cooked to al dente texture.
7. Stir in grated Parmesan cheese and season with salt and pepper to taste.
8. Garnish with chopped fresh parsley before serving.

Stuffed Portobello Mushrooms:

Ingredients:

- 4 large Portobello mushrooms, stems removed
- 1 cup spinach, chopped

- 1/2 cup sun-dried tomatoes, chopped
- 1/2 cup feta or goat cheese, crumbled
- 2 cloves garlic, minced
- 2 tablespoons balsamic vinegar
- 2 tablespoons olive oil
- Salt and pepper to taste
- Fresh basil, chopped (for garnish)

Instructions:

1. Preheat the oven to 375°F (190°C). Line a baking sheet with parchment paper.
2. In a bowl, mix chopped spinach, sun-dried tomatoes, crumbled cheese, minced garlic, balsamic vinegar, and olive oil. Season with salt and pepper.
3. Place the Portobello mushrooms on the prepared baking sheet.
4. Stuff each mushroom cap with the spinach and cheese mixture.
5. Bake in the preheated oven for about 20-25 minutes or until the mushrooms are tender.
6. Garnish with chopped fresh basil before serving.

These mushroom recipes showcase the versatility of this fungi, whether incorporated into a creamy and comforting risotto or transformed into a flavorful stuffed dish. Enjoy the rich and earthy flavors of mushrooms in these delicious and satisfying recipes.

Historical uses:

Mushrooms have a long history of use by various cultures around the world, both for culinary and medicinal purposes.

Culinary Use in Ancient Rome:

- Mushrooms were highly valued in Ancient Rome and were considered a delicacy among the elite. The Romans cultivated mushrooms, and they were often featured in extravagant banquets and feasts. The philosopher Pliny the Elder documented the cultivation of mushrooms in his natural history writings, highlighting their popularity among the Roman aristocracy. Mushrooms were often prepared in various dishes, such as sauces and stews, showcasing their versatility in Roman cuisine.

These historical uses of mushrooms reflect the diverse ways in which cultures have appreciated and integrated these fungi into their daily lives, whether for health-promoting purposes or culinary enjoyment. Over time, mushrooms have continued to be valued for their unique qualities and have become a staple in cuisines and traditional medicine practices across the globe.

Tips on Growing Mushrooms

The time it takes for mushrooms to grow from inoculation to harvest depends on various factors, including the species of mushroom, the growing method, and environmental conditions. Here's a detailed breakdown of the typical growth stages of mushrooms using the common example of cultivating button mushrooms (Agaricus bisporus), which are one of the most widely cultivated mushroom species:

1. **Spawn Run (2-4 weeks)**:
   - The process begins with the inoculation of a substrate (such as compost or sterilized organic material) with mushroom spawn.
   - During the spawn run phase, mycelium (the vegetative part of the fungus) colonizes the substrate. This stage usually takes 2 to 4 weeks, during which the mycelium spreads throughout the substrate, forming a network of fine white threads.
2. **Casing (1-2 weeks)**:
   - After the spawn run, the substrate is typically covered with a layer of casing material (such as peat moss or vermiculite) to provide moisture and support for fruiting.
   - During casing, the mycelium colonizes the casing layer and prepares for the formation of mushroom primordia (tiny mushroom pins).
3. **Pin Formation (1-2 weeks)**:
   - Once the casing layer is fully colonized, environmental conditions such as temperature, humidity, and light are manipulated to induce pin formation.
   - Mushroom primordia begin to form, appearing as small bumps or pins on the surface of the casing layer.
   - This stage typically lasts 1 to 2 weeks, during which the primordia develop into mature mushrooms.
4. **Fruiting (1-2 weeks)**:
   - The pins continue to develop into mature mushrooms during the fruiting stage.
   - Mushrooms grow rapidly, increasing in size and developing caps and stems.
   - Fruiting typically lasts 1 to 2 weeks, depending on the species and environmental conditions.
5. **Harvest**:
   - Mushrooms are ready for harvest once they reach the desired size and maturity.

- Harvesting is usually done by gently twisting or cutting the mushrooms at the base of the stem to avoid damaging the mycelium.
- Harvested mushrooms can be consumed fresh or processed for storage.

6. **Flushes**:

- After the initial harvest, some mushroom species may produce additional flushes of mushrooms over several weeks or months, depending on the species and growing conditions.
- Each flush may require adjustments to environmental conditions to promote optimal mushroom growth.

It's important to note that the timelines provided are approximate and can vary depending on factors such as mushroom species, growing method, substrate composition, and environmental conditions. Additionally, different species of mushrooms may have different growth requirements and timelines.

Conclusion:

Mushrooms, with their distinctive flavor and remarkable nutritional benefits, have rightfully earned their place as a culinary and health-promoting treasure. Whether enjoyed as a savory side dish, a hearty main course, or a nourishing addition to soups and stews, mushrooms offer a delectable way to enhance both the taste and nutritional value of your meals. If you have specific health concerns, allergies, or conditions, it's advisable to consult with a healthcare professional or a registered dietitian before making significant changes to your diet.

Embrace the magic of mushrooms and savor the diverse benefits they bring to your table and well-being.

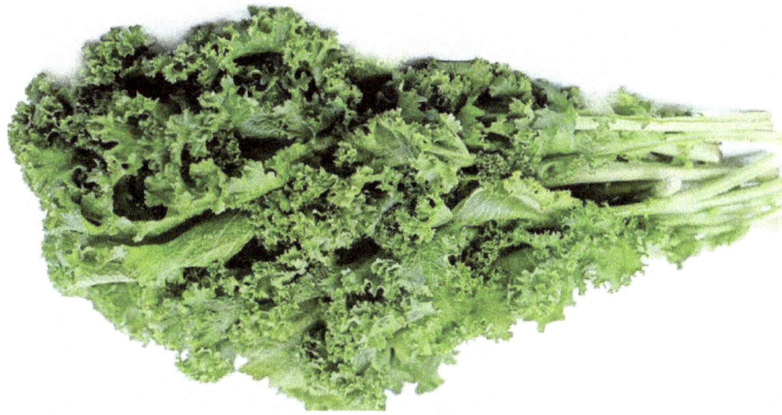

Mustard Greens

A Nutrient-Rich Powerhouse for Health and Culinary Delight

Mustard greens, with their bold flavor and robust nutritional profile, have earned their place as a staple in various cuisines around the world. These leafy greens, part of the Brassicaceae family, share a botanical lineage with kale, broccoli, and Brussels sprouts. Beyond their culinary versatility, mustard greens offer an array of health benefits, making them a valuable addition to a well-balanced diet. In this article, we'll explore the numerous advantages and creative uses that make mustard greens a nutritional powerhouse.

Nutrient-Rich Composition:

Mustard greens are celebrated for their dense concentration of essential nutrients, providing a wide array of vitamins, minerals, and antioxidants. Here's a closer look at the key components that make mustard greens a nutritional powerhouse:

Vitamins:

Vitamin K:

- Mustard greens are particularly rich in vitamin K, which plays a crucial role in blood clotting and bone metabolism.

Vitamin A:

- Mustard greens contain beta-carotene, a precursor to vitamin A, which is essential for vision, immune function, and skin health.

Vitamin C:

- Mustard greens are a good source of vitamin C, a powerful antioxidant that supports the immune system and promotes collagen synthesis.

Vitamin E:

- While present in smaller amounts compared to some other vitamins, mustard greens contribute to vitamin E intake, providing antioxidant benefits.

Vitamin B6 (Pyridoxine):

- Mustard greens contain vitamin B6, which is important for the metabolism of amino acids and the synthesis of neurotransmitters.

Folate (Vitamin B9):

- Folate is present in mustard greens and is essential for DNA synthesis and cell division.

Riboflavin (Vitamin B2):

- Mustard greens provide riboflavin, a B-vitamin involved in energy production and the metabolism of fats.

Thiamine (Vitamin B1):

- Thiamine is found in mustard greens and is essential for energy metabolism and nerve cell function.

Niacin (Vitamin B3):

- Mustard greens contain niacin, a B-vitamin important for energy metabolism and the health of the nervous system.

Vitamin C:

- Mustard greens are a good source of vitamin C, a powerful antioxidant that supports the immune system and promotes collagen synthesis.

Including mustard greens in your diet can contribute to meeting your daily vitamin needs and provide a wide range of health benefits associated with these essential nutrients. As with any food, it's important to consume a variety of nutrient-rich foods to ensure a balanced intake of vitamins and other essential nutrients.

Minerals:

Mustard greens are rich in various minerals that contribute to their nutritional value. Here is a list of minerals found in mustard greens:

Calcium:

- Mustard greens provide calcium, which is crucial for bone health, nerve function, and blood clotting.

Iron:

- Iron is present in mustard greens and is essential for the formation of hemoglobin, the protein responsible for carrying oxygen in the blood.

Magnesium:

- Magnesium in mustard greens supports muscle and nerve function, regulates blood pressure, and contributes to bone health.

Potassium:

- Mustard greens are a good source of potassium, an electrolyte that helps regulate fluid balance, nerve signals, and muscle contractions.

Phosphorus:

- Phosphorus is present in mustard greens and is essential for bone and teeth formation, DNA synthesis, and energy metabolism.

Manganese:

- Manganese is a trace mineral found in mustard greens, contributing to bone formation, blood clotting, and reducing inflammation.

Zinc:

- Mustard greens contain zinc, a trace mineral that plays a role in immune function, wound healing, and DNA synthesis.

Copper:

- Copper is present in mustard greens and is essential for the formation of red blood cells, maintenance of healthy bones and nerves, and immune system function.

Selenium:

- While present in smaller amounts compared to some other minerals, mustard greens contribute to selenium intake, supporting immune function and acting as an antioxidant.

Including mustard greens in your diet can help ensure a diverse intake of minerals, supporting various physiological functions and promoting overall health. As with any food, it's important to consume a variety of nutrient-rich foods to ensure a broad spectrum of minerals and other essential nutrients.

Antioxidants:

Mustard greens contain a variety of antioxidants, including beta-carotene, lutein, and zeaxanthin, which help combat oxidative stress and reduce inflammation.

Beta-Carotene:

- Beta-carotene is a precursor to vitamin A and acts as a powerful antioxidant. Mustard greens contain beta-carotene, contributing to eye health and overall antioxidant defense.

Lutein:

- Mustard greens are rich in lutein, a carotenoid that plays a crucial role in maintaining eye health and preventing age-related macular degeneration.

Zeaxanthin:

- Zeaxanthin, another carotenoid found in mustard greens, works alongside lutein to support eye health and protect against oxidative damage.

Quercetin:

- Quercetin is a flavonoid with antioxidant properties that may help reduce inflammation and lower the risk of chronic diseases. Mustard greens contain quercetin.

Kaempferol:

- Kaempferol is a flavonoid with antioxidant and anti-inflammatory properties. It is found in various leafy greens, including mustard greens.

Glucosinolates:

- Mustard greens belong to the Brassica family, known for its rich content of glucosinolates. These compounds have antioxidant and anti-cancer properties.

Vitamin E:

- While present in smaller amounts compared to some other antioxidants, mustard greens contribute to vitamin E intake, providing fat-soluble antioxidant benefits.

Selenium:

- Mustard greens contain selenium, a trace mineral with antioxidant properties that work in conjunction with other antioxidants to protect cells from oxidative stress.

Consuming a diet rich in antioxidants, such as those found in mustard greens, can help support overall health and may contribute to the prevention of chronic diseases associated with oxidative damage. As with any food, it's essential to include a variety of antioxidant-rich foods in your diet for optimal health benefits.

Fiber:

- A rich source of dietary fiber, mustard greens promote digestive health, regulate blood sugar levels, and contribute to a feeling of fullness.

Health Benefits:

Bone Health:

- The high vitamin K and calcium content in mustard greens supports bone health, aiding in bone density and strength.

Heart Health:

- Potassium, magnesium, and fiber contribute to heart health by regulating blood pressure, reducing cholesterol levels, and supporting overall cardiovascular function.

Anti-Inflammatory Properties:

- The antioxidants in mustard greens help combat inflammation, potentially reducing the risk of chronic diseases.

Vision Support:

- Lutein and zeaxanthin in mustard greens play a role in maintaining eye health and may reduce the risk of age-related macular degeneration.

Nutritional Content

The nutritional content in 1 cup (approximately 56 grams) of chopped mustard greens typically includes:

- Calories: Around 15 kcal
- Carbohydrates: Approximately 2 grams
- Protein: Roughly 1.5 grams
- Fiber: About 1.5 grams
- Fat: Approximately 0.2 grams
- Sugar: Less than 1 gram

Please note that these values are approximate and can vary slightly depending on factors such as the specific variety of mustard greens and whether they are cooked or raw. Mustard greens are low in calories and fat but are rich in vitamins, minerals, and antioxidants.

Culinary Uses:

Salads:

- Mustard greens add a peppery and slightly bitter kick to salads, providing a flavorful alternative to traditional greens.

Sautéed or Stir-Fried:

- Sauté mustard greens with garlic, olive oil, and a splash of lemon for a simple and delicious side dish.

Smoothies:

- Incorporate mustard greens into your morning smoothies for an extra nutrient boost without overpowering the flavor.

Soups and Stews:

- Add chopped mustard greens to soups, stews, or curries for a nutritional boost and a vibrant color.

Mustard greens can be used in a variety of recipes, either as a side dish or as a main component. Here are two delicious recipes featuring mustard greens:

Mustard Greens Stir Fry

Ingredients:

- 1 bunch of fresh mustard greens, washed and chopped
- 2 tablespoons sesame oil
- 3 cloves garlic, minced
- 1 tablespoon soy sauce
- 1 tablespoon rice vinegar
- 1 teaspoon honey or maple syrup
- Red pepper flakes (optional)
- Sesame seeds for garnish

Instructions:

1. Heat sesame oil in a large pan or wok over medium heat.
2. Add minced garlic and sauté for 1-2 minutes until fragrant.
3. Add chopped mustard greens to the pan and stir-fry until they begin to wilt, about 2-3 minutes.
4. In a small bowl, mix soy sauce, rice vinegar, and honey (or maple syrup). Pour the sauce over the mustard greens and toss to coat evenly.
5. Continue to stir-fry for an additional 2-3 minutes until the greens are tender but still vibrant.
6. Optionally, sprinkle red pepper flakes for a bit of heat.
7. Garnish with sesame seeds before serving.
8. Serve this flavorful mustard greens stir fry as a side dish or over rice for a quick and nutritious meal.

Lentil and Mustard Greens Soup

Ingredients:

- 1 cup dried green or brown lentils, rinsed
- 1 bunch of fresh mustard greens, stems removed and chopped
- 1 onion, chopped
- 2 carrots, diced
- 3 cloves garlic, minced
- 6 cups vegetable broth
- 1 teaspoon ground cumin
- 1 teaspoon ground coriander
- Salt and pepper to taste
- Olive oil for sautéing

Instructions:

1. In a large pot, heat olive oil over medium heat. Add chopped onions, carrots, and garlic. Sauté until onions are translucent.
2. Add lentils, cumin, and coriander to the pot. Stir to coat the lentils with the spices.
3. Pour in vegetable broth and bring the mixture to a boil. Reduce heat, cover, and simmer for about 20 minutes or until lentils are tender.
4. Add chopped mustard greens to the pot and cook for an additional 5-7 minutes until the greens are wilted.
5. Season the soup with salt and pepper to taste.
6. Serve this hearty lentil and mustard greens soup hot, garnished with a drizzle of olive oil or a sprinkle of fresh herbs if desired.

These recipes showcase the versatility of mustard greens, whether stir-fried for a quick side dish or incorporated into a hearty lentil soup for a wholesome meal. Enjoy experimenting with the vibrant flavors and nutrients that mustard greens bring to your table!

Tips on Growing Mustard Greens

Mustard greens are fast-growing leafy vegetables that can be harvested relatively quickly compared to many other crops. Here's a detailed overview of the growth stages and timeline for mustard greens:

1. **Germination (5-10 days)**:
    - Mustard greens seeds typically germinate within 5 to 10 days when planted in well-draining soil with temperatures between 45°F to 85°F (7°C to 29°C). Providing consistent moisture and warmth during this stage is crucial for successful germination.
2. **Seedling Stage (1-2 weeks)**:
    - After germination, mustard green seedlings emerge from the soil. During this stage, they develop their first true leaves and establish their root system. Seedlings should be thinned to allow adequate space for growth, typically leaving about 4 to 6 inches (10 to 15 centimeters) between plants.
3. **Vegetative Growth (3-4 weeks)**:
    - As the mustard green plants mature, they enter a phase of vegetative growth, focusing on developing foliage and stems. With adequate sunlight, water, and nutrients, mustard greens grow rapidly during this stage, reaching heights of 12 to 18 inches (30 to 45 centimeters).
4. **Maturity and Harvesting (6-8 weeks)**:
    - Mustard greens are typically ready for harvest about 6 to 8 weeks after planting. However, you can begin harvesting individual leaves as soon as they reach a suitable size, typically about 4 to 6 inches (10 to 15 centimeters) in length.
    - To harvest mustard greens, use scissors or garden shears to cut the outer leaves from the plant, leaving the inner leaves to continue growing. Harvesting in this manner allows the plants to continue producing new leaves for an extended harvest period.
5. **Bolting and Flowering (8-10 weeks)**:
    - If left to grow for an extended period without harvesting, mustard greens may begin to bolt, or produce flower stalks. Bolting typically occurs 8 to 10 weeks after planting, especially in warm weather.
    - Once mustard greens bolt and flower, the leaves become bitter and less palatable. To prevent bolting and prolong the harvest period, harvest the leaves regularly and plant mustard greens in cooler weather if possible.

By following this timeline and providing proper care and maintenance, you can enjoy a bountiful harvest of fresh mustard greens within a relatively short timeframe. Additionally, succession planting can help ensure a continuous supply of greens throughout the growing season.

Conclusion:

Mustard greens stand out not only for their culinary versatility but also for their impressive nutritional content. Whether you enjoy them raw in salads or cooked in a variety of dishes, incorporating mustard greens into your diet can contribute to overall health and well-being. If you have specific health concerns, allergies, or conditions, it's advisable to consult with a healthcare professional or a registered dietitian before making significant changes to your diet.

Embrace the peppery goodness of mustard greens and savor the benefits they bring to both your plate and your body.

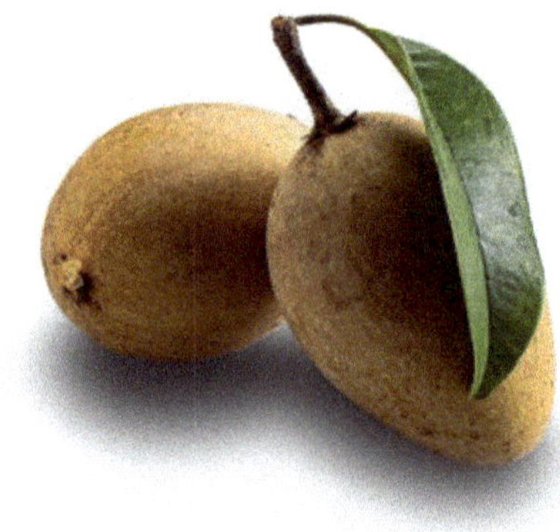

Naseberry

Unlocking the Delightful Naseberry: Exploring its Benefits and Uses

Naseberry, scientifically known as Manilkara zapota, is a tropical fruit native to Central America and Mexico. Also referred to as sapodilla, this fruit belongs to the Sapotaceae family and has been cherished for centuries for its sweet flavor, creamy texture, and various health benefits. Let's delve into the wonderful world of naseberry, uncovering its remarkable attributes and versatile uses.

Nutritional Profile

Naseberry is a nutrient-rich fruit, offering a range of vitamins, minerals, and phytonutrients essential for optimal health. Its potential to support immune function, promote cardiovascular health, aid digestion, and protect against oxidative stress and inflammation. It contains significant amounts of:

Fiber:

Naseberry is a good source of dietary fiber, which aids in digestion, promotes satiety, and supports heart health by helping to lower cholesterol levels.

Vitamins:

Vitamin C:

- **Benefits**: Boosts immune function, promotes collagen synthesis for healthy skin, aids in wound healing, and acts as an antioxidant to protect cells from damage caused by free radicals.

Vitamin A:

- **Benefits:** Supports vision health, promotes healthy skin and mucous membranes, boosts immune function, and acts as an antioxidant to protect against oxidative stress.

Vitamin E:

- **Benefits:** Acts as a powerful antioxidant, protecting cells from oxidative damage, supports immune function, and may have anti-inflammatory properties.

Vitamin K:

- **Benefits:** Essential for blood clotting, helps maintain bone health by supporting bone mineralization, and may have anti-inflammatory effects.

Vitamin B6:

- **Benefits:** Plays a crucial role in metabolism, including the synthesis of neurotransmitters, supports immune function, and helps maintain healthy nerve function.

Folate (Vitamin B9):

- **Benefits:** Important for DNA synthesis and cell division, supports red blood cell formation, and may help reduce the risk of neural tube defects during pregnancy.

Minerals:

Potassium:

- Benefits: Regulates fluid balance, supports nerve function and muscle contractions, helps maintain normal blood pressure, and may reduce the risk of stroke and kidney stones.

Calcium:

- Benefits: Essential for bone and teeth health, supports muscle function, nerve transmission, and blood clotting.

Phosphorus:

- Benefits: Works with calcium to build strong bones and teeth, supports energy metabolism, and plays a role in cell signaling and DNA/RNA synthesis.

Magnesium:

- Benefits: Supports bone health, muscle function, nerve transmission, energy production, and may help regulate blood pressure and blood sugar levels.

Iron:

- Benefits: Essential for the formation of hemoglobin and red blood cells, transports oxygen throughout the body, supports energy metabolism, and may help prevent iron deficiency anemia.

Zinc:

- Benefits: Supports immune function, wound healing, DNA synthesis, and cell division, and may have antioxidant properties to protect against oxidative stress.

Copper:

- Benefits: Necessary for the formation of red blood cells, supports iron absorption and utilization, helps maintain healthy connective tissues, and may have antioxidant properties.

Manganese:

- Benefits: Acts as a cofactor for various enzymes involved in metabolism, bone formation, and antioxidant defense.

Antioxidants and Other Phytonutrients:

Flavonoids:

- Benefits: Possess antioxidant and anti-inflammatory properties, support cardiovascular health, and may help reduce the risk of chronic diseases such as heart disease and cancer.

Polyphenols:

- Benefits: Act as antioxidants, protect against oxidative stress, support heart health, and may have anti-inflammatory effects.

Carotenoids (including lutein and zeaxanthin):

- Benefits: Support eye health, protect against age-related macular degeneration, and may have antioxidant properties to reduce the risk of chronic diseases.

Tannins:

- Benefits: Have antioxidant properties, support digestive health by promoting the growth of beneficial gut bacteria, and may have anti-inflammatory effects.

These vitamins, minerals, and antioxidants found in naseberry (sapodilla) contribute to its overall health benefits, including immune support, cardiovascular health, skin health, and protection against oxidative stress and inflammation. Incorporating naseberry into your diet can be a delicious and nutritious way to promote overall well-being.

Health Benefits

Consuming naseberry can offer several health benefits, thanks to its rich nutrient profile and bioactive compounds. Some of the notable advantages include:

Digestive Health: The fiber content in naseberry promotes healthy digestion, prevents constipation, and supports gastrointestinal function, aiding in the maintenance of a healthy digestive system.

Immune Support: Naseberry's vitamin C content helps bolster the immune system, strengthening the body's defenses against infections and illnesses.

Heart Health: Potassium in naseberry plays a role in regulating blood pressure and supporting heart function, potentially reducing the risk of cardiovascular diseases.

Antioxidant Protection: The presence of vitamins A and C, along with other antioxidants in naseberry, helps neutralize free radicals, reducing oxidative stress and inflammation in the body.

Skin and Vision Health: Vitamin A in naseberry supports healthy skin, promotes wound healing, and contributes to vision health, particularly night vision.

Nutritional Content

Naseberry, also known as sapodilla, is a tropical fruit native to southern Mexico, Central America, and the Caribbean. Here's the approximate nutritional content in 1 cup (approximately 200 grams) of naseberry:

- Calories: Around 230 kcal
- Carbohydrates: Approximately 60 grams
- Protein: Roughly 2 grams
- Fiber: About 10 grams
- Fat: Approximately 1 gram
- Sugar: Around 40 grams

Please note that these values are approximate and can vary slightly depending on factors such as the ripeness and variety of the naseberry. Naseberry is a delicious fruit rich in carbohydrates, fiber, and various vitamins and minerals.

Culinary Uses:

Naseberry's sweet and subtly aromatic flavor makes it a delightful addition to various culinary creations. Here are some popular ways to enjoy this tropical fruit:

Fresh Consumption: Enjoy naseberry fresh as a delicious and nutritious snack on its own or added to fruit salads for a burst of flavor and texture.

Smoothies and Juices: Incorporate naseberry into smoothies or freshly squeezed juices for a refreshing and nutritious beverage option.

Desserts: Use naseberry in desserts such as ice creams, sorbets, puddings, and custards to add natural sweetness and creaminess.

Baked Goods: Add chopped naseberry to muffins, cakes, bread, or pies for a unique twist on traditional baked goods.

Sauces and Chutneys: Prepare savory sauces or chutneys using naseberry as a base ingredient to accompany grilled meats, seafood, or vegetarian dishes.

Here are two delicious recipes that incorporate naseberry:

Naseberry Smoothie Bowl:

Ingredients:

- 2 ripe naseberries (sapodillas), peeled and seeds removed
- 1 frozen banana, sliced
- 1/2 cup frozen mixed berries (such as strawberries, blueberries, and raspberries)
- 1/2 cup plain Greek yogurt
- 1/4 cup almond milk (or any milk of your choice)
- 1 tablespoon honey or maple syrup (optional, adjust to taste)
- Toppings: sliced fresh fruit (such as banana, strawberries, or kiwi), granola, shredded coconut, chia seeds, nuts, or seeds

Instructions:

1. In a blender, combine the ripe naseberries, frozen banana slices, frozen mixed berries, Greek yogurt, almond milk, and honey or maple syrup (if using).
2. Blend until smooth and creamy, adding more almond milk if needed to reach your desired consistency.
3. Pour the smoothie into a bowl and top with your favorite toppings, such as sliced fresh fruit, granola, shredded coconut, chia seeds, nuts, or seeds.
4. Serve immediately and enjoy your refreshing and nutritious naseberry smoothie bowl!

Naseberry Salad with Citrus Dressing:

Ingredients:

- 2 ripe naseberries (sapodillas), peeled and seeds removed
- 4 cups mixed salad greens (such as baby spinach, arugula, and romaine lettuce)
- 1/2 cup cherry tomatoes, halved
- 1/4 cup cucumber, thinly sliced

- 1/4 cup red onion, thinly sliced
- 1/4 cup feta cheese, crumbled
- 2 tablespoons chopped fresh herbs (such as basil, mint, or cilantro)
- Citrus Dressing:
    - 2 tablespoons freshly squeezed orange juice
    - 1 tablespoon freshly squeezed lemon juice
    - 1 tablespoon extra-virgin olive oil
    - 1 teaspoon honey or maple syrup
    - Salt and freshly ground black pepper, to taste

Instructions:

1. Slice the ripe naseberries into thin wedges and set aside.
2. In a large mixing bowl, combine the mixed salad greens, cherry tomatoes, cucumber slices, red onion slices, crumbled feta cheese, and chopped fresh herbs.
3. In a small bowl, whisk together the freshly squeezed orange juice, lemon juice, extra-virgin olive oil, honey or maple syrup, salt, and freshly ground black pepper to make the citrus dressing.
4. Pour the citrus dressing over the salad and toss gently to coat the ingredients evenly.
5. Add the sliced naseberries to the salad and toss gently to combine.
6. Transfer the salad to serving plates or bowls and serve immediately as a refreshing and flavorful side dish or light meal.

These recipes showcase the delicious flavor and versatility of naseberry (sapodilla) and are perfect for enjoying its unique taste and nutritional benefits.

Conclusion:

Naseberry, with its delectable taste and array of health benefits, offers a delightful addition to any diet. Whether enjoyed fresh, blended into beverages, or incorporated into a variety of culinary creations, this tropical fruit provides a flavorful and nutritious experience. Embrace the goodness of naseberry and savor its many delights, knowing that each bite contributes to your well-being and culinary enjoyment.

If you have specific health concerns, allergies, or conditions, it's advisable to consult with a healthcare professional or a registered dietitian before making significant changes to your diet.

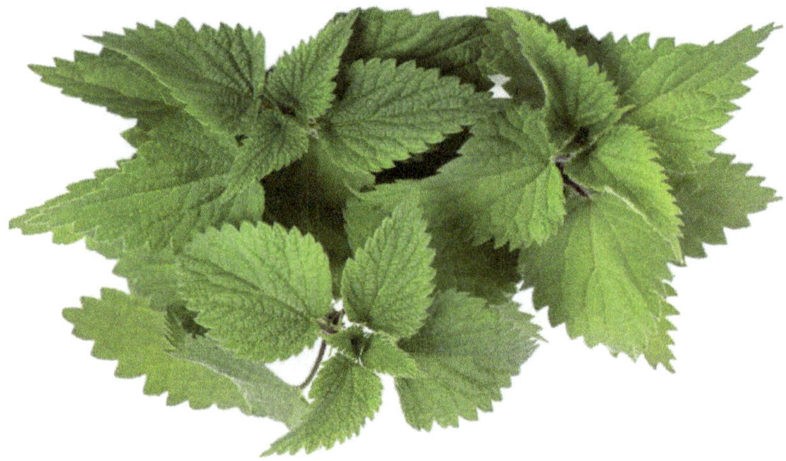

Nettle

Unveiling the Healing Power of Nettle

Nettle, scientifically known as Urtica dioica, is a perennial flowering plant that has been cherished for centuries for its numerous health benefits and versatile uses. Despite its reputation as a pesky weed due to its stinging hairs, nettle possesses remarkable medicinal properties and culinary potential that make it a valuable addition to any herbal medicine cabinet and kitchen pantry. Let's explore the myriad benefits and uses of this often-overlooked botanical marvel.

Nutritional Powerhouse:

Nettle leaves are rich in an array of essential nutrients, including vitamins, minerals, and antioxidants, making them a nutrient-dense addition to your diet.

- **Vitamins:** Nettle is a good source of vitamins A, C, and K, as well as several B vitamins, which play vital roles in supporting overall health and well-being.
- **Minerals:** It contains minerals such as calcium, magnesium, iron, and potassium, which are essential for maintaining strong bones, supporting muscle function, and regulating blood pressure.
- **Antioxidants:** Nettle is packed with antioxidants like flavonoids and carotenoids, which help protect cells from damage caused by free radicals and may reduce the risk of chronic diseases.

Here's a list of some of the key nutrients found in nettle and their associated benefits:

Vitamins:

Vitamin A:

- Benefits: Essential for maintaining healthy vision, supporting immune function, promoting skin health, and aiding in cell growth and development.

Vitamin C:

- Benefits: Boosts immune system function, acts as an antioxidant to protect cells from damage caused by free radicals, supports collagen production for healthy skin, and enhances iron absorption.

Vitamin K:

- Benefits: Plays a crucial role in blood clotting, bone metabolism, and cardiovascular health, and may help prevent bone fractures and osteoporosis.

Vitamin E:

- Benefits: Acts as an antioxidant, protecting cells from damage caused by free radicals, supports immune function, promotes skin health, and may help prevent age-related cognitive decline.

Minerals:

Calcium:

- Benefits: Essential for building and maintaining strong bones and teeth, supporting muscle function, and aiding in nerve transmission.

Magnesium:

- Benefits: Supports muscle and nerve function, regulates blood sugar levels, aids in energy production, promotes bone health, and contributes to heart health.

Iron:

- Benefits: Necessary for the production of hemoglobin, which carries oxygen in the blood, supports energy metabolism, and helps prevent iron deficiency anemia.

Potassium:

- Benefits: Regulates fluid balance, supports proper muscle function, helps maintain healthy blood pressure levels, and plays a role in nerve transmission.

Manganese:

- Benefits: Necessary for bone formation, wound healing, metabolism of carbohydrates and cholesterol, and antioxidant defense.

Antioxidants:

Flavonoids:

- Benefits: Possess antioxidant and anti-inflammatory properties, support cardiovascular health by improving blood flow and reducing the risk of blood clots, and may help lower blood pressure and cholesterol levels.

Carotenoids (including beta-carotene):

- Benefits: Function as antioxidants to protect cells from damage, support eye health, boost immune function, and may reduce the risk of chronic diseases such as heart disease and cancer.

Quercetin:

- Benefits: Acts as a powerful antioxidant and anti-inflammatory agent, supporting cardiovascular health, immune function, and respiratory health.

Chlorophyll:

- Benefits: Supports detoxification and cleansing of the body, promotes healthy digestion, and may have anti-inflammatory and antioxidant properties.

These vitamins, minerals, and antioxidants found in nettle contribute to its numerous health benefits, including immune support, improved bone health, enhanced skin health, and reduced inflammation. Incorporating nettle into your diet through teas, supplements, or culinary dishes can be a flavorful and nutritious way to reap these benefits and support overall health and well-being.

Health Benefits:

Anti-inflammatory Properties:

- Nettle has potent anti-inflammatory properties, making it effective in reducing inflammation associated with conditions such as arthritis, gout, and inflammatory bowel diseases.

Allergy Relief:

- Consuming nettle tea or supplements may help alleviate symptoms of seasonal allergies, such as sneezing, itching, and nasal congestion, due to its natural antihistamine properties.

Detoxification:

- Nettle acts as a diuretic, promoting the elimination of toxins from the body through increased urine production. It supports kidney function and may aid in detoxification.

Blood Sugar Regulation:

- Some studies suggest that nettle may help lower blood sugar levels and improve insulin sensitivity, making it potentially beneficial for individuals with diabetes or prediabetes.

Skin Health:

- Nettle extract or topical applications of nettle may help relieve symptoms of certain skin conditions, such as eczema, psoriasis, and acne, due to its anti-inflammatory and antimicrobial properties.

Nutritional Content

The nutritional content of 1 cup (approximately 89 grams) of raw nettles can vary slightly depending on factors such as the specific variety of nettle and its growing conditions. However, here's an approximate breakdown of the nutritional content in 1 cup of raw nettles:

- **Calories**: Approximately 37 calories
- **Carbohydrates**: Approximately 6.6 grams
- **Protein**: Approximately 2.4 grams
- **Fiber**: Approximately 2.4 grams
- **Fat**: Approximately 0.1 grams

It's important to note that these values are estimates and may vary based on factors such as serving size and preparation method. Additionally, cooking or drying nettles can slightly alter their nutritional content. Nonetheless, nettles are generally low in calories and fat while providing a good source of carbohydrates, protein, fiber, and various vitamins and minerals.

Culinary and Herbal Uses:

Culinary Delights:

- Nettle leaves can be cooked and consumed as a nutritious leafy green vegetable. They can be used in soups, stews, sauces, and stir-fries, similar to spinach or kale.
- Nettle leaves can also be dried and brewed into a flavorful and healthful tea, either on their own or blended with other herbs.

Herbal Remedies:

- Nettle tea is commonly used as a tonic to support overall health and vitality. It is believed to boost energy levels, improve digestion, and promote general well-being.
- Nettle supplements, available in various forms such as capsules, tinctures, and extracts, are often used to address specific health concerns, including allergies, joint pain, and urinary issues.

Here are two delicious recipes featuring nettle:

Nettle Soup:

Ingredients:

- 4 cups fresh nettle leaves (wear gloves when handling)
- 1 onion, chopped
- 2 cloves garlic, minced
- 2 medium potatoes, peeled and diced

- 4 cups vegetable or chicken broth
- 1 tablespoon olive oil
- Salt and pepper to taste
- Optional: cream or yogurt for serving

Instructions:

1. Begin by washing the nettle leaves thoroughly under cold water to remove any dirt or debris. Be sure to wear gloves to avoid stings.
2. In a large pot, heat the olive oil over medium heat. Add the chopped onion and minced garlic, and sauté until softened.
3. Add the diced potatoes and vegetable or chicken broth to the pot. Bring to a boil, then reduce heat and simmer for about 10 minutes, or until the potatoes are tender.
4. Add the nettle leaves to the pot and simmer for an additional 5 minutes, or until the nettles are wilted and tender.
5. Using an immersion blender or a regular blender, carefully blend the soup until smooth. Season with salt and pepper to taste.
6. Serve the nettle soup hot, optionally garnished with a swirl of cream or yogurt for added richness.

Nettle Pesto Pasta:

Ingredients:

- 4 cups fresh nettle leaves (wear gloves when handling)
- 2 cloves garlic
- 1/4 cup pine nuts or walnuts
- 1/4 cup grated Parmesan cheese
- 1/4 cup olive oil
- Salt and pepper to taste
- Cooked pasta of your choice (such as spaghetti or penne)

Instructions:

1. Wash the nettle leaves thoroughly under cold water and blanch them in boiling water for about 1-2 minutes to remove the sting. Drain and set aside to cool.
2. In a food processor, combine the blanched nettle leaves, garlic, pine nuts or walnuts, and Parmesan cheese. Pulse until coarsely chopped.

3. With the food processor running, slowly drizzle in the olive oil until the mixture forms a smooth paste. Season with salt and pepper to taste.
4. Cook the pasta according to package instructions until al dente. Drain, reserving some of the pasta cooking water.
5. In a large bowl, toss the cooked pasta with the nettle pesto until well coated, adding a splash of pasta cooking water if needed to loosen the sauce.
6. Serve the nettle pesto pasta hot, optionally garnished with additional grated Parmesan cheese and a sprinkle of pine nuts or walnuts.

These recipes showcase the versatility of nettle and its delicious culinary potential. Enjoy the unique flavor and nutritional benefits of this nutritious and flavorful ingredient!

Tips on Growing Nettle

Growing nettles (Urtica dioica) can be relatively easy, as they are hardy perennial plants that tolerate a wide range of growing conditions. Here's a detailed breakdown of the typical timeline for growing nettles from seed or cutting to harvest:

1. Seed Germination (7-21 days):

- Nettles can be grown from seeds, but they can also propagate readily from root cuttings or divisions.
- If starting from seeds, sow them indoors in early spring or directly in the garden after the last frost date.
- Keep the soil consistently moist and maintain a temperature between 60-70°F (15-21°C) for optimal germination.
- Nettle seeds typically germinate within 7 to 21 days, depending on conditions such as temperature and soil moisture.

2. Seedling Stage (2-4 weeks):

- Once the seeds have germinated, they will develop into seedlings with several sets of true leaves.
- Transplant the seedlings into larger pots or directly into the garden, spacing them about 12-18 inches apart to allow for growth.
- Keep the soil consistently moist and provide adequate sunlight or artificial light if growing indoors.

3. Vegetative Growth (6-8 weeks):

- Nettle plants will enter a period of vigorous vegetative growth, producing new leaves and stems.

- Maintain consistent watering to keep the soil evenly moist, but avoid waterlogging, as nettles prefer well-drained soil.
- Nettles thrive in rich, fertile soil, so amending the soil with compost or organic matter can promote healthy growth.

4. Harvesting (ongoing):

- Nettle leaves can be harvested once the plants have reached a height of about 12-18 inches. Harvesting can begin as early as 8 to 10 weeks after germination.
- Use scissors or gardening gloves to carefully harvest the top few inches of the young, tender leaves, as older leaves can become tough and fibrous.
- Harvesting can be done throughout the growing season, but it's best to avoid overharvesting to allow the plants to continue growing and producing new leaves.

Maturity: Nettle plants reach maturity within a few months, usually around 3 to 4 months after germination. At this point, they are fully established and capable of producing a continuous harvest throughout the growing season.

5. Maintenance (ongoing):

- Nettles are relatively low-maintenance plants but may benefit from occasional fertilization with a balanced fertilizer during the growing season.
- Remove any weeds or competing plants that may encroach on the nettle patch to give the nettles room to grow.
- In late fall or early winter, cut back the nettles to ground level to encourage regrowth in the following spring.

6. Propagation (optional):

- Nettles can be propagated by dividing mature plants or taking root cuttings.
- Divide mature plants in early spring or fall by carefully digging up the plant and separating the root ball into smaller sections, each containing a portion of the roots and stems.
- Root cuttings can be taken in late fall or early spring by cutting sections of the roots and planting them in moist soil to establish new plants.

By following these guidelines and providing proper care and attention, you can expect to enjoy a bountiful harvest of nettles throughout the growing season. These versatile plants can be used fresh in culinary dishes or dried for use in teas, tinctures, and herbal remedies.

Precautions:

While nettle is generally considered safe for most people when consumed in moderate amounts, it may cause side effects in some individuals, particularly those with certain medical conditions or allergies. It's always advisable to consult with a healthcare professional before incorporating nettle into your diet or using it for medicinal purposes, especially if you are pregnant, breastfeeding, or taking medications.

Conclusion:

Nettle is a remarkable plant with a wide range of health benefits and culinary uses. Whether enjoyed as a nourishing herbal tea, a flavorful addition to savory dishes, or a natural remedy for various ailments, nettle continues to captivate with its healing prowess and nutritional richness. Embrace the power of nettle and experience its transformative effects on your health and well-being.

Nori

The Nutrient-Rich Seaweed Offering Health Benefits and Culinary Delight

Nori, a type of edible seaweed commonly used in Asian cuisine, has gained global recognition for its unique flavor, versatility, and impressive nutritional profile. Derived from red algae, nori is not only a staple in sushi rolls but also a healthy addition to various dishes. In this article, we'll explore the benefits of nori and its diverse uses in the culinary world.

Nutrient-Rich Composition:

Nori stands out for being a nutrient-dense seaweed, packed with essential vitamins, minerals, and other bioactive compounds. Here are some key components that make nori a nutritional powerhouse:

Protein:

- Nori contains a surprisingly high amount of protein, making it a valuable source for plant-based protein, especially for those following vegetarian or vegan diets.

Iodine:

- As a seaweed, nori is an excellent source of iodine, a crucial mineral for thyroid function. Adequate iodine intake is essential for the production of thyroid hormones that regulate metabolism.

Vitamins:

Nori provides various vitamins, including vitamin A, vitamin C, and vitamin B12. Vitamin A supports vision and immune health, vitamin C is an antioxidant, and vitamin B12 is vital for nerve function and red blood cell formation.

Nori, a type of edible seaweed, contains various vitamins that contribute to its nutritional content. Here's a list of vitamins found in nori:

Vitamin A:

- Nori is a good source of vitamin A, particularly in the form of beta-carotene. Vitamin A is crucial for vision, immune function, and skin health.

Vitamin C:

- Nori contains vitamin C, an antioxidant that supports the immune system, promotes healthy skin, and helps the body absorb iron.

Vitamin E:

- While present in smaller amounts, nori provides vitamin E, an antioxidant that protects cells from oxidative damage.

Vitamin K:

- Nori is rich in vitamin K, which is essential for blood clotting and plays a role in bone health by contributing to bone mineralization.

Vitamin B1 (Thiamine):

- Thiamine is found in nori and is essential for energy metabolism and the proper functioning of the nervous system.

Vitamin B2 (Riboflavin):

- Nori contains riboflavin, which is important for energy production and supports the metabolism of fats, drugs, and steroids.

Vitamin B3 (Niacin):

- Niacin is present in nori and plays a role in energy metabolism, DNA repair, and the functioning of the nervous system.

Vitamin B5 (Pantothenic Acid):

- Pantothenic acid is found in nori and is involved in the synthesis of essential molecules in the body, including fatty acids and cholesterol.

Vitamin B6 (Pyridoxine):

- Nori provides vitamin B6, which is important for the metabolism of amino acids, the synthesis of neurotransmitters, and immune function.

Vitamin B12:

- Nori contains a form of vitamin B12, although it is debated whether it is in a bioavailable form for humans. Vitamin B12 is vital for nerve function and red blood cell formation.

Incorporating nori into your diet can contribute to a diverse intake of vitamins, supporting various physiological functions and promoting overall health. As with any food, it's important to consume a variety of nutrient-rich foods to ensure a balanced intake of vitamins and other essential nutrients.

Minerals:

Nori is rich in minerals such as iron, calcium, magnesium, and potassium, contributing to bone health, blood circulation, and overall well-being.

Iodine:

- Nori is an excellent source of iodine, a crucial mineral for the production of thyroid hormones that regulate metabolism.

Iron:

- Nori contains iron, which is essential for the formation of hemoglobin, the protein responsible for carrying oxygen in the blood.

Calcium:

- Nori provides calcium, an essential mineral for bone health, muscle function, and nerve transmission.

Magnesium:

- Magnesium in nori supports muscle and nerve function, regulates blood pressure, and contributes to overall cardiovascular health.

Potassium:

- Nori is a source of potassium, an electrolyte that helps regulate fluid balance, muscle contractions, and nerve signals.

Sodium:

- While seaweed naturally contains sodium, the sodium content in nori is generally lower compared to traditional table salt.

Phosphorus:

- Phosphorus is present in nori and is important for bone and teeth formation, energy metabolism, and DNA synthesis.

Zinc:

- Nori provides zinc, a trace mineral important for immune function, wound healing, and DNA synthesis.

Copper:

- Copper, a trace mineral present in nori, plays a role in the formation of red blood cells, maintenance of healthy bones and nerves, and immune system function.

Manganese:

- Nori contains manganese, a trace mineral involved in bone formation, blood clotting, and reducing inflammation.

Including nori in your diet can contribute to a diverse intake of minerals, supporting various physiological functions and promoting overall health. As with any food, it's essential to consume a variety of nutrient-rich foods to ensure a balanced intake of minerals and other essential nutrients.

Dietary Fiber:

- Nori contains dietary fiber, promoting digestive health and contributing to a feeling of satiety.

Health Benefits:

Thyroid Health:

- The iodine content in nori supports thyroid function, helping to maintain a healthy metabolism and prevent thyroid-related disorders.

Heart Health:

- The potassium and magnesium in nori contribute to heart health by regulating blood pressure and supporting cardiovascular function.

Antioxidant Properties:

- Nori contains antioxidants that help combat oxidative stress, inflammation, and reduce the risk of chronic diseases.

Bone Health:

- The calcium and magnesium in nori play a role in maintaining bone density, promoting strong and healthy bones.

Nutritional Content

Nori is a type of edible seaweed commonly used in Japanese cuisine, particularly for making sushi rolls. Here's the approximate nutritional content in 1 cup (approximately 8 grams) of dried nori sheets:

- Calories: Around 35 kcal
- Carbohydrates: Approximately 4.5 grams
- Protein: Roughly 4 grams
- Fiber: About 1 gram
- Fat: Approximately 0.5 grams
- Sugar: Less than 1 gram

Please note that these values are approximate and can vary slightly depending on factors such as the brand and processing method of the nori sheets. Nori is a nutritious food that is low in calories and fat but rich in protein, vitamins, and minerals, particularly iodine.

Culinary Uses:

Sushi Rolls (Maki):

- Nori is perhaps best known as the outer wrapping of sushi rolls. Maki rolls often combine nori with rice, vegetables, and various proteins.

Snack:

- Roasted nori sheets make for a delicious and nutritious snack. They can be enjoyed on their own or seasoned with a touch of soy sauce and sesame oil.

Soup and Salad Garnish:

- Crumbled or shredded nori can be used as a garnish for soups, salads, or noodle dishes, adding a savory umami flavor.

Homemade Seaweed Snacks:

- Bake nori sheets with seasonings to create homemade seaweed snacks. This provides a healthier alternative to traditional processed snacks.

Nori's unique flavor and versatility make it a fantastic ingredient for a variety of dishes. Here are two delicious recipes featuring nori:

Nori Rolls (Vegetarian Sushi Rolls):

Ingredients:

- 10 sheets nori seaweed
- 2 cups sushi rice, cooked and seasoned with rice vinegar, sugar, and salt
- Assorted vegetables (cucumber, avocado, carrot, bell pepper), julienned
- Sesame seeds
- Soy sauce and pickled ginger for serving

Instructions:

1. **Prepare the Ingredients:**
    - Lay a sheet of nori on a bamboo sushi rolling mat.
    - Wet your hands to prevent sticking, and spread a thin layer of sushi rice over the nori, leaving a small border at the top.
2. **Add Vegetables:**
    - Arrange the julienned vegetables horizontally along the center of the rice.

3. **Roll the Nori:**
    - Using the sushi rolling mat, carefully roll the nori and rice over the vegetables, applying gentle pressure to shape it into a cylinder.
4. **Slice and Serve:**
    - With a sharp, wet knife, slice the roll into bite-sized pieces. Repeat with the remaining nori sheets.
    - Serve the vegetarian sushi rolls with soy sauce, pickled ginger, and a sprinkle of sesame seeds.

Nori Chips:

Ingredients:

- Nori sheets
- Toasted sesame oil
- Soy sauce
- Sesame seeds
- Optional: Chili flakes or seasoning of your choice

Instructions:

1. **Preheat the Oven:**
    - Preheat your oven to 300°F (150°C).
2. **Prepare the Nori:**
    - Cut nori sheets into bite-sized squares or rectangles.
3. **Season the Nori:**
    - Lightly brush each piece of nori with toasted sesame oil and soy sauce. Sprinkle sesame seeds and optional chili flakes or other seasonings.
4. **Bake:**
    - Place the seasoned nori pieces on a baking sheet lined with parchment paper.
    - Bake in the preheated oven for about 10-15 minutes or until the nori becomes crispy.
5. **Cool and Enjoy:**
    - Allow the nori chips to cool before serving. They can be a delightful snack on their own or paired with dips like guacamole or hummus.

These recipes showcase the versatility of nori, whether used in classic sushi rolls or transformed into crispy and flavorful chips. Enjoy the unique taste and nutritional benefits of nori in these creative and delicious dishes!

Conclusion:

Nori's unique taste, versatility, and nutritional benefits make it a valuable addition to a balanced and diverse diet. Whether enjoyed in sushi, used as a garnish, or savored as a snack, nori brings a wealth of nutrients and flavors to the table. If you have specific health concerns, allergies, or conditions, it's advisable to consult with a healthcare professional or a registered dietitian before making significant changes to your diet.

Embrace the culinary possibilities of nori and indulge in a tasty journey that supports your well-being.

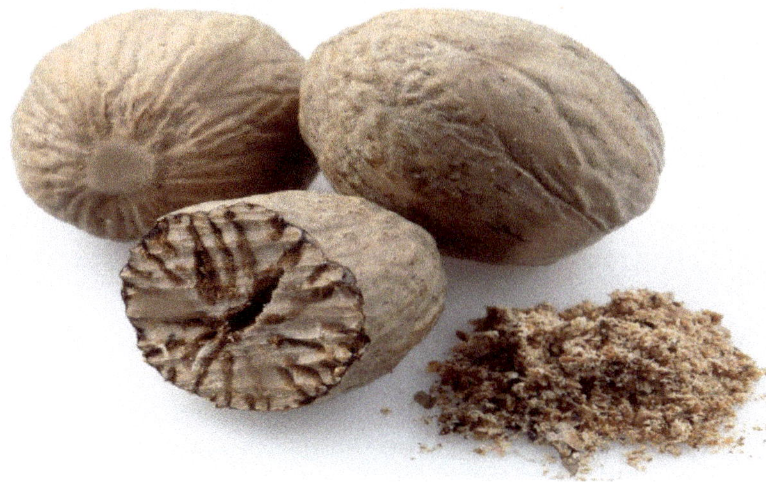

Nutmeg

Unveiling the Warmth: Nutmeg's Benefits and Diverse Culinary Uses

Nutmeg, with its warm and aromatic flavor, has been a prized spice for centuries, adding depth and richness to both sweet and savory dishes. Beyond its culinary allure, nutmeg boasts an array of health benefits that have been cherished in traditional medicine. In this article, we'll explore the nutritional advantages of nutmeg and its versatile uses in the kitchen.

Nutritional Content:

Nutmeg is a spice derived from the seed of the Myristica fragrans tree. While used sparingly due to its potent flavor, nutmeg offers various essential nutrients, including:

Dietary Fiber: Supports digestive health and helps maintain a feeling of fullness.

Magnesium: Essential for muscle and nerve function, as well as bone health.

Copper: Contributes to iron absorption, collagen formation, and overall metabolic function.

Zinc:

Benefits:

- ***Immune Support:*** Supports a healthy immune system.
- ***Wound Healing:*** Plays a role in wound healing and the maintenance of skin integrity.

Iron:

Benefits:

- ***Oxygen Transport:*** **Essential** for the formation of hemoglobin, which transports oxygen in the blood.

- ***Energy Metabolism:*** Involved in energy production and metabolism.

Phosphorus:

Benefits:

- ***Bone Health:*** Works in conjunction with calcium for the formation and maintenance of strong bones and teeth.
    - ***Energy Production:*** Plays a role in energy metabolism and the synthesis of ATP.

Health Benefits:

Anti-Inflammatory Properties:

- Nutmeg contains compounds like myristicin and elemicin, known for their anti-inflammatory effects, which may contribute to overall health.

Digestive Aid:

- Nutmeg has been traditionally used to alleviate digestive issues such as indigestion and bloating, thanks to its carminative properties.

Brain Health:

- Compounds in nutmeg have been linked to cognitive health, potentially improving memory and concentration.

Culinary Uses:

Baking and Desserts:

- Nutmeg is a key player in classic desserts like pumpkin pie, apple pie, and custards, imparting a warm and comforting flavor.

Savory Dishes:

- Used in various savory dishes, nutmeg adds depth to creamy sauces, soups, and vegetable gratins.

Spiced Beverages:

- Nutmeg enhances the flavor profile of spiced beverages like eggnog, chai tea, and mulled wine, providing a cozy and aromatic touch.

Homemade Spice Blends:

- Ground nutmeg is a staple in homemade spice blends, contributing to the complexity of flavors in dishes like curries and stews.

Infused Oils and Syrups:

- Nutmeg-infused oils and syrups are popular for adding a hint of warmth to both sweet and savory recipes.

Nutmeg is a versatile spice that adds warm, earthy flavor to both sweet and savory dishes.

Here are two recipes that incorporate nutmeg:

Homemade Eggnog:

- ***Ingredients:***
  - 4 cups whole milk
  - 1 cup heavy cream
  - 4 large eggs, separated
  - 2/3 cup granulated sugar
  - 1 teaspoon vanilla extract
  - 1/2 teaspoon ground nutmeg, plus extra for garnish
  - 1/4 teaspoon ground cinnamon
  - Optional: 1/4 cup rum or bourbon (for adults)
- ***Instructions:***
  1. In a large saucepan, combine the milk, heavy cream, and nutmeg. Heat over medium heat until steaming but not boiling.
  2. In a mixing bowl, whisk together the egg yolks and sugar until light and creamy.
  3. Slowly pour the hot milk mixture into the egg yolk mixture, whisking constantly to temper the eggs.
  4. Return the mixture to the saucepan and cook over low heat, stirring constantly, until slightly thickened. Do not let it boil.
  5. Remove from heat and stir in the vanilla extract and optional rum or bourbon, if using.
  6. Transfer the eggnog to a pitcher and refrigerate until chilled.
  7. Before serving, beat the egg whites until stiff peaks form. Gently fold the egg whites into the chilled eggnog.
  8. Pour the eggnog into glasses, sprinkle with additional nutmeg and cinnamon for garnish, and serve chilled.

Baked Apples with Nutmeg and Cinnamon:

- ***Ingredients:***

  0. 4 large apples (such as Granny Smith or Honeycrisp)
  1. 1/4 cup brown sugar
  2. 1 teaspoon ground cinnamon
  3. 1/4 teaspoon ground nutmeg
  4. 2 tablespoons unsalted butter, melted
  5. 1/2 cup water or apple cider
  6. Vanilla ice cream or whipped cream, for serving (optional)

- ***Instructions:***

  1. Preheat your oven to 375°F (190°C). Grease a baking dish large enough to hold the apples.
  2. Core the apples using an apple corer or a paring knife, leaving the bottoms intact.
  3. In a small bowl, mix together the brown sugar, cinnamon, and nutmeg.
  4. Place the cored apples in the prepared baking dish. Divide the melted butter evenly among the apples, brushing it over the tops and insides.
  5. Fill each apple cavity with the brown sugar mixture, pressing down gently.
  6. Pour the water or apple cider into the bottom of the baking dish.
  7. Cover the dish with aluminum foil and bake in the preheated oven for 25-30 minutes, or until the apples are tender but not mushy.
  8. Remove the foil and continue baking for an additional 5-10 minutes, or until the tops are lightly caramelized.
  9. Serve the baked apples warm, drizzled with any pan juices and topped with vanilla ice cream or whipped cream, if desired.

These recipes showcase the delightful flavor of nutmeg in both sweet and savory dishes. Enjoy!

Historical Uses:

Medieval Medicinal Uses:

- **Historical Use:**
  - In medieval times, nutmeg was highly valued for its perceived medicinal properties and was believed to have various health benefits.
  - Nutmeg was used as a remedy for digestive issues, including indigestion and flatulence, due to its carminative properties.
  - It was also believed to have aphrodisiac qualities and was used to address issues related to intimacy.

Culinary Spice Trade in the Age of Exploration:

- **Historical Use:**
  - During the Age of Exploration, nutmeg was a highly sought-after spice, leading to intense competition among European powers to control the nutmeg-producing islands in Southeast Asia.
  - Nutmeg was not only prized for its culinary uses but also for its perceived medicinal properties, including its ability to alleviate digestive discomfort.
  - The spice trade during this period had significant economic and geopolitical implications, making nutmeg a symbol of wealth and luxury.

These historical uses of nutmeg highlight its multifaceted role in both medicine and culinary pursuits. Whether utilized for its purported medicinal benefits in medieval times or as a sought-after culinary spice during the Age of Exploration, nutmeg has long been regarded as a valuable and versatile commodity with a rich history.

Conclusion:

Nutmeg's unique flavor profile and potential health benefits make it a treasured spice in kitchens worldwide. From its historical use in traditional medicine to its indispensable role in culinary creations, nutmeg continues to be a symbol of warmth and richness. Individuals with pre-existing medical conditions, such as liver problems, or allegic should consult with a healthcare professional before significantly increasing their nutmeg intake. As you savor the delightful taste of nutmeg in your favorite dishes, you're not just enjoying a spice – you're embracing a centuries-old tradition that has added depth and comfort to culinary experiences throughout the ages.

Essential Nutrients for Optimal Health

Optimal health requires a diverse array of nutrients that support various bodily functions and processes. Here's a comprehensive list of essential nutrients the body needs for optimal health:

Macronutrients:

Macronutrients are nutrients that the body requires in large amounts to provide energy and support vital functions. The three main macronutrients are **carbohydrates, proteins, and fats**, and they play essential roles in growth, metabolism, and overall health.

Types of Macronutrients and Their Functions

1. **Carbohydrates** – The body's primary source of energy.
    - Provides energy for cellular function, particularly for the brain and muscles.
    - Found in grains, fruits, vegetables, legumes, and dairy products.
2. **Proteins:**
    - Essential for building and repairing tissues, producing enzymes and hormones, and supporting immune function.
    - Found in meat, poultry, fish, eggs, dairy products, legumes, nuts, and seeds.
3. **Fats (Healthy Fats):**
    - Provides energy, support cell structure, assist in nutrient absorption, and help produce hormones.
    - Found in nuts, seeds, avocados, olive oil, fatty fish, and plant-based oils.

Balancing Macronutrients for Optimal Health

A well-balanced diet should include the right proportions of each macronutrient to support overall health:

- **Carbohydrates** – 45-65% of daily intake (focus on whole, unprocessed sources).
- **Proteins** – 10-35% of daily intake (include plant-based protein sources).
- **Fats** – 20-35% of daily intake (choose healthy fats like nuts, seeds, and avocados).

Micronutrients:

Micronutrients are essential vitamins and minerals that the body needs in small amounts to function properly. Unlike macronutrients (carbohydrates, proteins, and fats), which provide energy, micronutrients support various physiological processes, including immune function, brain development, bone health, and metabolism.

Types of Micronutrients

Vitamins – Organic compounds required for essential bodily functions.

1. **Water-Soluble Vitamins:**
    - Vitamin C: Supports immune function, collagen synthesis, and antioxidant activity.
    - B Vitamins (B1, B2, B3, B5, B6, B7, B9, B12): Essential for energy metabolism, nerve function, and red blood cell production.
2. **Fat-Soluble Vitamins:**
    - Vitamin A: Essential for vision, immune function, and skin health.
    - Vitamin D: Facilitates calcium absorption, supports bone health, and regulates immune function.
    - Vitamin E: Acts as an antioxidant, supports immune function, and protects cell membranes.
    - Vitamin K: Essential for blood clotting and bone metabolism.

Minerals – Inorganic elements crucial for various biological functions.

1. **Major Minerals:**
    - Calcium: Essential for bone and teeth health, muscle function, and nerve transmission.
    - Magnesium: Supports muscle and nerve function, bone health, and energy metabolism.
    - Phosphorus: Important for bone and teeth health, energy metabolism, and cell signaling.
2. **Trace Minerals:**
    - Iron: Necessary for oxygen transport, energy metabolism, and red blood cell production.
    - Zinc: Supports immune function, wound healing, and DNA synthesis.
    - Selenium: Acts as an antioxidant, supports thyroid function, and may reduce the risk of certain cancers.
    - Copper: Essential for iron metabolism, connective tissue formation, and antioxidant defense.

How to Get Enough Micronutrients?

The best way to obtain micronutrients is through a balanced diet rich in:

- Fruits and vegetables (rich in vitamins and antioxidants)
- Whole grains (contain B vitamins and minerals)
- Nuts and seeds (provide essential minerals like magnesium and zinc)
- Legumes and beans (great sources of iron and folate)
- Dairy or fortified plant-based alternatives (for calcium and vitamin D)

Other Essential Nutrients:

Water:

- Essential for hydration, digestion, nutrient transport, temperature regulation, and overall cellular function.

Fiber:

- Supports digestive health, promotes satiety, regulates blood sugar levels, and may reduce the risk of chronic diseases.

Phytonutrients:

- Found in plant-based foods, phytonutrients have antioxidant, anti-inflammatory, and other health-promoting properties.

Omega-3 Fatty Acids:

- Essential for brain health, heart health, and reducing inflammation.
- Found in fatty fish, flaxseeds, chia seeds, walnuts, and hemp seeds.

Incorporating a balanced diet rich in whole foods is crucial for obtaining these essential nutrients and supporting optimal health and well-being. Additionally, individual nutrient needs may vary based on factors such as age, gender, activity level, and health status. It's important to consult with a healthcare professional or registered dietitian for personalized nutrition recommendations.

What is Carbohydrate?

Carbohydrates are one of the three macronutrients, along with proteins and fats, that provide energy for the body. Chemically, carbohydrates are made up of carbon, hydrogen, and oxygen atoms, and they come in various forms, including sugars, starches, and fibers. Carbohydrates are found in a wide range of foods, including grains, fruits, vegetables, legumes, and dairy products.

Types of Carbohydrates:

1. **Simple Carbohydrates (Sugars):** These are composed of one or two sugar molecules and are quickly digested and absorbed into the bloodstream. Examples include glucose, fructose, and sucrose (table sugar), which are found in fruits, honey, and sweets.
2. **Complex Carbohydrates (Starches and Fibers):** These are composed of long chains of sugar molecules and take longer to digest, providing a steady source of energy. Examples include starches found in grains, legumes, and starchy vegetables, as well as dietary fibers found in fruits, vegetables, whole grains, and legumes.

Benefits of Carbohydrates:

1. **Energy Source:** Carbohydrates are the body's primary source of energy. When consumed, carbohydrates are broken down into glucose, which is transported to cells and used as fuel for cellular processes, physical activity, and metabolic functions.
2. **Brain Function:** Glucose derived from carbohydrates is the preferred source of energy for the brain. Adequate carbohydrate intake supports cognitive function, concentration, and mental alertness.
3. **Muscle Fuel:** Carbohydrates are essential for supporting muscle function and performance, especially during high-intensity exercise and endurance activities. Glycogen, the stored form of glucose in muscles, serves as a readily available energy source during physical exertion.
4. **Dietary Fiber:** Many carbohydrate-rich foods, such as fruits, vegetables, whole grains, and legumes, are excellent sources of dietary fiber. Fiber promotes digestive health, regulates bowel movements, aids in weight management by promoting satiety, and may reduce the risk of chronic diseases such as heart disease, diabetes, and certain cancers.
5. **Nutrient Dense:** Carbohydrate-rich foods often contain essential vitamins, minerals, and phytonutrients that contribute to overall health and well-being. Choosing whole food sources of carbohydrates, such as whole grains, fruits, and vegetables, provides a wide range of nutrients vital for optimal health.
6. **Blood Sugar Regulation:** Consuming carbohydrates along with fiber, protein, and healthy fats can help slow down the absorption of glucose into the bloodstream, preventing rapid spikes and crashes in blood sugar levels. This promotes stable energy levels and helps maintain insulin sensitivity.

Overall, carbohydrates play a crucial role in supporting energy production, brain function, muscle health, digestive health, and overall vitality. Including a variety of carbohydrate-rich foods as part of a balanced diet can help meet energy needs and support optimal health and well-being.

Plant-Based Foods High in Carbohydrates

Carbohydrates are one of the three macronutrients, along with proteins and fats, that provide energy for the body. Chemically, carbohydrates are made up of carbon, hydrogen, and oxygen atoms, and they come in various forms, including sugars, starches, and fibers. Carbohydrates are found in a wide range of foods, including grains, fruits, vegetables, legumes, and dairy products.

Grains and Grain Products:

1. **Bread:** Whole wheat bread, white bread, rye bread, sourdough bread, and multigrain bread.
2. **Cereal:** Oatmeal, granola, cornflakes, bran flakes, and muesli.
3. **Rice:** White rice, brown rice, basmati rice, jasmine rice, and wild rice.
4. **Pasta:** Spaghetti, penne, macaroni, fettuccine, and couscous.
5. **Quinoa:** A pseudo-grain that is high in protein and carbohydrates.
6. **Barley:** Pearl barley, hulled barley, and barley flakes.
7. **Bulgur:** A whole grain made from cracked wheat.
8. **Buckwheat:** Despite its name, buckwheat is not a wheat product and is gluten-free.

Starchy Vegetables:

1. **Potatoes:** Russet potatoes, sweet potatoes, white potatoes, and red potatoes.
2. **Corn:** Fresh corn on the cob, canned corn, and cornmeal.
3. **Peas:** Green peas, split peas, and chickpeas (also known as garbanzo beans).
4. **Winter Squash:** Butternut squash, acorn squash, and pumpkin.
5. **Plantains:** A starchy fruit commonly used in savory dishes.

Legumes:

1. **Beans:** Black beans, kidney beans, pinto beans, navy beans, and cannellini beans.
2. **Lentils:** Green lentils, red lentils, brown lentils, and French lentils.
3. **Chickpeas:** Also known as garbanzo beans, commonly used in dishes like hummus and falafel.
4. **Peas:** Split peas, green peas, and yellow peas.

Fruits:

1. **Bananas:** Known for their high carbohydrate content and potassium.
2. **Apples:** A good source of fiber and natural sugars.

3. **Oranges:** Rich in vitamin C and natural sugars.
4. **Grapes:** Red and green grapes are naturally sweet and contain carbohydrates.
5. **Mangoes:** A tropical fruit high in carbohydrates and vitamin C.
6. **Pineapples:** Sweet and tangy, pineapples are a good source of carbohydrates.

Dairy Products:

1. **Milk:** Cow's milk, soy milk, almond milk, and oat milk.
2. **Yogurt:** Greek yogurt, regular yogurt, and flavored yogurts.
3. **Kefir:** A fermented dairy beverage similar to drinkable yogurt.

These are just some examples of foods high in carbohydrates. Incorporating a variety of these foods into your diet can provide you with the energy and nutrients necessary for optimal health and well-being.

What is Protein?

Protein is one of the three macronutrients essential for human health, alongside carbohydrates and fats. Proteins are made up of amino acids, which are the building blocks of tissues, organs, enzymes, hormones, and various other molecules in the body. Protein is found in a wide range of foods, including animal-based sources such as meat, poultry, fish, eggs, and dairy products, as well as plant-based sources such as legumes, nuts, seeds, and grains.

Benefits of Protein:

1. **Muscle Growth and Repair:** Protein is crucial for building and repairing muscle tissues. During physical activity, muscle fibers undergo microscopic damage, and consuming protein helps repair and rebuild these tissues, leading to muscle growth and recovery.
2. **Supports Immune Function:** Many components of the immune system, including antibodies and immune cells, are made up of proteins. Adequate protein intake is essential for maintaining a strong and healthy immune system, which helps defend the body against infections and illnesses.
3. **Enzyme Function:** Enzymes are proteins that catalyze biochemical reactions in the body, facilitating processes such as digestion, metabolism, and cellular energy production. Without proteins, many essential metabolic reactions would occur at a much slower rate or not at all.
4. **Hormone Regulation:** Proteins play a role in hormone synthesis and signaling, helping regulate various physiological processes such as growth, metabolism, appetite, and mood. Hormones such as insulin, growth hormone, and thyroid hormones are all made up of proteins.

5. **Structural Support:** Proteins provide structural support to cells, tissues, and organs throughout the body. Collagen, for example, is a protein that forms the structural framework of skin, bones, tendons, and ligaments, contributing to their strength and elasticity.

6. **Transport and Storage:** Certain proteins serve as carriers, transporting essential molecules such as oxygen (in the form of hemoglobin) and nutrients (such as iron and vitamin A) throughout the body. Additionally, proteins are involved in storing and releasing nutrients and other molecules for use as energy or building blocks.

7. **Satiety and Weight Management:** Protein is the most satiating macronutrient, meaning it helps promote feelings of fullness and satisfaction after meals. Including protein-rich foods in your diet can help curb hunger, reduce overall calorie intake, and support weight management efforts.

8. **Maintains Hair, Skin, and Nails:** Proteins are vital for maintaining the health and integrity of hair, skin, and nails. Keratin, a structural protein found in these tissues, provides strength and resilience, contributing to healthy hair, skin, and nails.

In summary, protein plays a crucial role in supporting muscle health, immune function, enzyme activity, hormone regulation, structural integrity, nutrient transport, satiety, and overall health and well-being. Including adequate protein sources in your diet is essential for meeting nutrient needs and maintaining optimal health throughout life.

Plant-Based Foods High in Protein

Protein is one of the three macronutrients essential for human health, alongside carbohydrates and fats. Proteins are made up of amino acids, which are the building blocks of tissues, organs, enzymes, hormones, and various other molecules in the body. Protein is found in a wide range of foods, including animal-based sources such as meat, poultry, fish, eggs, and dairy products, as well as plant-based sources such as legumes, nuts, seeds, and grains.

1. **Legumes:**

    - **Lentils:** Lentils are a rich source of protein, with approximately 18 grams of protein per cooked cup. They are versatile and can be used in soups, salads, stews, and veggie burgers.

    - **Chickpeas:** Also known as garbanzo beans, chickpeas provide about 15 grams of protein per cooked cup. They are commonly used in hummus, curries, salads, and roasted as a crunchy snack.

    - **Black Beans:** Black beans offer approximately 15 grams of protein per cooked cup. They are a staple in Latin American cuisine and can be used in burritos, tacos, soups, and salads.

- **Kidney Beans:** Kidney beans provide around 15 grams of protein per cooked cup. They are often used in chili, bean salads, soups, and stews.

2. **Soy Products:**

    - **Tofu:** Tofu is made from soybeans and contains about 20 grams of protein per cooked cup. It is a versatile ingredient that can be used in stir-fries, soups, salads, and sandwiches.
    - **Tempeh:** Tempeh is a fermented soy product that offers approximately 30 grams of protein per cooked cup. It has a nutty flavor and can be grilled, sautéed, or crumbled into dishes.
    - **Edamame:** Edamame are young soybeans that provide around 17 grams of protein per cooked cup. They can be boiled or steamed and served as a snack or added to salads, stir-fries, and pasta dishes.

3. **Quinoa:**

    - Quinoa is a pseudo-grain that contains all nine essential amino acids, making it a complete protein source. It offers approximately 8 grams of protein per cooked cup and can be used as a base for salads, stir-fries, pilafs, and breakfast bowls.

4. **Seitan:**

    - Seitan, also known as wheat gluten, is made from wheat protein and provides about 21 grams of protein per cooked 3-ounce serving. It has a meat-like texture and is commonly used in vegetarian and vegan dishes such as stir-fries, sandwiches, and stews.

5. **Nuts and Seeds:**

    - **Almonds:** Almonds offer approximately 6 grams of protein per ounce. They can be eaten as a snack, added to salads, or used to make almond butter.
    - **Chia Seeds:** Chia seeds provide about 5 grams of protein per ounce. They can be sprinkled on yogurt, oatmeal, or salads, or used to make chia pudding.
    - **Hemp Seeds:** Hemp seeds offer approximately 10 grams of protein per ounce. They can be added to smoothies, salads, or granola, or used to make hemp milk.

6. **Green Peas:**

    - Green peas provide around 8 grams of protein per cooked cup. They can be added to soups, salads, stir-fries, or mashed as a side dish.

These plant-based foods are excellent sources of protein and can be incorporated into a balanced diet to meet protein needs and support overall health and well-being.

Fats (Healthy Fats)

What are Healthy Fats?

Healthy fats, also known as unsaturated fats, are essential components of a balanced diet and play numerous roles in promoting overall health and well-being. Unlike saturated fats and trans fats, which are considered less healthy, healthy fats provide a range of health benefits. Here are some examples of healthy fats and their benefits:

Types of Healthy Fats:

1. **Monounsaturated Fats:**
    - Found in foods such as olive oil, avocado, nuts (e.g., almonds, peanuts, cashews), and seeds (e.g., pumpkin seeds, sesame seeds).
    - Benefits: Monounsaturated fats can help reduce levels of LDL (bad) cholesterol and lower the risk of heart disease. They also provide energy, support cell growth and development, and help maintain healthy skin and hair.
2. **Polyunsaturated Fats:**
    - Includes omega-3 fatty acids and omega-6 fatty acids, both of which are essential fatty acids that the body cannot produce on its own.
    - **Omega-3 Fatty Acids:** Found in fatty fish (e.g., salmon, mackerel, sardines), flaxseeds, chia seeds, walnuts, and hemp seeds.
        - Benefits: Omega-3 fatty acids have anti-inflammatory properties and are crucial for heart health, brain function, and reducing the risk of chronic diseases such as heart disease, stroke, and certain cancers.
    - **Omega-6 Fatty Acids:** Found in vegetable oils (e.g., soybean oil, sunflower oil, corn oil), nuts, seeds, and certain grains.
        - Benefits: Omega-6 fatty acids are important for skin health, hormone production, and immune function. However, excessive consumption of omega-6 fatty acids relative to omega-3s may contribute to inflammation and increase the risk of chronic diseases.

Benefits of Healthy Fats:

Heart Health:

Healthy fats can help improve cholesterol levels by increasing HDL (good) cholesterol and decreasing LDL (bad) cholesterol. They also help reduce triglyceride levels and lower the risk of heart disease, stroke, and hypertension.

Brain Function:

Omega-3 fatty acids, in particular, are essential for brain health and cognitive function. They support the development and maintenance of brain cells, enhance memory and learning, and may reduce the risk of neurodegenerative diseases such as Alzheimer's disease.

Inflammation Reduction:

Omega-3 fatty acids have anti-inflammatory properties that help reduce inflammation in the body, which is associated with various chronic diseases, including heart disease, arthritis, and diabetes.

Skin and Hair Health:

Monounsaturated and polyunsaturated fats help maintain healthy skin and hair by providing essential fatty acids that support cell membranes and promote moisture retention. They also have antioxidant properties that protect against skin damage caused by UV radiation and environmental factors.

Nutrient Absorption:

Healthy fats are essential for the absorption of fat-soluble vitamins (A, D, E, and K) and other fat-soluble nutrients. They help transport these nutrients through the bloodstream and facilitate their uptake into cells.

Satiety and Weight Management:

Including healthy fats in meals can help promote satiety, reduce hunger, and stabilize blood sugar levels, which can aid in weight management efforts by preventing overeating and cravings.

Incorporating sources of healthy fats into your diet, such as olive oil, avocado, fatty fish, nuts, seeds, and plant-based oils, can contribute to overall health and well-being. Aim to include a variety of healthy fats in your meals while being mindful of portion sizes to support optimal health outcomes.

Plant-Based Foods Contains Fats (Healthy Fats)

Healthy fats, also known as unsaturated fats, are essential components of a balanced diet and play numerous roles in promoting overall health and well-being. Unlike saturated fats and trans fats, which are considered less healthy, healthy fats provide a range of health benefits. Here are some examples of healthy fats and their benefits:

1. **Avocado:**
    - Avocado is one of the richest sources of healthy fats among plant-based foods. It is high in monounsaturated fats, particularly oleic acid.
    - Benefits: Avocado consumption is associated with improved heart health, reduced inflammation, better nutrient absorption, and enhanced skin and hair health.

2. **Nuts:**
    - Various nuts such as almonds, walnuts, cashews, pistachios, and pecans are rich in healthy fats, predominantly monounsaturated and polyunsaturated fats.
    - Benefits: Nuts are associated with lower risk of heart disease, improved cholesterol levels, reduced inflammation, and better cognitive function.
3. **Seeds:**
    - Seeds like chia seeds, flaxseeds, hemp seeds, pumpkin seeds, and sunflower seeds are excellent sources of healthy fats, particularly omega-3 fatty acids and monounsaturated fats.
    - Benefits: Seeds contribute to heart health, brain function, reduced inflammation, improved digestion, and enhanced skin health.
4. **Olives:**
    - Olives and olive oil are rich in monounsaturated fats, particularly oleic acid, as well as other beneficial compounds like polyphenols.
    - Benefits: Olive consumption is associated with reduced risk of heart disease, improved cholesterol levels, lower blood pressure, and reduced inflammation.
5. **Coconut:**
    - Coconut, including coconut meat, coconut oil, and coconut milk, contains healthy saturated fats, particularly medium-chain triglycerides (MCTs).
    - Benefits: Coconut consumption is linked to improved heart health, weight management, enhanced brain function, and antimicrobial properties.
6. **Soybeans and Soy Products:**
    - Soybeans and soy-based products like tofu, tempeh, and edamame are good sources of healthy fats, including polyunsaturated and monounsaturated fats.
    - Benefits: Soy consumption is associated with improved heart health, reduced cholesterol levels, better bone health, and reduced risk of certain cancers.
7. **Dark Chocolate:**
    - Dark chocolate with a high cocoa content is a source of healthy fats, particularly monounsaturated fats. It also contains flavonoids with antioxidant properties.
    - Benefits: Dark chocolate consumption is linked to improved heart health, reduced inflammation, better cognitive function, and enhanced mood.

Incorporating these plant-based foods high in healthy fats into your diet can contribute to overall health and well-being. It's important to consume them in moderation as part of a balanced diet to reap their benefits while maintaining a healthy weight and lifestyle.

Other Foods Contain Healthy Fats:

Fatty Fish:

- Fatty fish like salmon, mackerel, sardines, trout, and herring are high in omega-3 fatty acids, particularly EPA and DHA.
- Benefits: Fatty fish consumption is linked to reduced risk of heart disease, improved cognitive function, and better mood.

What is Vitamin A?

Vitamin A is a fat-soluble vitamin that plays a critical role in various physiological functions in the human body. It exists in several forms, including retinol, retinal, retinoic acid, and provitamin A carotenoids.

Vitamin A is essential for various functions in the body, including vision, immune function, and skin health. While animal products are rich sources of preformed vitamin A (retinol), some plant-based foods provide provitamin A carotenoids, which the body can convert into active vitamin A.

Vitamin A is essential for:

Vision: One of the most well-known functions of vitamin A is its role in maintaining healthy vision. Retinal, a derivative of vitamin A, is a key component of rhodopsin, a protein found in the retina of the eye that is essential for low-light and color vision. Adequate vitamin A intake helps prevent night blindness and supports overall visual health.

Immune Function: Vitamin A plays a crucial role in supporting the immune system by promoting the production and function of white blood cells, which help the body fight off infections and diseases. It also helps maintain the integrity of mucosal surfaces in the respiratory, digestive, and urinary tracts, which serve as barriers against pathogens.

Skin Health: Vitamin A is involved in the growth and repair of skin cells, making it essential for maintaining healthy skin. It promotes cell turnover, supports the production of collagen, and helps prevent dryness, flakiness, and roughness of the skin. Topical retinoids derived from vitamin A are commonly used in skincare products to treat acne, wrinkles, and other skin conditions.

Reproduction and Growth: Vitamin A is important for reproductive health and fertility in both men and women. It is also necessary for normal growth and development, particularly in children, as it supports bone growth, tissue repair, and overall growth processes.

Gene Expression and Cell Differentiation: Vitamin A regulates gene expression and cell differentiation, influencing the development and function of various tissues and organs throughout the body. It plays a role in embryonic development, organ formation, and the maintenance of tissue integrity.

Vitamin A is found in a variety of foods, including liver, fish liver oils, dairy products, eggs, and fortified foods. It is also abundant in colorful fruits and vegetables, particularly those rich in provitamin A carotenoids such as beta-carotene, which the body can convert into active vitamin A. Consuming a balanced diet that includes a variety of foods rich in vitamin A is essential for maintaining optimal health and preventing deficiency-related health issues.

Plant-Based Foods High in Vitamin A

Here is a list of plant-based foods high in vitamin A or its precursors:

1. **Sweet Potatoes:**
    - High in beta-carotene, a provitamin A carotenoid.
2. **Carrots:**
    - Rich in beta-carotene, contributing to their orange color.
3. **Butternut Squash:**
    - Contains beta-carotene, providing both vitamin A and antioxidants.
4. **Pumpkin:**
    - Another excellent source of beta-carotene.
5. **Spinach:**
    - Contains beta-carotene and other carotenoids, contributing to its green color.
6. **Kale:**
    - Rich in beta-carotene and other carotenoids.
7. **Broccoli:**
    - Contains beta-carotene and is a good source of various nutrients.
8. **Mango:**
    - Provides beta-carotene, along with a sweet and tropical flavor.

9. **Cantaloupe:**
    - High in beta-carotene and provides a refreshing taste.
10. **Red and Yellow Bell Peppers:**
    - Contain beta-carotene, as well as vitamin C.
11. **Apricots (Dried):**
    - A good source of beta-carotene, especially when dried.
12. **Papaya:**
    - Contains beta-carotene and is rich in vitamin C.
13. **Tomatoes:**
    - Provide beta-carotene and other carotenoids, along with lycopene.
14. **Chili Peppers:**
    - Contain beta-carotene, especially in the red and orange varieties.
15. **Turnip Greens:**
    - Rich in beta-carotene, as well as other vitamins and minerals.

It's important to note that while these plant-based foods contain provitamin A carotenoids, the conversion efficiency to active vitamin A (retinol) may vary among individuals. Including a variety of colorful fruits and vegetables in your diet can contribute to overall health and help meet your vitamin A needs.

Vitamin B1 (Thiamine)

What is Vitamin B1 (Thiamine)?

Vitamin B1, also known as thiamine, is a water-soluble vitamin that plays a crucial role in energy metabolism and nerve function. It is one of the eight B vitamins that collectively form the vitamin B complex. Thiamine is essential for various physiological processes in the body, including:

1. **Energy Metabolism**: Thiamine is a coenzyme in the metabolism of carbohydrates, fats, and proteins. It helps convert carbohydrates into glucose, the body's primary source of energy. Thiamine is involved in the production of adenosine triphosphate (ATP), a molecule that stores and transports energy within cells.
2. **Nerve Function**: Thiamine is important for maintaining the health and function of the nervous system. It plays a role in the synthesis of neurotransmitters, which are chemical messengers that transmit signals between nerve cells. Thiamine deficiency can lead to nerve damage, resulting in symptoms such as numbness, tingling, muscle weakness, and impaired reflexes.
3. **Heart Health**: Thiamine is necessary for the proper functioning of the heart muscle. It helps regulate the contraction and relaxation of cardiac muscle cells, which is essential for maintaining normal heart rhythm and pumping blood throughout the body. Thiamine deficiency can lead to cardiovascular problems, including heart failure and enlarged heart.
4. **Brain Function**: Thiamine is important for cognitive function and mental health. It is involved in the synthesis of acetylcholine, a neurotransmitter that plays a role in memory, learning, and mood regulation. Thiamine deficiency has been associated with neurological disorders such as Wernicke-Korsakoff syndrome, characterized by confusion, memory loss, and impaired coordination.
5. **Digestive Health**: Thiamine is necessary for the production of stomach acid and the proper functioning of the digestive system. It helps convert carbohydrates into energy and supports the metabolism of nutrients in the gastrointestinal tract. Thiamine deficiency can lead to digestive issues such as poor appetite, constipation, and bloating.

Good dietary sources of thiamine include whole grains, fortified cereals, legumes, nuts, seeds, pork, beef, poultry, fish, and eggs. Cooking methods such as boiling and milling can deplete thiamine content in foods, so it's important to consume a varied diet that includes a mix of thiamine-rich foods to meet daily requirements. Additionally, certain factors such as alcohol consumption, certain medications, and certain medical conditions can increase the risk of thiamine deficiency, so it's important to be mindful of overall nutritional intake and health status.

Plant-Based Foods High in Vitamin B1 (Thiamine)

Vitamin B1, also known as thiamine, is crucial for energy metabolism and the proper functioning of the nervous system. For individuals following a plant-based or vegan diet, it's important to be aware of plant-based sources of vitamin B1 (thiamine). While animal products are typically rich in this vitamin, several plant-based foods also contain significant amounts of vitamin B1. Here is a list of plant-based foods high in vitamin B1:

Whole Grains:

- Brown rice
- Whole wheat
- Barley
- Quinoa
- Oats

Legumes:

- Lentils
- Black beans
- Kidney beans
- Chickpeas
- Green peas

Nuts and Seeds:

- Sunflower seeds
- Pecans
- Pistachios
- Flaxseeds
- Sesame seeds

Nutritional Yeast:

- Nutritional yeast is a popular ingredient in plant-based diets and is often fortified with vitamin B1 and other B-vitamins.

Fortified Foods:

- Some plant-based foods, especially breakfast cereals and plant-based milk alternatives (like almond, soy, or rice milk), are fortified with vitamin B1.

Whole Wheat Bread and Pasta:

- Choose whole wheat or whole grain bread and pasta for a vitamin B1 boost.

Leafy Greens:

- Spinach
- Kale
- Collard greens
- Swiss chard

Avocado:

- Avocado is not only a good source of healthy fats but also contains vitamin B1.

Dried Fruits:

- Raisins
- Apricots
- Dates

Brown Rice Syrup:

- Brown rice syrup, a sweetener derived from brown rice, can be a source of vitamin B1.

Incorporating a variety of these plant-based foods into your meals can help ensure an adequate intake of vitamin B1. It's essential to maintain a balanced and varied diet to meet overall nutritional needs. If you have specific dietary concerns or are considering a significant change in your diet, consulting with a healthcare professional or a registered dietitian is advisable.

Vitamin B2 (Riboflavin)

What is Vitamin B2 (Riboflavin)?

Vitamin B2, also known as riboflavin, is an essential water-soluble vitamin that plays a crucial role in energy metabolism and the maintenance of healthy skin, eyes, and nerve functions. It is one of the eight B vitamins that collectively form the vitamin B complex. Riboflavin is involved in numerous biochemical reactions, and its functions include:

Energy Metabolism: Riboflavin serves as a precursor for two important coenzymes involved in energy metabolism: flavin mononucleotide (FMN) and flavin adenine dinucleotide (FAD). These coenzymes participate in the electron transport chain, where they help convert carbohydrates, fats, and proteins into adenosine triphosphate (ATP), the body's primary source of energy.

Antioxidant Defense: Riboflavin functions as an antioxidant, helping to neutralize harmful free radicals and reactive oxygen species (ROS) that can damage cells and contribute to oxidative stress. As part of the antioxidant system, riboflavin helps protect cells and tissues from oxidative damage, which is associated with aging and various chronic diseases.

Cell Growth and Development: Riboflavin is necessary for normal cell growth, development, and repair. It plays a role in the synthesis of DNA, RNA, and proteins, which are essential for cellular processes such as replication, transcription, and translation. Riboflavin also contributes to the maintenance of healthy skin, hair, and nails.

Eye Health: Riboflavin is important for maintaining optimal vision and eye health. It is a component of flavoproteins involved in the production of glutathione, an antioxidant that protects the lens of the eye from oxidative damage. Riboflavin deficiency has been associated with eye disorders such as cataracts and photophobia (sensitivity to light).

Nervous System Function: Riboflavin plays a role in the functioning of the nervous system, including the synthesis of neurotransmitters and the maintenance of myelin sheaths, which protect and insulate nerve fibers. Adequate riboflavin intake is important for normal nerve function and transmission of nerve impulses.

Good dietary sources of riboflavin include dairy products (such as milk, yogurt, and cheese), eggs, lean meats, poultry, fish, nuts, seeds, and fortified cereals and grains. Riboflavin is relatively stable during cooking and food processing, but it can be destroyed by exposure to light. To ensure adequate riboflavin intake, it's important to consume a balanced diet that includes a variety of riboflavin-rich foods. Additionally, certain factors such as alcohol consumption, certain medications, and certain medical conditions can increase the risk of riboflavin deficiency, so it's important to be mindful of overall nutritional intake and health status.

Plant Based Foods High in Vitamin B2 (Riboflavin)

Here is a list of plant-based foods that are high in vitamin B2:

1. **Almonds:**
   - Almonds are not only a good source of healthy fats and protein but also contain significant amounts of vitamin B2.
2. **Sunflower Seeds:**
   - Sunflower seeds are rich in various nutrients, including vitamin B2. They make for a nutritious and convenient snack.
3. **Soybeans:**
   - Soybeans and soy-based products, such as tofu and tempeh, provide a substantial amount of vitamin B2 along with other essential nutrients.
4. **Spinach:**
   - Dark leafy greens like spinach are not only high in iron but also contain notable levels of vitamin B2.
5. **Mushrooms:**
   - Mushrooms, especially crimini and shiitake varieties, are good plant-based sources of vitamin B2.
6. **Whole Grains (Brown Rice, Quinoa, and Whole Wheat):**
   - Whole grains are rich in several B-vitamins, including vitamin B2. Opt for whole grains over refined grains for maximum nutritional benefits.
7. **Avocado:**
   - Avocado is a nutrient-dense fruit that contains various vitamins, including vitamin B2.
8. **Asparagus:**
   - Asparagus is a vegetable that not only provides fiber but also contributes to your vitamin B2 intake.
9. **Broccoli:**
   - Broccoli is a cruciferous vegetable that offers a good amount of vitamin B2 along with other vitamins and minerals.
10. **Fortified Plant-Based Milk:**
    - Many plant-based milk alternatives, such as almond milk, soy milk, and oat milk, are fortified with vitamin B2.

11. **Whole Grain Cereals:**

    - Choose whole grain cereals that are fortified with vitamins, including vitamin B2, for a nutritious breakfast option.

12. **Edamame:**

    - Edamame, or young soybeans, is a tasty and vitamin B2-rich snack or addition to salads and stir-fries.

Incorporating these plant-based foods into your diet can help ensure an adequate intake of vitamin B2. A well-balanced and varied plant-based diet provides the necessary nutrients for overall health and well-being.

Vitamin B3 (Niacin)

What is Vitamin B3?

Vitamin B3, also known as niacin, is a water-soluble vitamin that plays essential roles in various physiological processes within the body. It is one of the eight B vitamins that collectively form the vitamin B complex. Niacin is involved in numerous biochemical reactions, and its functions include:

Energy Metabolism: Niacin is a precursor for two coenzymes, nicotinamide adenine dinucleotide (NAD) and nicotinamide adenine dinucleotide phosphate (NADP), which are involved in energy metabolism. These coenzymes participate in the conversion of carbohydrates, fats, and proteins into adenosine triphosphate (ATP), the body's primary source of energy.

Cellular Respiration: Niacin plays a critical role in cellular respiration, the process by which cells convert glucose and oxygen into ATP through a series of biochemical reactions. NAD and NADP serve as electron carriers in these reactions, facilitating the transfer of electrons and the production of ATP.

DNA Repair and Synthesis: Niacin is necessary for the repair and synthesis of DNA, the genetic material found in cells. It plays a role in maintaining the integrity of the genome and preventing mutations that can lead to genetic disorders and cancer.

Regulation of Gene Expression: Niacin influences the expression of genes involved in various cellular processes, including metabolism, inflammation, and cell growth. It acts as a signaling molecule that modulates gene transcription and protein synthesis in response to physiological and environmental cues.

Cholesterol and Lipid Metabolism: Niacin has been shown to help regulate cholesterol and lipid levels in the blood. It can increase levels of high-density lipoprotein (HDL) cholesterol, often referred to as "good" cholesterol, while decreasing levels of low-density lipoprotein (LDL) cholesterol and triglycerides. This may help reduce the risk of cardiovascular disease.

Skin Health: Niacin can improve skin health by supporting the production of ceramides, which are lipid molecules that help maintain the skin's barrier function and prevent moisture loss. Niacin supplementation has been shown to benefit individuals with conditions such as acne, eczema, and aging-related skin changes.

Good dietary sources of niacin include meat (such as poultry, beef, and pork), fish, nuts, seeds, legumes, whole grains, and fortified cereals. Niacin can also be synthesized in the body from the amino acid tryptophan, although the conversion rate is relatively low. To ensure adequate niacin intake, it's important to consume a balanced diet that includes a variety of niacin-rich foods. Additionally, certain factors such as alcohol consumption, certain medications, and certain medical conditions can increase the risk of niacin deficiency, so it's important to be mindful of overall nutritional intake and health status.

Plant Based Foods High in Vitamin B3 (Niacin)

Here is a list of plant-based foods that are high in Vitamin B3:

1. **Mushrooms:**
    - Mushrooms, especially shiitake and portobello varieties, are a good source of niacin.
2. **Whole Grains:**
    - Whole grains such as brown rice, quinoa, and whole wheat are rich in niacin. Brown rice, in particular, contains more niacin than white rice.
3. **Legumes:**
    - Legumes like lentils, chickpeas, and black beans provide a good amount of niacin. They are also high in protein and fiber.
4. **Nuts and Seeds:**
    - Peanuts, sunflower seeds, and almonds contain niacin. These nuts and seeds are not only a great source of niacin but also provide healthy fats and other essential nutrients.
5. **Fortified Foods:**
    - Some plant-based foods, such as certain fortified cereals and nutritional yeast, are enriched with niacin. Check the product labels for information on added vitamins.
6. **Green Leafy Vegetables:**
    - Certain green leafy vegetables like spinach, kale, and broccoli contain niacin. While the levels may not be as high as in some other foods, they contribute to overall niacin intake.
7. **Avocado:**
    - Avocado is a nutrient-dense fruit that contains small amounts of niacin along with other essential vitamins and minerals.
8. **Sweet Potatoes:**
    - Sweet potatoes are not only rich in niacin but also provide a good dose of other vitamins and minerals.
9. **Bananas:**
    - Bananas contain niacin and are a convenient and portable snack.

10. **Whole Wheat Bread:**
    - Opting for whole wheat bread instead of refined white bread can contribute to your niacin intake.

It's essential to maintain a well-balanced diet that includes a variety of foods to ensure an adequate intake of all essential nutrients, including Vitamin B3. If you have specific dietary concerns or restrictions, consulting with a healthcare professional or a registered dietitian can help you plan a nutritionally balanced plant-based diet.

Vitamin B5 (Pantothenic Acid):

What is Vitamin B5?

Vitamin B5, also known as pantothenic acid, is a water-soluble vitamin that plays essential roles in various physiological processes within the body. It is one of the eight B vitamins that collectively form the vitamin B complex. Pantothenic acid is involved in numerous biochemical reactions, and its functions include:

Energy Metabolism: Pantothenic acid is a precursor for coenzyme A (CoA), which is essential for the metabolism of carbohydrates, fats, and proteins. CoA serves as a cofactor in key enzymatic reactions involved in the breakdown of nutrients to produce energy in the form of adenosine triphosphate (ATP).

Synthesis of Fatty Acids: Pantothenic acid is necessary for the synthesis of fatty acids, which are building blocks of cell membranes, hormones, and other lipid molecules. CoA is required for the activation of fatty acids and their incorporation into triglycerides, phospholipids, and cholesterol esters.

Synthesis of Acetylcholine: Pantothenic acid is involved in the synthesis of acetylcholine, a neurotransmitter that plays a role in nerve impulse transmission, muscle contraction, and cognitive function. Acetylcholine is synthesized from acetyl-CoA, a derivative of pantothenic acid.

Synthesis of Steroid Hormones: Pantothenic acid is required for the synthesis of steroid hormones, such as cortisol, aldosterone, and testosterone, which regulate various physiological processes, including metabolism, stress response, fluid balance, and reproductive function.

Detoxification: Pantothenic acid is involved in the detoxification of harmful substances in the body. CoA participates in the metabolism of drugs, alcohol, and environmental toxins, facilitating their breakdown and elimination from the body.

Wound Healing: Pantothenic acid plays a role in wound healing and tissue repair. It is involved in the synthesis of collagen, a protein that provides structure and support to tissues, and in the formation of new blood vessels that deliver oxygen and nutrients to injured tissues.

Good dietary sources of pantothenic acid include meat (such as chicken, beef, and pork), fish, eggs, dairy products (such as milk, yogurt, and cheese), whole grains, legumes, nuts, seeds, and vegetables (such as avocados, broccoli, and sweet potatoes). Pantothenic acid is relatively stable during cooking and food processing, so it is present in a wide variety of foods. To ensure adequate pantothenic acid intake, it's important to consume a balanced diet that includes a variety of pantothenic acid-rich foods. Additionally, certain factors such as alcohol consumption, certain medications, and certain medical conditions can increase the risk of pantothenic acid deficiency, so it's important to be mindful of overall nutritional intake and health status.

Plant-Based Foods High in Vitamin B5 (Pantothenic Acid):

Here is a list of plant-based foods that are high in Vitamin B5:

1. **Mushrooms:**
    - Mushrooms, especially shiitake and portobello varieties, contain pantothenic acid.
2. **Avocado:**
    - Avocado is a nutrient-dense fruit that provides a good amount of Vitamin B5 along with healthy fats.
3. **Sweet Potatoes:**
    - Sweet potatoes are not only rich in Vitamin B5 but also offer a range of other vitamins and minerals.
4. **Legumes:**
    - Lentils, chickpeas, and other legumes are excellent sources of pantothenic acid. They are also rich in protein and fiber.
5. **Whole Grains:**
    - Whole grains such as brown rice, quinoa, and whole wheat contain Vitamin B5. These grains are also valuable sources of other essential nutrients.
6. **Broccoli:**
    - Broccoli is a cruciferous vegetable that provides Vitamin B5 along with a variety of other vitamins and minerals.
7. **Sunflower Seeds:**
    - Sunflower seeds are a nutrient-dense snack that contains Vitamin B5 as well as healthy fats and other essential nutrients.
8. **Cauliflower:**
    - Cauliflower is another cruciferous vegetable that contributes to Vitamin B5 intake.
9. **Potatoes:**
    - Potatoes, especially with the skin on, contain pantothenic acid. They are also a good source of carbohydrates and fiber.
10. **Whole Wheat Bread:**
    - Opting for whole wheat bread instead of refined white bread can contribute to your Vitamin B5 intake.

Including a variety of these plant-based foods in your diet can help ensure an adequate intake of Vitamin B5, supporting energy metabolism and overall health. Keep in mind that a well-balanced and varied diet is essential for meeting all your nutritional needs.

Vitamin B6 (Pyridoxine):

What is Vitamin B6?

Vitamin B6, also known as pyridoxine, is a crucial water-soluble vitamin that plays a vital role in various bodily functions, including metabolism, immune function, and neurotransmitter synthesis. It is one of the eight B vitamins that collectively form the vitamin B complex. Pyridoxine is involved in numerous biochemical reactions, and its functions include:

Amino Acid Metabolism: Vitamin B6 is necessary for the metabolism of amino acids, the building blocks of proteins. It is involved in the synthesis and breakdown of amino acids, as well as the conversion of one amino acid into another. Pyridoxine helps ensure that amino acids are available for protein synthesis, as well as for the production of other important molecules such as neurotransmitters, hormones, and enzymes.

Glycogen Metabolism: Pyridoxine plays a role in glycogen metabolism, the process by which glycogen, the storage form of glucose, is broken down into glucose to provide energy for the body. It helps activate enzymes involved in glycogenolysis, the breakdown of glycogen, and gluconeogenesis, the synthesis of glucose from non-carbohydrate sources.

Neurotransmitter Synthesis: Vitamin B6 is involved in the synthesis of several neurotransmitters, including serotonin, dopamine, norepinephrine, and gamma-aminobutyric acid (GABA). These neurotransmitters play important roles in mood regulation, cognition, sleep, and stress response. Pyridoxine helps convert the amino acid tryptophan into serotonin, and it is involved in the synthesis of other neurotransmitters from amino acid precursors.

Hemoglobin Synthesis: Pyridoxine is necessary for the synthesis of hemoglobin, the protein in red blood cells that carries oxygen from the lungs to tissues throughout the body. It helps convert the amino acid glycine into heme, the iron-containing component of hemoglobin. Vitamin B6 deficiency can lead to impaired hemoglobin synthesis and a type of anemia called sideroblastic anemia.

Immune Function: Vitamin B6 plays a role in immune function by supporting the production and activity of immune cells, such as lymphocytes and macrophages. It helps regulate immune responses to infections and inflammation, and it is involved in the production of antibodies that recognize and neutralize pathogens.

Good dietary sources of vitamin B6 include poultry, fish, meat (such as pork and beef), eggs, dairy products, whole grains, nuts, seeds, bananas, avocados, and potatoes. Pyridoxine is relatively stable during cooking and food processing, so it is present in a wide variety of foods. To ensure adequate vitamin B6 intake, it's important to consume a balanced diet that includes a variety of pyridoxine-rich foods. Additionally, certain factors such as alcohol consumption, certain medications, and certain medical conditions can increase the risk of vitamin B6 deficiency, so it's important to be mindful of overall nutritional intake and health status.

Plant-Based Foods High in Vitamin B6 (Pyridoxine):

While animal products are common sources of vitamin B6, there are also plenty of plant-based foods that can help you meet your daily requirements. Here's a list of plant-based foods high in vitamin B6:

1. **Sunflower Seeds:** These tiny seeds are not only rich in vitamin E but also contain a good amount of vitamin B6. They make for a nutritious and crunchy snack.
2. **Pistachio Nuts:** Pistachios are not only delicious but also provide a decent amount of vitamin B6. Snack on them or use them as a topping for salads and desserts.
3. **Bananas:** Along with being a great source of potassium, bananas also contain vitamin B6. They make for a convenient and portable snack.
4. **Avocado:** Avocados are not only creamy and rich in healthy fats but also contain vitamin B6. Enjoy them in salads, sandwiches, or as a topping on toast.
5. **Potatoes:** Potatoes, especially when consumed with the skin, are a good source of vitamin B6. Opt for baked or boiled potatoes for a healthier preparation.
6. **Chickpeas (Garbanzo Beans):** Chickpeas are versatile legumes that can be used in salads, soups, or as the main ingredient in dishes like hummus. They are also a good source of vitamin B6.
7. **Spinach:** Leafy greens like spinach are not only rich in iron but also contain vitamin B6. Add spinach to salads, smoothies, or lightly sauté it as a side dish.
8. **Fortified Plant-Based Milk:** Some plant-based milk alternatives, such as almond, soy, or rice milk, are fortified with vitamins, including B6. Check the labels to ensure they contain added nutrients.
9. **Whole Grains (Brown Rice, Quinoa):** Whole grains like brown rice and quinoa contain vitamin B6. They are excellent additions to a balanced plant-based diet.
10. **Bell Peppers:** Bell peppers, especially the red variety, contain a good amount of vitamin B6. Enjoy them raw in salads or as a crunchy snack.
11. **Watermelon:** This refreshing fruit not only helps keep you hydrated but also provides a small amount of vitamin B6. Enjoy it on its own or add it to fruit salads.
12. **Carrots:** Carrots are not only a good source of vitamin A but also contain vitamin B6. Snack on raw carrot sticks or add them to soups and stews.
13. **Hazelnuts:** Hazelnuts are not only delicious but also contain vitamin B6. Enjoy them as a snack or use them in baking and cooking.
14. **Fortified Cereals:** Many breakfast cereals are fortified with vitamins, including B6. Check the nutritional labels to find fortified cereals that can contribute to your vitamin B6 intake.

Including a variety of these plant-based foods in your diet can help ensure an adequate intake of vitamin B6, supporting overall health and well-being.

Vitamin B7 *(Biotin)*

What is Vitamin B7 *(Biotin)*?

Vitamin B7, also known as biotin, is a water-soluble vitamin that plays a key role in energy metabolism and the maintenance of healthy skin, hair, and nails. It is one of the eight B vitamins that collectively form the vitamin B complex. Biotin is involved in numerous biochemical reactions, and its functions include:

Metabolism of Carbohydrates, Fats, and Proteins: Biotin serves as a cofactor for several enzymes involved in the metabolism of macronutrients. It helps convert carbohydrates, fats, and proteins into energy that the body can use for various functions. Biotin assists in the breakdown of glucose for energy production, the synthesis of fatty acids and cholesterol, and the metabolism of amino acids.

Synthesis of Fatty Acids and Gluconeogenesis: Biotin is necessary for the synthesis of fatty acids, which are important components of cell membranes and storage forms of energy. It helps activate enzymes involved in fatty acid synthesis and elongation. Additionally, biotin is involved in gluconeogenesis, the process by which glucose is synthesized from non-carbohydrate sources such as amino acids and glycerol.

Hair, Skin, and Nail Health: Biotin is often referred to as the "beauty vitamin" because of its role in promoting healthy hair, skin, and nails. It contributes to the maintenance of strong and resilient hair follicles, the formation of keratin (the protein that makes up hair and nails), and the renewal of skin cells. Biotin deficiency can lead to symptoms such as thinning hair, brittle nails, and dry, scaly skin.

Regulation of Gene Expression: Biotin influences the expression of genes involved in various cellular processes, including metabolism, cell growth, and differentiation. It acts as a cofactor for enzymes that regulate gene transcription and protein synthesis. Biotin deficiency can disrupt normal gene expression patterns and contribute to metabolic disorders.

Blood Sugar Regulation: Biotin may play a role in regulating blood sugar levels by enhancing insulin sensitivity and glucose uptake in cells. It helps activate enzymes involved in glucose metabolism and insulin signaling pathways. Biotin supplementation has been shown to improve glucose tolerance and reduce insulin resistance in some studies.

Good dietary sources of biotin include egg yolks, liver, nuts (such as almonds, peanuts, and walnuts), seeds (such as sunflower seeds), whole grains, legumes, avocado, sweet potatoes, and certain fruits (such as bananas). Biotin is also produced by bacteria in the gut, although the amount synthesized is thought to be relatively small compared to dietary intake. To ensure adequate biotin intake, it's important to consume a balanced diet that includes a variety of biotin-rich foods. Additionally, certain factors such as pregnancy, breastfeeding, certain medications, and certain medical conditions can increase the need for biotin, so it's important to be mindful of overall nutritional intake and health status.

Plant-Based Foods High in Vitamin B7 (Biotin):

While biotin deficiency is rare, incorporating foods rich in this vitamin into a plant-based diet can contribute to overall well-being. Here is a list of plant-based foods high in vitamin B7 (biotin):

1. **Nuts (especially peanuts and almonds):** Peanuts and almonds are excellent sources of biotin. Snack on them or add them to your salads and meals for a biotin boost.
2. **Seeds (especially sunflower seeds):** Sunflower seeds are rich in biotin and can be sprinkled on salads, yogurt, or enjoyed on their own as a snack.
3. **Legumes (especially lentils):** Lentils, chickpeas, and other legumes are good sources of biotin. Incorporate them into soups, stews, and salads for a nutrient-packed meal.
4. **Whole Grains (especially oats and barley):** Whole grains like oats and barley contain biotin. Enjoy them as part of your breakfast or in various dishes to increase your biotin intake.
5. **Sweet Potatoes:** Sweet potatoes not only provide a healthy dose of biotin but also offer other essential nutrients. Roast, mash, or bake sweet potatoes for a nutritious side dish.
6. **Bananas:** Bananas are not only a convenient and portable snack but also contain biotin. Add them to your smoothies or enjoy them as a quick energy boost.
7. **Avocado:** Avocado is a nutrient-rich fruit that contains biotin. Use it in salads, sandwiches, or as a topping for toast.
8. **Broccoli:** Broccoli is a cruciferous vegetable that is not only high in biotin but also offers various vitamins and minerals. Steam or stir-fry broccoli to retain its nutritional value.
9. **Spinach:** Spinach is a leafy green vegetable that provides biotin along with other essential nutrients. Add spinach to salads, smoothies, or sauté it as a side dish.
10. **Mushrooms:** Certain types of mushrooms, such as shiitake and portobello, contain biotin. Incorporate them into your meals for an umami flavor and a biotin boost.
11. **Tomatoes:** Tomatoes are not only a tasty addition to various dishes but also contain biotin. Include them in salads, sauces, or enjoy them fresh.
12. **Carrots:** Carrots are a good source of biotin and can be enjoyed raw as a snack, in salads, or cooked in various dishes.

Including a variety of these plant-based foods in your diet can help ensure an adequate intake of biotin, supporting the health of your skin, hair, and nails, as well as overall energy metabolism.

Vitamin B9 (Folate or Folic Acid):

What is vitamin B9?

Vitamin B9, commonly known as folate or folic acid, is a crucial nutrient for various bodily functions, including DNA synthesis, cell division, and the formation of red blood cells. It is particularly important during pregnancy for fetal development. It is one of the eight B vitamins that collectively form the vitamin B complex. Folate is crucial for several functions, including:

DNA Synthesis and Repair: Folate is essential for the synthesis and repair of DNA, the genetic material found in every cell of the body. It is particularly important during periods of rapid cell division and growth, such as during pregnancy and infancy. Folate helps ensure that cells can replicate and repair their DNA accurately, preventing mutations and abnormalities.

Cell Division and Growth: Folate plays a key role in cell division and growth by supporting the formation of new cells. It is necessary for the production of nucleotides, the building blocks of DNA and RNA, which are required for cell replication and proliferation. Adequate folate intake is important for normal development and growth, especially in fetuses, infants, and children.

Red Blood Cell Formation: Folate is involved in the production of red blood cells, which are responsible for carrying oxygen from the lungs to tissues throughout the body. Folate is necessary for the maturation of red blood cell precursors in the bone marrow and for the synthesis of hemoglobin, the protein that binds and transports oxygen in the blood. Folate deficiency can lead to a type of anemia called megaloblastic anemia, characterized by large, immature red blood cells.

Homocysteine Metabolism: Folate plays a role in the metabolism of homocysteine, an amino acid that can accumulate in the blood if not properly metabolized. High levels of homocysteine are associated with an increased risk of cardiovascular disease, stroke, and other health problems. Folate helps convert homocysteine into methionine, a process that requires vitamin B12 and vitamin B6 as cofactors.

Neurological Function: Folate is important for normal neurological function and brain health. It is involved in the synthesis of neurotransmitters such as serotonin, dopamine, and norepinephrine, which play key roles in mood regulation, cognition, and behavior. Adequate folate intake is important for maintaining mental and emotional well-being.

Good dietary sources of folate include leafy green vegetables (such as spinach, kale, and collard greens), legumes (such as lentils, chickpeas, and black beans), fruits (such as oranges, strawberries, and avocado), fortified grains and cereals, nuts, seeds, and liver. Folate is also available in supplement form, and folic acid is the synthetic form of folate used in fortified foods and supplements. Pregnant women, women of childbearing age, and individuals with certain medical conditions may require additional folate supplementation to meet their needs.

Plant-Based Foods High in Vitamin B9 (Folate or Folic Acid):

Here is a list of plant-based foods high in vitamin B9:

1. **Leafy Greens (Spinach, Kale, Collard Greens):** Leafy greens are rich sources of folate. Add spinach or kale to your salads, smoothies, or stir-fries to boost your folate intake.
2. **Legumes (Lentils, Chickpeas, Black Beans):** Lentils, chickpeas, and black beans are excellent plant-based sources of folate. Incorporate them into soups, stews, and salads for a nutrient-rich meal.
3. **Asparagus:** Asparagus is a tasty vegetable that provides a good amount of folate. Roast or steam asparagus as a side dish or add it to pasta dishes.
4. **Avocado:** Avocado is not only a creamy and nutritious fruit but also contains folate. Enjoy avocado in salads, sandwiches, or as a topping for toast.
5. **Broccoli:** Broccoli is a cruciferous vegetable that offers a significant amount of folate. Include broccoli in your meals by steaming, roasting, or adding it to stir-fries.
6. **Citrus Fruits (Oranges, Grapefruits):** Citrus fruits are known for their vitamin C content, but they also provide folate. Enjoy oranges, grapefruits, or their juices as part of your daily fruit intake.
7. **Brussels Sprouts:** Brussels sprouts are a cruciferous vegetable that contributes to your folate intake. Roast or sauté Brussels sprouts for a flavorful side dish.
8. **Papaya:** Papaya is a tropical fruit that not only provides a burst of sweetness but also contains a good amount of folate. Enjoy fresh papaya or add it to fruit salads.
9. **Sunflower Seeds:** Sunflower seeds are a nutrient-dense snack that contains folate. Sprinkle them on salads, yogurt, or eat them on their own for a crunchy treat.
10. **Edamame:** Edamame, or young soybeans, is a tasty and protein-rich snack that also offers folate. Boil or steam edamame and enjoy them as a snack or appetizer.
11. **Cauliflower:** Cauliflower is a versatile vegetable that can be used in various dishes. Roast, mash, or include cauliflower in curries to increase your folate intake.
12. **Beets:** Beets are not only colorful and flavorful but also provide a good amount of folate. Roast, boil, or grate beets for salads or side dishes.

Incorporating a variety of these plant-based foods into your diet can help ensure an adequate intake of vitamin B9, supporting overall health and well-being. If you are pregnant or planning to become pregnant, it's crucial to consult with a healthcare professional to ensure you meet your folate requirements for optimal fetal development.

Vitamin B12 (Cobalamin)

What is Vitamin B12?

Vitamin B12, also known as cobalamin. This plays a crucial role in various bodily functions, including the formation of red blood cells and maintenance of the nervous system. It is one of the eight B vitamins that collectively form the vitamin B complex. Vitamin B12 is crucial for several functions, including:

Red Blood Cell Formation: Vitamin B12 is essential for the production of red blood cells, which are responsible for carrying oxygen from the lungs to tissues throughout the body. B12 is required for the synthesis of DNA and RNA in red blood cell precursors in the bone marrow, as well as for the maturation of red blood cells. Vitamin B12 deficiency can lead to a type of anemia called megaloblastic anemia, characterized by large, immature red blood cells.

Nervous System Function: Vitamin B12 plays a critical role in the functioning of the nervous system. It is involved in the maintenance of myelin, a protective sheath that surrounds and insulates nerve fibers, allowing for efficient transmission of nerve impulses. B12 is also necessary for the synthesis of neurotransmitters such as serotonin, dopamine, and norepinephrine, which play key roles in mood regulation, cognition, and behavior.

DNA Synthesis and Repair: Vitamin B12 is required for the synthesis and repair of DNA, the genetic material found in every cell of the body. It is particularly important during periods of rapid cell division and growth, such as during pregnancy, infancy, and adolescence. B12 helps ensure that cells can replicate and repair their DNA accurately, preventing mutations and abnormalities.

Homocysteine Metabolism: Vitamin B12 is involved in the metabolism of homocysteine, an amino acid that can accumulate in the blood if not properly metabolized. High levels of homocysteine are associated with an increased risk of cardiovascular disease, stroke, and other health problems. B12 helps convert homocysteine into methionine, a process that requires folate and vitamin B6 as cofactors.

Cellular Energy Production: Vitamin B12 plays a role in energy metabolism by aiding in the conversion of certain fatty acids and amino acids into energy. It is involved in the synthesis of succinyl-CoA, a compound that participates in the citric acid cycle, a series of biochemical reactions that generate ATP, the body's primary source of energy.

Good dietary sources of vitamin B12 include animal products such as meat (particularly liver and shellfish), poultry, fish, eggs, dairy products (such as milk, cheese, and yogurt), and fortified foods (such as breakfast cereals, plant-based milk alternatives, and nutritional yeast). Vitamin B12 is not found in plant foods unless they are fortified with the vitamin. Individuals following a vegan or vegetarian diet may need to supplement with vitamin B12 to ensure adequate intake. Additionally, certain factors such as age, digestive disorders, and certain medications can impair the absorption of vitamin B12, so it's important to be mindful of overall nutritional intake and health.

Plant-Based Foods High in Vitamin B12 (Cobalamin)

It is primarily found in animal products making it challenging for individuals following a strict plant-based diet to obtain adequate amounts. However, there are some plant-based foods that may contain small amounts of B12 or are fortified with synthetic B12. It's important to note that these sources may not provide sufficient B12 for everyone, and supplementation or fortified foods may be necessary. Always consult with a healthcare professional for personalized advice. Here are some plant-based sources of vitamin B12:

1. **Cranberries:**
    - Cranberries may contain trace amounts of vitamin B12, but they are not a reliable source.
2. **Dates:**
    - Dates may contain small amounts of B12, but they are not considered a significant source.
3. **Mulberries:**
    - Mulberries are reported to contain minimal amounts of vitamin B12.
4. **Fortified Foods:**
    - Many plant-based foods are fortified with synthetic vitamin B12, such as:
        - Fortified plant-based milk (soy, almond, coconut, etc.)
        - Fortified breakfast cereals
        - Fortified nutritional yeast
5. **Algae/Spirulina:**
    - Some algae and spirulina products are claimed to contain B12; however, the B12 analogs found in these sources may not be readily absorbed or utilized by the human body. Therefore, they are not considered reliable sources of active B12.
6. **Fortified Plant-Based Meat Alternatives:**
    - Some plant-based meat substitutes are fortified with vitamin B12.

7. **Supplements:**
    - Vitamin B12 supplements are a reliable way for individuals following a plant-based diet to meet their B12 requirements. Always consult with a healthcare professional before starting any supplementation.

It's crucial for individuals following a strict plant-based or vegan diet to monitor their B12 levels regularly and consider supplementation or fortified foods to ensure they meet their nutritional needs. Vitamin B12 is essential for neurological health, red blood cell formation, and overall well-being, and a deficiency can lead to serious health issues over time.

Other Foods High in Vitamin B12 (Cobalamin)

Vitamin B12 is primarily found in animal products, and it plays a crucial role in various bodily functions, including the formation of red blood cells and maintenance of the nervous system. For individuals following a vegetarian or vegan diet, it's essential to obtain vitamin B12 from fortified foods or supplements, as natural sources are limited. Here is a list of foods rich in vitamin B12:

1. **Meat:**
    - Beef
    - Chicken
    - Pork
    - Lamb
2. **Fish:**
    - Salmon
    - Trout
    - Tuna
    - Sardines
    - Mackerel
    - Herring
3. **Shellfish:**
    - Clams
    - Oysters
    - Crab

- Mussels

4. **Dairy Products:**
    - Milk
    - Cheese
    - Yogurt
5. **Eggs:**
    - Eggs, particularly the yolk
6. **Fortified Plant-Based Foods:**
    - Fortified plant-based milk (soy, almond, coconut, etc.)
    - Fortified breakfast cereals
    - Fortified nutritional yeast
    - Fortified plant-based yogurt
7. **Organ Meats:**
    - Liver (beef, chicken, pork)
8. **Supplements:**
    - Vitamin B12 supplements, available in various forms such as cyanocobalamin or methylcobalamin.

It's important to note that while some plant-based foods may claim to contain B12, the B12 found in these sources is often in the form of analogs, which are structurally similar to B12 but not effectively utilized by the human body. Therefore, individuals following a plant-based or vegan diet should prioritize fortified foods or supplements to ensure adequate B12 intake.

Always consult with a healthcare professional for personalized advice on meeting your nutritional needs, especially if you are following a specific diet or have any health concerns.

Vitamin C (Ascorbic Acid)

What is Vitamin C?

Vitamin C, also known as ascorbic acid, is a water-soluble vitamin and is an essential nutrient that plays a crucial role in various bodily functions, including the formation of collagen, absorption of iron, the immune system, and antioxidant protection. It is a potent antioxidant and is necessary for several functions, including:

Antioxidant Defense: Vitamin C acts as an antioxidant, helping to neutralize harmful free radicals and reactive oxygen species (ROS) that can damage cells and contribute to oxidative stress. As an antioxidant, vitamin C helps protect cells and tissues from oxidative damage caused by environmental toxins, pollutants, UV radiation, and metabolic processes.

Collagen Synthesis: Vitamin C is essential for the synthesis of collagen, a structural protein found in connective tissues, skin, bones, cartilage, and blood vessels. Collagen provides strength and support to tissues, and it is necessary for wound healing, tissue repair, and the maintenance of healthy skin, hair, and nails. Vitamin C plays a critical role in the hydroxylation of proline and lysine residues during collagen synthesis.

Immune Function: Vitamin C is important for supporting the immune system and defending the body against infections and diseases. It enhances the function of various immune cells, including neutrophils, macrophages, and lymphocytes, and it helps promote the production and activity of antibodies that recognize and neutralize pathogens such as bacteria, viruses, and fungi.

Iron Absorption: Vitamin C enhances the absorption of non-heme iron, the form of iron found in plant-based foods and iron supplements. It helps convert ferric iron ($Fe3+$) into ferrous iron ($Fe2+$), which is more readily absorbed in the intestine. By improving iron absorption, vitamin C helps prevent and treat iron deficiency anemia, a common nutritional deficiency worldwide.

Neurotransmitter Synthesis: Vitamin C is involved in the synthesis of neurotransmitters such as serotonin, dopamine, and norepinephrine, which play key roles in mood regulation, cognition, and behavior. It acts as a cofactor for enzymes involved in the conversion of amino acids into neurotransmitters and in the metabolism of catecholamines.

Antiviral Properties: Vitamin C has been shown to exhibit antiviral properties and may help reduce the severity and duration of viral infections such as the common cold, influenza, and COVID-19. It supports the immune response to viral pathogens and may inhibit viral replication and spread.

Good dietary sources of vitamin C include citrus fruits (such as oranges, lemons, and grapefruits), strawberries, kiwi fruit, guava, papaya, pineapple, bell peppers (particularly red and yellow peppers), broccoli, Brussels sprouts, kale, and tomatoes. Vitamin C is also available in supplement form, including ascorbic acid and other vitamin C derivatives. It's important to consume a balanced diet that includes a variety of vitamin C-rich foods to ensure adequate intake of this essential nutrient. Additionally, certain factors such as smoking, alcohol consumption, stress, and certain medical conditions can increase the need for vitamin C, so it's important to be mindful of overall nutritional intake and health status.

Plant-Based Foods High in Vitamin C (Ascorbic Acid)

Here is a list of plant-based foods that are high in Vitamin C:

1. **Citrus Fruits:**
    - Oranges
    - Grapefruits
    - Lemons
    - Limes
    - Clementines
2. **Berries:**
    - Strawberries
    - Blueberries
    - Raspberries
    - Blackberries
    - Cranberries
3. **Tropical Fruits:**
    - Pineapple
    - Mango
    - Papaya
    - Guava
    - Kiwi

4. **Melons:**
    - Cantaloupe
    - Honeydew
5. **Citrus-Like Fruits:**
    - Acerola cherries
    - Kiwi (although it's not a citrus fruit, it has a high Vitamin C content)
6. **Cruciferous Vegetables:**
    - Broccoli
    - Brussels sprouts
    - Cauliflower
7. **Leafy Greens:**
    - Kale
    - Spinach
    - Swiss chard
    - Collard greens
8. **Bell Peppers:**
    - Red, green, or yellow bell peppers
9. **Tomatoes:**
    - Fresh tomatoes
    - Tomato juice
    - Tomato sauce
10. **Tropical Root Vegetables:**
    - Sweet potatoes
11. **Berries:**
    - Strawberries
    - Blueberries
    - Raspberries
    - Blackberries

- Cranberries

12. Paprika:

- This spice, derived from ground peppers, is a potent source of Vitamin C.

13. Guava:

- Guava is an exceptionally rich source of Vitamin C.

14. Pineapple:

- Besides being a tropical delight, pineapple is high in Vitamin C.

15. Mango:

- Mangoes not only offer a sweet taste but also contribute to your Vitamin C intake.

Including a variety of these plant-based foods in your diet can help ensure an adequate intake of Vitamin C, supporting your overall health and well-being.

Vitamin D

What is Vitamin D?

Vitamin D is a fat-soluble vitamin that plays a crucial role in various physiological processes within the human body. It is unique among vitamins in that it can be synthesized by the body in response to sunlight exposure as well as obtained from dietary sources and supplements. Vitamin D is essential for overall health and is involved in several important functions, including:

1. **Calcium absorption and bone health:** One of the primary functions of vitamin D is its role in promoting the absorption of calcium from the intestines into the bloodstream. Calcium is essential for maintaining strong bones and teeth, and adequate vitamin D levels are necessary for optimal calcium absorption. Vitamin D also helps regulate calcium levels in the blood by promoting calcium reabsorption in the kidneys and supporting bone mineralization.

2. **Bone growth and remodeling:** Vitamin D is important for bone growth and development, particularly during childhood and adolescence. It helps regulate the activity of osteoblasts, the cells responsible for building new bone tissue, and osteoclasts, the cells responsible for breaking down and resorbing old bone tissue. Vitamin D deficiency can lead to impaired bone mineralization, weakened bones, and an increased risk of fractures and bone disorders such as rickets in children and osteomalacia in adults.

3. **Immune function:** Vitamin D plays a role in modulating the immune system and has been shown to have anti-inflammatory and immunomodulatory effects. Adequate vitamin D levels may help reduce the risk of infections, autoimmune diseases, and chronic inflammatory conditions. Vitamin D receptors are found on various immune cells, and vitamin D regulates the expression of genes involved in immune response and inflammation.

4. **Regulation of cell growth and differentiation:** Vitamin D is involved in regulating cell growth, proliferation, and differentiation in various tissues throughout the body. It plays a role in controlling the expression of genes involved in cell cycle regulation, apoptosis (programmed cell death), and differentiation of cells into specialized cell types. Vitamin D may have implications for cancer prevention and treatment, as abnormal cell growth and differentiation are hallmarks of cancer development.

5. **Mood regulation and mental health:** There is growing evidence suggesting a link between vitamin D deficiency and mood disorders such as depression and seasonal affective disorder (SAD). Vitamin D receptors are found in areas of the brain involved in mood regulation, and vitamin D may influence neurotransmitter levels and neuronal function. Adequate vitamin D levels may help support mental well-being and reduce the risk of mood disorders.

Sources of vitamin D include sunlight exposure, dietary sources such as fatty fish (e.g., salmon, mackerel, tuna), fortified foods (e.g., fortified dairy products, breakfast cereals, and orange juice), and vitamin D supplements. However, many people may have difficulty obtaining sufficient vitamin D from sunlight and diet alone, especially during the winter months or in regions with limited sunlight exposure. Therefore, supplementation may be necessary for individuals at risk of vitamin D deficiency, particularly those with limited sun exposure, dark skin, older adults, individuals with certain medical conditions, or those who follow strict vegetarian or vegan diets.

While vitamin D is essential for overall health, it's important to maintain balanced levels, as excessive intake of vitamin D can lead to toxicity, known as hypervitaminosis D, which can cause symptoms such as nausea, vomiting, weakness, and hypercalcemia (elevated calcium levels in the blood). Therefore, it's important to consult with a healthcare professional for personalized guidance on vitamin D supplementation and monitoring of vitamin D levels.

Natural Foods High in Vitamin D

Vitamin D is unique because it can be synthesized by the body through exposure to sunlight. However, there are also some foods that naturally contain vitamin D. Here is a list of natural foods high in vitamin D:

1. **Fatty Fish:**
    - Salmon (wild-caught)
    - Mackerel
    - Sardines
    - Herring
    - Trout
    - Tuna (particularly canned in oil)
2. **Cod Liver Oil:**
    - Cod liver oil is an excellent source of vitamin D, but it should be consumed in moderation due to its high vitamin A content.
3. **Egg Yolks:**
    - Egg yolks contain small amounts of vitamin D. Choose eggs from pasture-raised or omega-3 enriched sources for higher vitamin D levels.
4. **Beef Liver:**
    - Beef liver is a good source of vitamin D, but it should be eaten in moderation due to its high vitamin A content.

5. **Mushrooms:**

    - Some mushrooms, when exposed to sunlight or ultraviolet (UV) light during growth, can produce vitamin D2. This includes maitake and UV-exposed portobello mushrooms.

6. **Fortified Foods:**

    - Certain foods are fortified with vitamin D, which means the vitamin is added during processing. This includes:
        - Fortified dairy products (milk, yogurt, cheese)
        - Fortified plant-based milk (soy, almond, rice, oat)
        - Fortified orange juice
        - Fortified breakfast cereals

It's essential to note that the amount of vitamin D in food sources can vary, and sunlight exposure remains a crucial factor in maintaining adequate vitamin D levels in the body. The recommended dietary allowance (RDA) for vitamin D can vary based on factors such as age, sex, and individual health conditions. If you have concerns about your vitamin D levels, it's advisable to consult with a healthcare professional for personalized advice.

Vitamin E (Tocopherol)

What is Vitamin E?

Vitamin E is a fat-soluble antioxidant that plays essential roles in various physiological processes within the body. It exists in several forms, with alpha-tocopherol being the most biologically active form. Vitamin E acts primarily as an antioxidant, protecting cells and tissues from oxidative damage caused by free radicals and reactive oxygen species. Its functions include:

Antioxidant Protection: Vitamin E scavenges free radicals and reactive oxygen species (ROS) that can damage cell membranes, DNA, proteins, and lipids, leading to oxidative stress and cellular damage. By neutralizing free radicals, vitamin E helps prevent oxidative damage and supports overall health and well-being.

Cell Membrane Stability: Vitamin E helps maintain the integrity and stability of cell membranes by protecting polyunsaturated fatty acids (PUFAs) from lipid peroxidation. It incorporates into cell membranes, where it acts as a lipid-soluble antioxidant, preventing oxidative damage to membrane lipids and preserving membrane structure and function.

Immune Function: Vitamin E supports the function of the immune system by enhancing the activity of immune cells, such as T cells, B cells, natural killer (NK) cells, and macrophages. It helps regulate immune responses to infections, inflammation, and tissue injury, and it plays a role in modulating cytokine production and signaling pathways involved in immune regulation.

Cardiovascular Health: Vitamin E may help protect against cardiovascular disease by reducing oxidative stress, inflammation, and endothelial dysfunction. It inhibits the oxidation of low-density lipoprotein (LDL) cholesterol, a process that contributes to the development of atherosclerosis and coronary artery disease. Vitamin E also helps improve blood vessel function and reduce platelet aggregation and thrombosis.

Skin Health: Vitamin E is often used in skincare products and supplements due to its potential benefits for skin health. It helps protect the skin from UV radiation, environmental pollutants, and oxidative stress, which can cause premature aging, wrinkles, and skin damage. Vitamin E promotes skin hydration, elasticity, and regeneration, and it may help reduce inflammation and promote wound healing.

Neurological Function: Vitamin E plays a role in neurological function and brain health. It protects nerve cells from oxidative damage and supports the integrity of myelin, the fatty substance that insulates nerve fibers and facilitates efficient nerve impulse transmission. Vitamin E may help reduce the risk of neurodegenerative diseases such as Alzheimer's disease and Parkinson's disease.

Good dietary sources of vitamin E include nuts (such as almonds, hazelnuts, and sunflower seeds), seeds (such as pumpkin seeds and flaxseeds), vegetable oils (such as wheat germ oil, sunflower oil, and safflower oil), green leafy vegetables (such as spinach and kale), avocados, and fortified foods (such as cereals and spreads). Vitamin E supplements are also available, but it's important to consult with a healthcare professional before starting supplementation, as excessive intake of vitamin E supplements may have adverse effects in some individuals. Additionally, vitamin E works synergistically with other antioxidants, such as vitamin C, so it's important to consume a balanced diet rich in a variety of antioxidants to support overall health and well-being.

Plant-Based Foods High in Vitamin E (Tocopherol)

Here is a list of plant-based foods that are high in vitamin E:

1. **Nuts:**
    - Almonds
    - Sunflower seeds
    - Hazelnuts
    - Pine nuts
    - Brazil nuts
    - Peanuts (and peanut butter)
2. **Seeds:**
    - Sunflower seeds
    - Pumpkin seeds
    - Sesame seeds
3. **Plant Oils:**
    - Sunflower oil
    - Wheat germ oil
    - Olive oil
    - Almond oil
    - Hazelnut oil
4. **Leafy Green Vegetables:**
    - Spinach
    - Swiss chard
    - Kale

- Collard greens
- Turnip greens

5. **Fruits:**
    - Avocado
    - Kiwi
    - Blackberries
    - Blueberries
6. **Fortified Foods:**
    - Some processed and fortified foods, like cereals and plant-based milk, may contain added vitamin E.
7. **Whole Grains:**
    - Wheat germ
    - Brown rice
    - Oats
8. **Legumes:**
    - Chickpeas
    - Lentils

Including a variety of these vitamin E-rich plant-based foods in your diet can contribute to meeting your daily vitamin E needs. Keep in mind that vitamin E is found in different forms, such as tocopherols and tocotrienols, and a diverse diet helps ensure you get a range of these beneficial compounds. As with any nutrient, it's always a good idea to achieve a balance in your diet rather than relying on a single source. If you have specific dietary concerns or conditions, consider consulting with a healthcare professional or a registered dietitian for personalized advice.

Vitamin K

What is Vitamin K?

Vitamin K is a fat-soluble vitamin that plays essential roles in blood clotting, bone metabolism, and cardiovascular health. There are two main forms of vitamin K: vitamin K1 (phylloquinone) and vitamin K2 (menaquinone).

Blood Clotting: Vitamin K is necessary for the synthesis of clotting factors in the liver, particularly factors II (prothrombin), VII, IX, and X. These clotting factors are essential for the blood coagulation process, which helps stop bleeding when blood vessels are injured. Vitamin K promotes the conversion of precursor proteins into active forms that participate in the clotting cascade, leading to the formation of blood clots.

Bone Metabolism: Vitamin K plays a role in bone metabolism by supporting the activation of osteocalcin, a protein involved in bone mineralization. Osteocalcin helps bind calcium ions to the bone matrix, promoting bone formation and strength. Vitamin K also regulates the activity of matrix Gla protein (MGP), which inhibits the calcification of soft tissues, such as blood vessels and cartilage, thus helping prevent arterial calcification and maintaining cardiovascular health.

Cardiovascular Health: Vitamin K2, in particular, has been associated with cardiovascular health benefits beyond its role in blood clotting. It helps prevent arterial calcification by activating matrix Gla protein (MGP), which inhibits the deposition of calcium in arterial walls and reduces the risk of atherosclerosis and cardiovascular disease. Adequate vitamin K intake has been linked to a lower risk of coronary artery calcification and cardiovascular events.

Brain and Nervous System: Emerging research suggests that vitamin K may play a role in brain and nervous system health. Vitamin K-dependent proteins are found in the brain, where they may contribute to neuronal function and protect against neurodegenerative diseases such as Alzheimer's disease. Further studies are needed to elucidate the specific mechanisms by which vitamin K influences brain health.

Immune Function: Vitamin K may modulate immune function by regulating the production of cytokines and inflammatory mediators. Some studies suggest that vitamin K deficiency may impair immune responses and increase susceptibility to infections and inflammatory diseases. However, more research is needed to fully understand the role of vitamin K in immune function.

Good dietary sources of vitamin K1 include green leafy vegetables (such as kale, spinach, collard greens, and Swiss chard), broccoli, Brussels sprouts, cabbage, and other cruciferous vegetables. Vitamin K2 is found in fermented foods (such as natto, a traditional Japanese dish made from fermented soybeans), cheese, egg yolks, and animal products (such as meat and liver). Additionally, vitamin K is synthesized by bacteria in the gut, but the extent of absorption varies among individuals. Adequate vitamin K intake is important for overall health and well-being, and deficiencies can lead to bleeding disorders, osteoporosis, and other health problems.

Plant-Based Foods High in Vitamin K

Here is a list of plant-based foods that are high in vitamin K:

1. **Leafy Greens:**
    - Kale
    - Spinach
    - Swiss chard
    - Collard greens
    - Mustard greens
    - Turnip greens
    - Beet greens
2. **Cruciferous Vegetables:**
    - Broccoli
    - Brussels sprouts
    - Cabbage
    - Cauliflower
3. **Herbs:**
    - Parsley
    - Basil
    - Thyme
    - Cilantro
    - Sage
4. **Lettuce Varieties:**
    - Romaine lettuce
    - Iceberg lettuce
    - Green leaf lettuce

5. **Green Vegetables:**
    - Asparagus
    - Green beans
    - Peas
    - Zucchini
6. **Natto:**
    - Natto, a traditional Japanese dish made from fermented soybeans, is particularly high in vitamin K2.
7. **Seaweed:**
    - Nori
    - Kelp
    - Wakame
8. **Avocado:**
    - Avocado provides a moderate amount of vitamin K.
9. **Brussels Sprouts:**
    - These cruciferous vegetables deserve a separate mention due to their notable vitamin K content.
10. **Kiwi:**
    - Kiwi fruit contains a modest amount of vitamin K.

Remember that vitamin K is fat-soluble, so consuming these foods with a source of healthy fat may enhance its absorption. Including a variety of these plant-based foods in your diet can help ensure an adequate intake of vitamin K, promoting overall health and well-being. Always consult with a healthcare professional or nutritionist to determine your specific nutritional needs.

Essential Minerals

What are Minerals?

Minerals are naturally occurring inorganic substances that are essential for various physiological functions in the human body. These substances cannot be synthesized by the body and must be obtained from dietary sources. Minerals play crucial roles in processes such as bone formation, nerve transmission, muscle function, fluid balance, and energy metabolism.

There are two main categories of minerals:

Macrominerals: These are minerals that are required by the body in larger amounts. Common macrominerals include calcium, phosphorus, magnesium, sodium, potassium, chloride, and sulfur. These minerals are vital for maintaining healthy bones, teeth, muscles, and electrolyte balance.

Microminerals (Trace Minerals): Microminerals are required by the body in smaller amounts compared to macrominerals. Examples of trace minerals include iron, zinc, copper, selenium, iodine, manganese, chromium, and molybdenum. Despite their lower concentration in the body, trace minerals play crucial roles in enzyme function, hormone synthesis, immune function, and antioxidant defense.

Minerals are found in a variety of foods, including fruits, vegetables, whole grains, legumes, nuts, seeds, dairy products, and lean meats. The bioavailability of minerals can vary depending on factors such as the form of the mineral, the presence of other nutrients, and individual factors such as age and health status.

Here is a comprehensive list of crucial minerals that our body needs, along with their respective functions:

1. **Calcium:**
    - Functions: Bone and teeth health, blood clotting, nerve function, and muscle contraction.
2. **Phosphorus:**
    - Functions: Bone health, energy metabolism, and DNA and RNA synthesis.
3. **Potassium:**
    - Functions: Fluid balance, nerve function, muscle contraction, and blood pressure regulation.
4. **Sodium:**
    - Functions: Fluid balance, nerve function, muscle contraction, and blood pressure regulation.

5. **Magnesium:**
   - Functions: Muscle and nerve function, bone health, energy metabolism, and DNA synthesis.
6. **Sulfur:**
   - Functions: Component of certain amino acids and vitamins, supports protein structure.
7. **Iron:**
   - Functions: Oxygen transport (hemoglobin), energy metabolism, and immune function.
8. **Zinc:**
   - Functions: Immune function, wound healing, DNA synthesis, and cell division.
9. **Copper:**
   - Functions: Red blood cell formation, connective tissue health, and enzyme activity.
10. **Manganese:**
    - Functions: Bone formation, blood clotting, and antioxidant defense.
11. **Selenium:**
    - Functions: Antioxidant activity, thyroid function, and immune response.
12. **Iodine:**
    - Functions: Essential for thyroid hormone synthesis, which regulates metabolism.
13. **Fluoride:**
    - Functions: Dental health, prevents tooth decay, and strengthens tooth enamel.
14. **Chromium:**
    - Functions: Enhances insulin activity, supports glucose metabolism.
15. **Molybdenum:**
    - Functions: Enzyme activity, including those involved in amino acid metabolism.
16. **Cobalt:**
    - Functions: Component of vitamin B12, involved in red blood cell formation.
17. **Nickel:**
    - Functions: Enzyme activity, though its essential role in humans is not well-established.

These minerals are crucial for a wide range of physiological functions, and maintaining an adequate intake is essential for overall health. A balanced and varied diet that includes nutrient-dense foods is the best way to ensure proper mineral intake. If there are concerns about mineral levels or specific health conditions, consulting with a healthcare professional can provide personalized guidance.

Calcium

What is Calcium?

Calcium is a chemical element with the symbol Ca and atomic number 20. It is an essential mineral that plays a crucial role in various physiological processes within the human body. Calcium is the most abundant mineral in the body, with about 99% of it stored in bones and teeth, where it provides strength and structure. The remaining 1% of calcium circulates in the bloodstream and is involved in numerous vital functions, including:

Bone Health: Calcium is a key component of bone tissue, contributing to bone density and strength. Adequate calcium intake during childhood and adolescence is crucial for optimal bone development and growth. Throughout adulthood, calcium helps maintain bone mass and prevents osteoporosis, a condition characterized by weakened and porous bones.

Teeth Health: Calcium is also essential for dental health, as it helps build and maintain the structure of tooth enamel, the outer layer of the teeth. Tooth enamel is primarily composed of hydroxyapatite, a calcium phosphate mineral that provides protection against decay and erosion.

Muscle Contraction: Calcium ions play a central role in muscle contraction, including both skeletal muscle (voluntary muscle) and smooth muscle (involuntary muscle). When stimulated by nerve impulses, calcium is released from storage sites within muscle cells, triggering a series of biochemical reactions that result in muscle contraction.

Nerve Function: Calcium ions are involved in nerve transmission and signaling. They help regulate the release of neurotransmitters, which are chemical messengers that transmit signals between nerve cells. Calcium ions also participate in the generation and propagation of action potentials, the electrical impulses that allow nerve cells to communicate with each other.

Blood Clotting: Calcium is essential for the process of blood clotting (coagulation), which helps prevent excessive bleeding when blood vessels are injured. Calcium ions interact with various proteins and enzymes involved in the coagulation cascade, leading to the formation of fibrin, a fibrous protein that forms blood clots and stops bleeding.

Cell Signaling: Calcium ions serve as universal signaling molecules within cells, regulating a wide range of cellular processes, including gene expression, enzyme activity, hormone secretion, and cell proliferation. Calcium signaling pathways are involved in the control of cell growth, differentiation, and apoptosis (programmed cell death).

Good dietary sources of calcium include dairy products (such as milk, cheese, and yogurt), fortified plant-based milk alternatives (such as almond milk and soy milk), leafy green vegetables (such as kale, broccoli, and collard greens), tofu, sardines, salmon, almonds, and calcium-fortified foods (such as breakfast cereals and orange juice). In addition to dietary sources, calcium supplements may be recommended for individuals who have difficulty meeting their calcium needs through diet alone. However, it's important to consult with a healthcare professional before starting any supplement regimen, as excessive calcium intake can have adverse effects.

Plant-Based Foods High in Calcium

Calcium is an essential mineral for bone health, muscle function, and nerve transmission. While dairy products are a well-known source of calcium, there are plenty of plant-based foods that provide this vital nutrient. Here is a list of plant-based foods that are high in calcium:

1. **Leafy Green Vegetables:**
    - Kale
    - Collard greens
    - Turnip greens
    - Bok choy
    - Broccoli
2. **Fortified Plant Milks:**
    - Soy milk (fortified)
    - Almond milk (fortified)
    - Oat milk (fortified)
    - Coconut milk (fortified)
    - Rice milk (fortified)
3. **Tofu and Tempeh:**
    - Tofu, especially firm or extra-firm varieties
    - Tempeh
4. **Nuts and Seeds:**
    - Almonds
    - Chia seeds
    - Sesame seeds
    - Poppy seeds

5. **Legumes:**
    - Chickpeas
    - Lentils
    - Black beans
    - White beans
6. **Whole Grains:**
    - Amaranth
    - Quinoa
    - Oats (especially fortified oatmeal)
    - Teff
7. **Fortified Foods:**
    - Certain plant-based foods are fortified with calcium. Check labels for added calcium in products like breakfast cereals, energy bars, and plant-based yogurt.
8. **Dried Fruits:**
    - Figs (dried)
    - Apricots (dried)
9. **Seaweed:**
    - Wakame and hijiki seaweed are good sources of calcium. However, their consumption should be moderated due to their iodine content.
10. **Oranges and Figs:**
    - Oranges and figs contain some calcium and can contribute to your overall intake.

Remember that the absorption of calcium can be influenced by other nutrients in your diet. Consuming foods rich in vitamin D, magnesium, and vitamin K, as well as maintaining a well-balanced diet, can optimize calcium absorption. If you have specific dietary concerns or restrictions, it's advisable to consult with a healthcare professional or a registered dietitian for personalized advice on meeting your calcium needs.

Magnesium

What is Magnesium?

Magnesium is a chemical element with the symbol Mg and atomic number 12. It is a vital mineral that plays numerous essential roles in the human body. Magnesium is involved in over 300 biochemical reactions, making it crucial for various physiological functions. Some key functions of magnesium include:

Muscle Function: Magnesium is necessary for proper muscle function, including muscle contraction and relaxation. It works in concert with calcium to regulate muscle contractions by activating and deactivating muscle proteins.

Nerve Function: Magnesium plays a role in nerve transmission and neuromuscular conduction. It helps regulate the flow of calcium ions across nerve cell membranes, which is essential for transmitting nerve impulses.

Energy Metabolism: Magnesium is involved in the production and utilization of ATP (adenosine triphosphate), the primary energy currency of cells. It participates in various enzymatic reactions involved in carbohydrate, protein, and fat metabolism.

Protein Synthesis: Magnesium is required for the synthesis of proteins, including enzymes and structural proteins. It helps stabilize the structure of ribosomes, the cellular machinery responsible for protein synthesis.

DNA and RNA Synthesis: Magnesium is essential for the replication and transcription of DNA and RNA. It facilitates the binding of enzymes involved in DNA replication and repair, as well as the assembly of ribonucleotides into RNA molecules.

Bone Health: Magnesium is a component of bone tissue and contributes to bone density and strength. It works synergistically with calcium and vitamin D to support bone mineralization and prevent osteoporosis.

Cardiovascular Health: Magnesium plays a role in maintaining normal heart rhythm and function. It helps regulate the contraction and relaxation of the heart muscle and supports the function of the cardiovascular system.

Blood Pressure Regulation: Magnesium helps regulate blood pressure by relaxing blood vessels and improving blood flow. It inhibits the constriction of blood vessels and counteracts the effects of calcium, which can promote vasoconstriction.

Good dietary sources of magnesium include green leafy vegetables (such as spinach, kale, and Swiss chard), nuts and seeds (such as almonds, pumpkin seeds, and sunflower seeds), legumes (such as beans, lentils, and chickpeas), whole grains (such as brown rice, quinoa, and oats), avocados, bananas, and dark chocolate. In addition to dietary sources, magnesium supplements are available and may be recommended for individuals who have difficulty meeting their magnesium needs through diet alone. However, it's important to consult with a healthcare professional before starting any supplement regimen, as excessive magnesium intake can have adverse effects, particularly in individuals with kidney problems.

Plant-Based Foods High in Magnesium

Magnesium is an essential mineral that plays a crucial role in various bodily functions, including muscle and nerve function, blood sugar regulation, and bone health. Here is a list of plant-based foods that are high in magnesium:

1. **Leafy Green Vegetables:**
    - Spinach
    - Swiss chard
    - Kale
    - Collard greens
    - Turnip greens
2. **Nuts and Seeds:**
    - Almonds
    - Cashews
    - Pumpkin seeds
    - Sunflower seeds
    - Flaxseeds
    - Chia seeds
3. **Whole Grains:**
    - Brown rice
    - Quinoa
    - Oats
    - Buckwheat
    - Barley
    - Whole wheat
4. **Legumes:**
    - Black beans

- Chickpeas
- Lentils
- Kidney beans
- Edamame

5. **Fruits:**
    - Bananas
    - Avocados
    - Figs
    - Prunes
    - Raisins
6. **Vegetables:**
    - Potatoes (with skin)
    - Sweet potatoes
    - Broccoli
    - Brussels sprouts
    - Zucchini
7. **Tofu:**
    - Tofu and other soy products can be good sources of magnesium.
8. **Dark Chocolate:**
    - Dark chocolate with a high cocoa content is not only a delicious treat but also contains magnesium.
9. **Whole Plant Foods:**
    - Eating a variety of whole, plant-based foods in your diet ensures a balanced intake of magnesium. Include a colorful array of fruits, vegetables, nuts, seeds, and whole grains to meet your nutritional needs.

It's important to note that the magnesium content in foods can vary based on factors such as soil quality and processing methods. Additionally, some plant-based foods contain compounds that may affect magnesium absorption. Consuming a diverse and balanced plant-based diet is key to obtaining not only magnesium but also a wide range of essential nutrients for overall health. If you have specific dietary concerns or health conditions, consider consulting with a healthcare professional or a registered dietitian.

Phosphorus

What is Phosphorus?

Phosphorus is a chemical element with the symbol P and atomic number 15. It is an essential mineral that plays critical roles in various biological processes within the human body. Phosphorus is the second most abundant mineral in the body, after calcium, and is primarily found in bones and teeth, where it provides structural support and strength. Some key functions of phosphorus include:

Bone and Teeth Health: Phosphorus is a major component of bone mineral hydroxyapatite, along with calcium. It contributes to bone density, strength, and rigidity, making it essential for bone formation and maintenance. Phosphorus is also present in tooth enamel, where it helps protect against decay and erosion.

Energy Metabolism: Phosphorus is a crucial component of adenosine triphosphate (ATP), the primary energy currency of cells. ATP is involved in various cellular processes that require energy, including muscle contraction, nerve transmission, and biochemical reactions involved in metabolism.

Cellular Structure and Function: Phosphorus is a key structural component of cell membranes, where it forms phospholipids, a type of lipid molecule. Phospholipids help maintain the integrity and fluidity of cell membranes and play roles in cell signaling, transport, and cell-to-cell communication.

DNA and RNA Synthesis: Phosphorus is an essential component of nucleic acids, including DNA (deoxyribonucleic acid) and RNA (ribonucleic acid). It forms the backbone of the nucleic acid molecules, providing structural stability and serving as a template for genetic information.

Buffering System: Phosphorus participates in the body's acid-base balance as a component of buffer systems, such as phosphate buffers. Buffer systems help maintain the pH (acidity or alkalinity) of bodily fluids within a narrow range, which is essential for proper cellular function and physiological processes.

Cellular Signaling and Communication: Phosphorus-containing molecules, such as phosphorylated proteins and second messengers like cyclic adenosine monophosphate (cAMP) and inositol triphosphate (IP3), play crucial roles in cellular signaling pathways. They regulate various cellular processes, including gene expression, enzyme activity, hormone secretion, and cell growth and differentiation.

Good dietary sources of phosphorus include dairy products (such as milk, cheese, and yogurt), meat, poultry, fish, eggs, nuts, seeds, legumes (such as beans and lentils), whole grains (such as wheat, oats, and barley), and fortified foods (such as breakfast cereals and beverages). Most people obtain an adequate amount of phosphorus through a balanced diet, and deficiencies are rare in healthy individuals. However, excessive phosphorus intake from phosphorus-rich processed foods and additives may contribute to health issues, particularly in individuals with kidney problems or certain medical conditions.

Plant-Based Foods High in Phosphorus

Phosphorus is an essential mineral that plays a crucial role in various bodily functions, including bone and teeth health, energy metabolism, and kidney function. While animal products are often rich sources of phosphorus, several plant-based foods also contain significant amounts of this essential nutrient. Here is a list of plant-based foods high in phosphorus:

1. **Sunflower Seeds:**
   - Sunflower seeds are not only a tasty snack but also a good source of phosphorus. They can be sprinkled on salads, yogurt, or enjoyed on their own.
2. **Pumpkin Seeds:**
   - Pumpkin seeds, also known as pepitas, are rich in phosphorus and make a nutritious addition to salads, granola, or trail mix.
3. **Soybeans:**
   - Soybeans and soy-based products, such as tofu and tempeh, contain significant amounts of phosphorus. Incorporate soy-based foods into your diet for a plant-based phosphorus boost.
4. **Lentils:**
   - Lentils are a versatile legume that provides not only protein and fiber but also phosphorus. They can be used in soups, stews, salads, or as a side dish.
5. **Chickpeas:**
   - Chickpeas, whether cooked and tossed into salads or blended into hummus, are a good plant-based source of phosphorus.
6. **Quinoa:**
   - Quinoa, a protein-rich pseudo-grain, contains phosphorus. It can be used as a base for salads, bowls, or served as a side dish.
7. **Nuts (Almonds, Cashews, Walnuts):**
   - Various nuts, including almonds, cashews, and walnuts, contain phosphorus. Enjoy them as a snack or incorporate them into your meals and desserts.
8. **Whole Grains (Brown Rice, Oats):**

- Whole grains such as brown rice and oats provide not only complex carbohydrates but also phosphorus. They can be used in a variety of dishes, from breakfast porridge to savory meals.

9. **Spinach:**
    - Leafy greens like spinach contain phosphorus, along with other essential nutrients. Add spinach to salads, smoothies, or sauté it as a side dish.
10. **Broccoli:**
    - Broccoli is a cruciferous vegetable that is not only rich in vitamins but also contains phosphorus. Include broccoli in stir-fries, salads, or as a side dish.
11. **Brussels Sprouts:**
    - Brussels sprouts are another cruciferous vegetable that contributes to your phosphorus intake. Roast or sauté them for a delicious side dish.
12. **Sweet Potatoes:**
    - Sweet potatoes provide not only a healthy dose of beta-carotene but also contain phosphorus. Bake or roast sweet potatoes for a nutritious side dish.

It's important to note that the phosphorus content in plant-based foods may vary, and factors like cooking methods can influence nutrient availability. Maintaining a well-balanced and varied plant-based diet can help ensure an adequate intake of essential nutrients, including phosphorus. If you have specific dietary concerns or conditions, it's advisable to consult with a healthcare professional or a registered dietitian.

Sodium

What is Sodium?

Sodium is a chemical element with the symbol Na and atomic number 11. It is an essential mineral that plays crucial roles in various physiological processes within the human body. Sodium is primarily known for its role in regulating fluid balance, blood pressure, and nerve function. Some key functions of sodium include:

Fluid Balance: Sodium is one of the main electrolytes in the body and plays a central role in maintaining fluid balance. It works in conjunction with other electrolytes, such as potassium and chloride, to regulate the distribution of water inside and outside of cells. Sodium helps maintain proper hydration levels and prevents dehydration by facilitating the movement of water across cell membranes through osmosis.

Blood Pressure Regulation: Sodium plays a key role in regulating blood pressure by controlling blood volume and fluid balance. It helps maintain the proper concentration of electrolytes in the blood and extracellular fluid, which influences blood volume and vascular tone. High sodium intake can lead to increased blood volume and fluid retention, raising blood pressure and increasing the risk of hypertension and cardiovascular disease.

Nerve Function: Sodium ions are essential for the generation and propagation of nerve impulses (action potentials) along nerve cells (neurons). When stimulated, sodium channels in the cell membrane open, allowing sodium ions to flow into the cell and depolarize the membrane. This depolarization triggers an action potential, which is transmitted along the length of the neuron to communicate signals between cells.

Muscle Contraction: Sodium ions also play a role in muscle contraction, particularly in skeletal muscle (voluntary muscle) and smooth muscle (involuntary muscle). During muscle contraction, sodium ions enter muscle cells, triggering the release of calcium ions from intracellular stores and initiating the contraction process.

Acid-Base Balance: Sodium bicarbonate (NaHCO3) is an important buffer in the body that helps regulate acid-base balance. It acts as a base to neutralize excess acids in the blood and maintain the pH (acidity or alkalinity) within a narrow range. Sodium bicarbonate is produced by the kidneys and helps prevent acidosis (excess acidity) by removing hydrogen ions from the bloodstream.

Good dietary sources of sodium include table salt (sodium chloride), processed foods (such as canned soups, snack foods, condiments, and ready-to-eat meals), cured meats (such as bacon and ham), cheese, pickled foods, and restaurant meals. While sodium is essential for health, excessive sodium intake can have adverse effects on blood pressure and cardiovascular health. Therefore, it's important to consume sodium in moderation and to choose whole, unprocessed foods whenever possible.

Plant-Based Foods Contain Sodium

While excessive sodium intake is generally discouraged due to its association with health issues like high blood pressure, some plant-based foods naturally contain sodium. It's important to note that the sodium content in plant-based foods is typically lower compared to processed and animal-based products. Here are some plant-based foods that naturally contain sodium:

1. **Vegetables:**
    - Many vegetables contain small amounts of sodium. Examples include:
        - Spinach
        - Beets
        - Celery
        - Carrots
        - Tomatoes
2. **Legumes:**
    - Legumes are a good source of plant-based protein and may contain some sodium. Examples include:
        - Lentils
        - Chickpeas
        - Black beans
        - Kidney beans
3. **Whole Grains:**
    - Some whole grains naturally contain small amounts of sodium. Examples include:
        - Quinoa
        - Brown rice
        - Oats
4. **Nuts and Seeds:**
    - Nuts and seeds may contain trace amounts of sodium. Examples include:
        - Almonds
        - Sunflower seeds
        - Chia seeds

5. **Fruits:**
    - While fruits are generally low in sodium, certain fruits like avocados may contain small amounts.
6. **Seaweed:**
    - Seaweed, such as nori or dulse, naturally contains sodium due to its marine environment.
7. **Plant-Based Condiments:**
    - Some plant-based condiments and seasonings can contribute sodium to your diet. Examples include:
        - Soy sauce (choose low-sodium options if available)
        - Tamari
        - Miso paste
        - Pickles

It's important to emphasize that while these plant-based foods contain some sodium, they are generally much lower in sodium than processed foods and animal products. For individuals aiming to reduce their sodium intake, focusing on a diet rich in whole, minimally processed plant-based foods is a recommended approach. Always consult with a healthcare professional or nutritionist for personalized dietary advice.

Potassium

What is Potassium?

Potassium is a chemical element with the symbol K and atomic number 19. It is an essential mineral that plays numerous critical roles in various physiological processes within the human body. Potassium is one of the most abundant electrolytes in the body and is primarily found inside cells, where it helps maintain fluid balance, regulate muscle function, and support nerve transmission. Some key functions of potassium include:

Fluid Balance: Potassium is a major intracellular cation and plays a crucial role in maintaining fluid balance inside cells. It works in conjunction with sodium, another electrolyte, to regulate osmotic pressure and water distribution across cell membranes. Potassium helps prevent cellular dehydration and maintains proper hydration levels, which is essential for cell function and overall health.

Nerve Function: Potassium is essential for nerve transmission and impulse conduction. It helps regulate the electrical excitability of nerve cells (neurons) by maintaining the resting membrane potential and repolarizing the cell membrane after an action potential. Potassium ions move across nerve cell membranes through specialized channels, contributing to the generation and propagation of nerve impulses.

Muscle Contraction: Potassium plays a crucial role in muscle function, including skeletal muscle (voluntary muscle) and smooth muscle (involuntary muscle). It helps regulate muscle contraction by controlling the resting membrane potential and action potential in muscle cells. Potassium ions flow into muscle cells during repolarization, allowing muscles to relax after contraction.

Heart Function: Potassium is essential for maintaining normal heart rhythm and function. It plays a key role in regulating the electrical activity of cardiac muscle cells (cardiomyocytes) and coordinating the contraction and relaxation of the heart muscle. Potassium ions contribute to the generation of action potentials in cardiac cells and help propagate electrical impulses throughout the heart, ensuring coordinated heartbeats.

Blood Pressure Regulation: Potassium helps regulate blood pressure by counteracting the effects of sodium on blood volume and vascular tone. High potassium intake can help lower blood pressure by promoting sodium excretion through the kidneys and relaxing blood vessel walls (vasodilation). Adequate potassium intake is associated with a reduced risk of hypertension and cardiovascular disease.

Good dietary sources of potassium include fruits (such as bananas, oranges, kiwi, and avocados), vegetables (such as potatoes, sweet potatoes, spinach, and broccoli), legumes (such as beans, lentils, and peas), nuts, seeds, whole grains, dairy products, and fish. Most people obtain adequate potassium through a balanced diet rich in fruits, vegetables, and whole foods. However, certain medical conditions, medications, and dietary factors can affect potassium levels in the body, so it's important to consult with a healthcare professional for personalized guidance on potassium intake and supplementation.

Plant-Based Foods High Potassium

Potassium is an essential mineral that plays a crucial role in maintaining proper heart, muscle, and nerve function. Including potassium-rich foods in your diet is important for overall health. Here is a list of plant-based foods that are high in potassium:

1. **Bananas:**
    - Bananas are perhaps one of the most well-known potassium-rich fruits. They are convenient and make for a great portable snack.
2. **Sweet Potatoes:**
    - Sweet potatoes are not only delicious but also packed with potassium. Roasted, baked, or mashed, they offer a versatile and nutritious addition to your meals.
3. **Spinach:**
    - Dark leafy greens, such as spinach, are excellent sources of potassium. Whether eaten raw in salads or cooked in various dishes, spinach is a nutrient powerhouse.
4. **Avocado:**
    - Avocado is not only a good source of healthy fats but also contains a substantial amount of potassium. Enjoy it sliced on toast, in salads, or as guacamole.
5. **Oranges:**
    - Oranges and other citrus fruits like grapefruits and mandarins are not only rich in vitamin C but also provide a decent amount of potassium.
6. **Potatoes:**
    - Potatoes, whether white or sweet, are reliable sources of potassium. Be sure to eat the skin, as it contains additional nutrients.
7. **Beans and Lentils:**
    - Legumes, including kidney beans, black beans, lentils, and chickpeas, are excellent plant-based sources of potassium. They are also high in fiber and protein.
8. **Tomatoes and Tomato Products:**
    - Tomatoes, tomato sauce, and tomato paste are good sources of potassium. They can be included in a variety of dishes, from salads to sauces.

9. **Coconut Water:**
    - Coconut water is not only a hydrating beverage but also contains potassium. It's a natural and refreshing option to help meet your potassium needs.
10. **Mushrooms:**
    - Mushrooms, especially white button mushrooms and shiitake mushrooms, contain potassium and can be a tasty addition to various dishes.
11. **Cantaloupe:**
    - Cantaloupe and other melons, such as honeydew, provide a sweet and hydrating way to increase potassium intake.
12. **Broccoli:**
    - Broccoli is a nutrient-rich vegetable that contains potassium along with vitamins, fiber, and other minerals.

Including a variety of these potassium-rich plant-based foods in your diet can contribute to maintaining a healthy balance of electrolytes and supporting overall well-being. As with any dietary changes, it's advisable to consult with a healthcare professional, especially if you have specific health concerns or conditions.

Chloride

What is Chloride?

Chloride is an essential mineral and an electrolyte that plays important roles in various physiological processes within the human body. It is an anion, meaning it carries a negative electrical charge, and is often found in the form of chloride ions (Cl-) dissolved in bodily fluids. Chloride is the major negatively charged ion in extracellular fluid, working in tandem with other electrolytes like sodium and potassium to maintain fluid balance, regulate pH, and support nerve function. Some key functions of chloride include:

Fluid Balance: Chloride ions help maintain the balance of fluids inside and outside of cells. Together with sodium, chloride regulates osmotic pressure and water distribution across cell membranes. This balance is critical for proper cell hydration and overall cellular function.

Acid-Base Balance: Chloride ions are involved in the body's acid-base balance, helping to regulate pH levels in bodily fluids. Chloride serves as a component of the bicarbonate buffer system, which helps neutralize excess acids or bases in the blood and maintain the body's pH within a narrow, optimal range.

Digestion: Chloride ions play a role in the production of hydrochloric acid (HCl) in the stomach. Hydrochloric acid is essential for the breakdown of food in the stomach, aiding in digestion and the absorption of nutrients such as proteins, minerals, and vitamins.

Nerve Function: Chloride ions contribute to the transmission of nerve impulses (action potentials) along nerve cells (neurons). They help maintain the resting membrane potential and regulate the excitability of nerve cells, influencing nerve signaling and communication throughout the nervous system.

Electrolyte Balance: Chloride ions, along with sodium and potassium, help maintain the balance of electrolytes in the body. These electrolytes play critical roles in cellular function, muscle contraction, nerve transmission, and fluid balance, among other physiological processes.

Good dietary sources of chloride include table salt (sodium chloride), seaweed, olives, celery, tomatoes, lettuce, and other vegetables. Chloride is also present in many processed foods, as salt (sodium chloride) is commonly used as a flavoring and preservative. Most people obtain adequate chloride through their diet, and deficiencies are rare in healthy individuals. However, excessive intake of sodium chloride (salt) can contribute to health issues such as high blood pressure and cardiovascular disease, so it's important to consume salt in moderation and to focus on a balanced diet rich in whole, unprocessed foods.

Plant-Based Foods Contain Chloride

Plant-based foods that contain chloride include:

1. **Celery:** Celery is a crunchy vegetable that contains a moderate amount of chloride.
2. **Tomatoes:** Tomatoes are a versatile fruit (often consumed as a vegetable) that contain chloride.
3. **Lettuce:** Various types of lettuce, such as romaine, iceberg, and leaf lettuce, contain chloride.
4. **Olives:** Olives, whether green or black, are a source of chloride.
5. **Seaweed:** Certain types of seaweed, such as nori, kombu also known as Kelp, and wakame, contain chloride.
6. **Spinach:** Spinach is a leafy green vegetable that contains chloride, among other nutrients.
7. **Swiss Chard:** Swiss chard, a leafy green vegetable similar to spinach, contains chloride.
8. **Kale:** Kale, a nutrient-rich leafy green vegetable, contains chloride.
9. **Arugula:** Arugula, also known as rocket or rucola, contains chloride and other essential nutrients.
10. **Cabbage:** Various types of cabbage, including green cabbage, red cabbage, and Napa cabbage, contain chloride.

These plant-based foods provide a variety of essential nutrients, including chloride, as part of a balanced diet. Incorporating a diverse range of fruits, vegetables, whole grains, legumes, nuts, and seeds into meals can help ensure adequate intake of essential minerals like chloride, along with other vitamins, minerals, fiber, and phytonutrients.

Iron

What is Iron?

Iron is a crucial mineral that plays a vital role in various physiological processes within the human body. It is classified as a trace mineral because the body requires it in relatively small amounts compared to other nutrients, but its importance cannot be overstated. Iron is essential for the formation of hemoglobin, a protein found in red blood cells that is responsible for transporting oxygen from the lungs to the rest of the body's tissues and organs. Additionally, iron is a key component of myoglobin, a protein found in muscles that helps store and transport oxygen for muscle function.

There are two main forms of dietary iron: heme iron and non-heme iron. Heme iron is found in animal-based foods, such as meat, poultry, and fish, and is more easily absorbed by the body. Non-heme iron is found in plant-based foods, such as beans, lentils, fortified grains, and leafy green vegetables, but it is not as readily absorbed by the body as heme iron.

Iron deficiency is one of the most common nutritional deficiencies worldwide and can lead to a condition known as iron deficiency anemia. Symptoms of iron deficiency anemia may include fatigue, weakness, pale skin, shortness of breath, dizziness, headaches, and cold hands and feet. It is particularly prevalent among pregnant women, infants, young children, adolescents, menstruating individuals, and individuals following vegetarian or vegan diets.

To prevent iron deficiency, it is important to consume an adequate amount of iron-rich foods in your diet. Additionally, consuming vitamin C-rich foods alongside iron-rich foods can enhance the absorption of non-heme iron. In cases of severe iron deficiency or anemia, supplementation with iron supplements may be necessary under the guidance of a healthcare professional.

In summary, iron is an essential mineral that plays a critical role in oxygen transport, energy production, and overall health. Consuming a balanced diet that includes iron-rich foods is essential for preventing iron deficiency and maintaining optimal health and well-being.

Plant-Based Foods High in Iron

Iron is also involved in energy metabolism, DNA synthesis, and the production of neurotransmitters. Some key benefits of iron are Oxygen Transport, Energy Metabolism, Immune Function, Cognitive Function, Muscle Function, Healthy Pregnancy, Healthy Skin, Hair and Nails.

Here is a list of plant-based foods that are high in iron:

1. **Legumes:**
    - Lentils
    - Chickpeas (garbanzo beans)
    - Black beans
    - Kidney beans
    - Soybeans (including tofu and tempeh)
    - Peas (green peas, split peas)
2. **Leafy Greens:**
    - Spinach
    - Kale
    - Swiss chard
    - Collard greens
    - Beet greens
3. **Seeds:**
    - Pumpkin seeds (pepitas)
    - Sesame seeds (including tahini)
    - Hemp seeds
    - Flaxseeds
4. **Nuts:**
    - Cashews
    - Pine nuts
    - Almonds
    - Pistachios
5. **Whole Grains:**
    - Quinoa
    - Oats (including oatmeal)
    - Brown rice

- Amaranth
- Buckwheat

6. **Fortified Foods:**
    - Fortified breakfast cereals
    - Fortified plant-based milk (such as almond milk, soy milk, or oat milk)
    - Fortified tofu
7. **Dried Fruits:**
    - Apricots
    - Raisins
    - Prunes
    - Dates
8. **Herbs and Spices:**
    - Thyme
    - Cumin
    - Parsley
    - Turmeric
    - Coriander

Incorporating these iron-rich plant-based foods into your diet can help meet your daily iron needs and support overall health. Pairing iron-rich foods with sources of vitamin C can enhance iron absorption, so consider including citrus fruits, bell peppers, strawberries, or tomatoes in your meals to maximize iron absorption. Additionally, soaking, sprouting, fermenting, or cooking certain plant-based foods can help improve the bioavailability of iron. If you have concerns about your iron intake or suspect iron deficiency, consult with a healthcare professional for personalized advice.

Zinc

What is Zinc?

Zinc is an essential mineral that is vital for numerous physiological functions in the human body. It plays a crucial role in various enzymatic reactions, immune function, protein synthesis, wound healing, DNA synthesis, and cell division. Zinc is classified as a trace mineral, meaning that the body requires only small amounts of it for optimal health, but its importance cannot be understated.

One of the primary functions of zinc is its role as a cofactor for over 300 enzymes involved in various biochemical processes. These enzymes are involved in tasks such as metabolism, digestion, and the synthesis of DNA and proteins. Zinc also plays a key role in maintaining the integrity of cell membranes and supporting the function of the immune system, helping to defend the body against infections and diseases.

Zinc deficiency is relatively common, particularly in populations with inadequate dietary intake or impaired absorption of zinc. Symptoms of zinc deficiency may include impaired growth and development, delayed wound healing, hair loss, skin rashes, loss of appetite, and weakened immune function. Severe zinc deficiency can lead to more serious health problems, including immune system dysfunction and impaired neurological function.

Good dietary sources of zinc include meat, poultry, seafood (especially oysters), dairy products, nuts, seeds, and whole grains. Plant-based sources of zinc, such as legumes and grains, contain phytates, which can inhibit the absorption of zinc. However, soaking, sprouting, or fermenting these foods can help reduce phytate levels and enhance zinc absorption.

In some cases, supplementation with zinc may be necessary to address deficiency or support specific health conditions. However, excessive intake of zinc can lead to adverse effects, including nausea, vomiting, diarrhea, and impaired immune function. Therefore, it's important to consult with a healthcare professional before starting any zinc supplementation regimen.

In conclusion, zinc is an essential mineral that plays a vital role in numerous physiological processes in the body. Consuming a balanced diet that includes zinc-rich foods is crucial for maintaining optimal health and well-being, while supplementation may be necessary in cases of deficiency or certain health conditions, under the guidance of a healthcare professional.

Plant-Based Foods High in Zinc

Zinc is an essential mineral that plays a crucial role in various physiological processes, including immune function, wound healing, and DNA synthesis. While animal products like meat and seafood are rich sources of zinc, there are also several plant-based foods that provide this important nutrient. Here are some plant-based foods that are relatively high in zinc:

Legumes:

1. **Chickpeas (Garbanzo Beans):** Chickpeas are an excellent source of zinc, providing approximately 2.5 milligrams of zinc per 1 cup serving when cooked. They are versatile legumes commonly used in salads, stews, curries, and hummus.
2. **Lentils:** Lentils are rich in zinc, offering around 2 milligrams of zinc per 1 cup serving when cooked. They come in various colors, including green, brown, red, and black, and can be used in soups, stews, salads, and side dishes.
3. **Black Beans:** Black beans contain a moderate amount of zinc, providing approximately 1.8 milligrams of zinc per 1 cup serving when cooked. They are commonly used in Latin American, Caribbean, and Tex-Mex cuisines, in dishes such as black bean soup, burritos, and salads.
4. **Kidney Beans:** Kidney beans are another legume with a decent zinc content, offering around 1.5 milligrams of zinc per 1 cup serving when cooked. They are often used in chili, bean salads, bean dips, and casseroles.
5. **White Beans (Navy Beans/Cannellini Beans):** White beans are relatively high in zinc, providing approximately 1.4 milligrams of zinc per 1 cup serving when cooked. They have a mild flavor and creamy texture, making them suitable for soups, stews, casseroles, and salads.
6. **Adzuki Beans:** Adzuki beans contain a moderate amount of zinc, offering approximately 1.2 milligrams of zinc per 1 cup serving when cooked. They are commonly used in Asian cuisine, particularly in sweet red bean paste for desserts, as well as in savory dishes like soups and stews.
7. **Soybeans (Edamame):** Soybeans are rich in zinc, providing approximately 1.1 milligrams of zinc per 1 cup serving when cooked. They are used to make various soy products, including tofu, tempeh, soy milk, and edamame, and are also used in Asian dishes such as stir-fries and salads.

Seeds:

1. **Pumpkin Seeds (Pepitas):** Pumpkin seeds are one of the best plant-based sources of zinc. They provide approximately 7.5 milligrams of zinc per 1 ounce (28 grams) serving. Pumpkin seeds are versatile and can be enjoyed roasted as a snack, added to salads, soups, granola, or used as a topping for yogurt or oatmeal.
2. **Hemp Seeds:** Hemp seeds are rich in zinc, providing around 5 milligrams of zinc per 3 tablespoon serving. These nutritious seeds have a slightly nutty flavor and can be sprinkled on salads, blended into smoothies, or incorporated into baked goods like bread and muffins.
3. **Sesame Seeds:** Sesame seeds contain a good amount of zinc, offering approximately 2.8 milligrams of zinc per 1 ounce (28 grams) serving. They are commonly used in Asian,

Middle Eastern, and Mediterranean cuisines to add flavor and texture to dishes like tahini (sesame seed paste), hummus, salads, stir-fries, and baked goods.

4. **Sunflower Seeds:** Sunflower seeds are a decent source of zinc, providing around 1.5 milligrams of zinc per 1 ounce (28 grams) serving. They can be enjoyed roasted as a snack, added to salads, trail mix, granola, or used as a garnish for soups and stir-fries.
5. **Flaxseeds:** Flaxseeds contain a moderate amount of zinc, offering approximately 1.2 milligrams of zinc per 2 tablespoon serving. These tiny seeds are rich in omega-3 fatty acids and fiber, and they can be ground and added to smoothies, yogurt, oatmeal, or used in baking recipes like bread, muffins, and cookies.
6. **Chia Seeds:** Chia seeds contain a small amount of zinc, providing around 1 milligram of zinc per 1 ounce (28 grams) serving. These nutritious seeds are high in fiber, protein, and omega-3 fatty acids, and they can be soaked in water or milk to make chia pudding, added to smoothies, yogurt, oatmeal, or used as an egg substitute in baking.

Nuts:

1. **Cashews:** Cashews are one of the best plant-based sources of zinc among nuts. They provide approximately 1.6 milligrams of zinc per 1 ounce (28 grams) serving. Cashews are creamy and versatile, making them a popular snack on their own or used in recipes like cashew cheese, sauces, and desserts.
2. **Pine Nuts:** Pine nuts contain a good amount of zinc, offering approximately 1.3 milligrams of zinc per 1 ounce (28 grams) serving. They have a sweet, buttery flavor and are commonly used in Mediterranean and Middle Eastern cuisines in dishes like pesto, salads, pilafs, and baked goods.
3. **Almonds:** Almonds are a decent source of zinc, providing around 0.9 milligrams of zinc per 1 ounce (28 grams) serving. They are crunchy and nutritious, making them a popular snack and ingredient in recipes like almond butter, almond milk, granola, and baked goods.
4. **Brazil Nuts:** Brazil nuts contain a moderate amount of zinc, offering approximately 0.8 milligrams of zinc per 1 ounce (28 grams) serving. They are also rich in selenium, another essential mineral with antioxidant properties. Brazil nuts have a rich, creamy flavor and can be enjoyed on their own or added to trail mix, salads, and desserts.
5. **Pecans:** Pecans contain a small amount of zinc, providing around 0.7 milligrams of zinc per 1 ounce (28 grams) serving. They have a sweet, buttery flavor and are commonly used in baked goods like pies, cookies, and bars, as well as salads and savory dishes.

Whole Grains:

1. **Wheat Germ:** Wheat germ is one of the best whole grain sources of zinc. It provides approximately 4.7 milligrams of zinc per 100 grams. Wheat germ can be sprinkled on yogurt, oatmeal, or smoothies, or used as an ingredient in baked goods like bread, muffins, and pancakes.

2. **Quinoa:** Quinoa contains a decent amount of zinc, providing around 2 milligrams of zinc per 100 grams. It is a versatile whole grain that can be used as a base for salads, pilafs, stir-fries, and breakfast porridge. Quinoa is also gluten-free and high in protein, making it a popular choice among health-conscious individuals.

3. **Oats:** Oats contain a moderate amount of zinc, offering approximately 3 milligrams of zinc per 100 grams. They are a nutritious whole grain that can be enjoyed as oatmeal, granola, overnight oats, or added to baked goods like cookies, bread, and muffins.

4. **Brown Rice:** Brown rice contains a small amount of zinc, providing around 1.2 milligrams of zinc per 100 grams. It is a whole grain alternative to white rice and can be used in various dishes, including stir-fries, pilafs, casseroles, and sushi rolls.

5. **Barley:** Barley contains a modest amount of zinc, offering approximately 1.1 milligrams of zinc per 100 grams. It is commonly used in soups, stews, salads, and risottos, and can also be ground into flour for baking or used as a substitute for rice or pasta.

Tofu: Tofu, made from **soybeans**, is a good source of zinc. It is also a versatile ingredient that can be used in a variety of dishes, including stir-fries, soups, and sandwiches.

Tempeh: Tempeh, another soy-based product, is high in zinc. It is a fermented food that offers protein, probiotics, and other nutrients along with zinc.

Vegetables: Some vegetables contain small amounts of zinc, although they are not as high as other plant-based foods. Examples include **spinach, kale, peas**, and **Brussels sprouts**. While these vegetables may not be significant sources of zinc individually, they can contribute to overall zinc intake when consumed regularly as part of a balanced diet.

Incorporating a variety of these plant-based foods into meals and snacks can help individuals following a vegetarian or vegan diet meet their zinc requirements. It's important to note that plant-based sources of zinc may have lower bioavailability compared to animal sources, so consuming a diverse range of zinc-rich foods and including sources of vitamin C, which enhances zinc absorption, can help optimize zinc intake from plant-based sources.

Copper

What is Copper?

Copper is an essential trace mineral that plays a crucial role in various physiological processes within the human body. It is involved in the formation of red blood cells, maintenance of connective tissues, energy production, and functioning of the nervous and immune systems. Copper is also a cofactor for several enzymes involved in antioxidant defense, iron metabolism, and the synthesis of neurotransmitters and collagen.

One of the primary functions of copper is its role in the synthesis of hemoglobin, the protein in red blood cells that carries oxygen from the lungs to the body's tissues and organs. Copper is also involved in the production of collagen and elastin, which are essential for the formation and maintenance of connective tissues, such as bones, cartilage, and skin.

In addition to its structural and enzymatic roles, copper plays a key role in antioxidant defense. Copper-containing enzymes, such as superoxide dismutase (SOD), help neutralize harmful free radicals and protect cells from oxidative damage. This antioxidant activity is essential for maintaining cellular health and reducing the risk of chronic diseases associated with oxidative stress, such as cardiovascular disease, cancer, and neurodegenerative disorders.

Copper deficiency is relatively rare but can occur in individuals with inadequate dietary intake, malabsorption disorders, or excessive zinc intake, which can interfere with copper absorption. Symptoms of copper deficiency may include anemia, fatigue, weakness, impaired immune function, bone abnormalities, and neurological disturbances.

On the other hand, excessive intake of copper can lead to toxicity, resulting in symptoms such as nausea, vomiting, diarrhea, abdominal pain, liver damage, and neurological symptoms. Chronic copper toxicity can also lead to Wilson's disease, a rare genetic disorder characterized by the accumulation of copper in the liver, brain, and other organs.

Good dietary sources of copper include organ meats (such as liver), shellfish (such as oysters and crab), nuts, seeds, whole grains, legumes, and dark leafy greens. Consuming a balanced diet that includes copper-rich foods is essential for maintaining optimal health and well-being.

In summary, copper is an essential trace mineral that plays a crucial role in numerous physiological processes within the body. Consuming a balanced diet that includes copper-rich foods is important for ensuring adequate intake of this vital nutrient and supporting overall health and well-being. However, excessive intake of copper should be avoided to prevent toxicity and adverse health effects.

Plant-Based Foods High in Copper

While copper is predominantly found in animal-based foods like liver and shellfish, several plant-based foods also contain significant amounts of this mineral. Here is a list of plant-based foods that are high in copper:

1. **Nuts and Seeds:**
    - Sunflower seeds
    - Sesame seeds
    - Pumpkin seeds (Pepitas)
    - Cashews
    - Almonds
    - Pine nuts
    - Hemp seeds
    - Flaxseeds
2. **Legumes:**
    - Lentils
    - Chickpeas (Garbanzo beans)
    - Soybeans
    - Black beans
    - Lima beans
    - Navy beans
    - Pinto beans
3. **Whole Grains:**
    - Quinoa
    - Buckwheat
    - Oats
    - Barley
    - Brown rice
    - Wild rice

4. **Leafy Greens and Vegetables:**
    - Spinach
    - Kale
    - Swiss chard
    - Asparagus
    - Mushrooms (especially shiitake mushrooms)
    - Sweet potatoes
    - Avocado
5. **Dried Fruits:**
    - Dried apricots
    - Prunes (Dried plums)
    - Raisins
    - Dates
6. **Cocoa and Dark Chocolate:**
    - Cocoa powder
    - Dark chocolate (with high cocoa content)
7. **Tofu:**
    - Firm tofu
    - Silken tofu
8. **Whole Grains:**
    - Whole wheat
    - Spelt
    - Millet

Incorporating these plant-based foods into your diet can help ensure an adequate intake of copper, supporting overall health and well-being. It's essential to consume a variety of nutrient-rich foods to meet your body's copper requirements and maintain optimal health.

Selenium

What is Selenium?

Selenium is a trace mineral that is essential for human health. It acts primarily as an antioxidant, helping to protect cells from damage caused by free radicals and oxidative stress. Selenium is also involved in various physiological processes, including thyroid function, immune system regulation, and reproduction.

One of the key functions of selenium is its role in the production of selenoproteins, a group of proteins that contain selenium in the form of the amino acid selenocysteine. These selenoproteins play important roles in antioxidant defense, thyroid hormone metabolism, DNA synthesis and repair, and immune function.

As an antioxidant, selenium helps neutralize harmful free radicals and reduce oxidative stress, which can damage cells and contribute to chronic diseases such as heart disease, cancer, and neurodegenerative disorders. Selenium works in concert with other antioxidants, such as vitamin E, to protect cells and tissues from oxidative damage.

Selenium is also important for thyroid function, as it is required for the conversion of the inactive thyroid hormone thyroxine (T4) to the active form triiodothyronine (T3). Adequate selenium levels are essential for maintaining proper thyroid hormone levels and supporting metabolic function, energy production, and overall health.

In addition, selenium plays a role in immune system regulation by modulating inflammation and promoting immune cell function. It helps regulate the production of cytokines, which are signaling molecules involved in the immune response, and supports the activity of white blood cells, which are responsible for fighting off infections and pathogens.

Selenium deficiency is relatively rare in healthy individuals, as selenium is widely distributed in foods and is present in trace amounts in many soils. However, certain factors, such as poor dietary intake, gastrointestinal disorders, and soil depletion, can increase the risk of deficiency. Symptoms of selenium deficiency may include fatigue, weakness, hair loss, poor immune function, and cognitive impairment.

Conversely, excessive intake of selenium can lead to toxicity, known as selenosis, which can cause symptoms such as nausea, vomiting, diarrhea, hair loss, brittle nails, and neurological abnormalities. Chronic selenium toxicity can also lead to more serious health problems, including liver and kidney damage.

Good dietary sources of selenium include seafood (such as fish, shellfish, and seaweed), Brazil nuts, organ meats (such as liver and kidney), whole grains, eggs, poultry, and dairy products. Consuming a balanced diet that includes selenium-rich foods is important for maintaining optimal selenium levels and supporting overall health and well-being.

In summary, selenium is an essential trace mineral that plays important roles in antioxidant defense, thyroid function, immune regulation, and overall health. Consuming a varied diet that includes selenium-rich foods is essential for ensuring adequate selenium intake and supporting optimal health and well-being. However, excessive intake of selenium should be avoided to prevent toxicity and adverse health effects.

Plant-Based Foods High in Selenium

Selenium is an essential mineral that plays a critical role in various bodily functions, including thyroid function, antioxidant defense, and immune system health. While selenium is primarily found in animal-based foods like seafood, there are several plant-based sources available. Here are some plant-based foods high in selenium:

1. **Brazil Nuts:**
    - Brazil nuts are one of the richest sources of selenium. Just one or two nuts can provide your daily recommended intake of selenium.
2. **Sunflower Seeds:**
    - Sunflower seeds are a nutritious snack and a good source of selenium. They can be enjoyed on their own, added to salads, or incorporated into baked goods.
3. **Chia Seeds:**
    - Chia seeds are not only high in fiber and omega-3 fatty acids but also contain selenium. They can be added to smoothies, yogurt, oatmeal, or used as an egg substitute in baking.
4. **Flaxseeds:**
    - Flaxseeds are rich in alpha-linolenic acid (ALA) and also contain selenium. They can be ground and added to baked goods, sprinkled over salads, or mixed into smoothies.
5. **Mushrooms (especially Shiitake Mushrooms):**
    - Certain varieties of mushrooms, such as shiitake mushrooms, contain selenium. Incorporating mushrooms into stir-fries, soups, or pasta dishes can boost your selenium intake.
6. **Whole Grains (especially Whole Wheat Bread and Brown Rice):**
    - Whole grains like whole wheat bread, brown rice, oats, and barley contain small amounts of selenium. Enjoying whole grain foods as part of your meals can contribute to your selenium intake.

7. **Legumes (especially Lentils and Chickpeas):**
    - Legumes such as lentils, chickpeas, and kidney beans contain selenium. They are versatile ingredients that can be used in soups, stews, salads, or as a base for vegetarian patties or burgers.
8. **Spinach:**
    - Spinach is a nutrient-rich leafy green vegetable that contains selenium. Enjoy spinach raw in salads, cooked in stir-fries, soups, or as a side dish.

Incorporating these plant-based foods high in selenium into your diet can help ensure you meet your daily selenium needs and support overall health and wellbeing. Remember to consume a varied and balanced diet to obtain a wide range of essential nutrients.

Iodine

What is Iodine?

Iodine is a chemical element that is essential for human health. It is primarily known for its role in the production of thyroid hormones, which are critical for regulating metabolism, growth, and development. The human body does not produce iodine on its own, so it must be obtained from dietary sources.

The thyroid gland, located in the neck, absorbs iodine from the bloodstream and uses it to produce thyroid hormones, primarily thyroxine (T4) and triiodothyronine (T3). These hormones play a crucial role in regulating various metabolic processes, including energy production, temperature regulation, heart rate, and digestion. They are also important for proper growth and development, particularly during infancy and childhood.

Iodine deficiency can lead to inadequate production of thyroid hormones, resulting in a condition known as hypothyroidism. Symptoms of hypothyroidism may include fatigue, weight gain, cold intolerance, dry skin, hair loss, constipation, and cognitive impairment. Severe iodine deficiency during pregnancy can also lead to developmental abnormalities in the fetus, including intellectual disabilities and impaired growth.

To prevent iodine deficiency, it is important to consume an adequate amount of iodine-rich foods in the diet. Good dietary sources of iodine include iodized salt, seafood (such as fish, shellfish, and seaweed), dairy products, eggs, and fortified foods. In regions where iodine deficiency is common, iodine supplementation may be recommended, particularly for pregnant women and infants.

While iodine deficiency is a concern in certain parts of the world, excessive iodine intake can also have adverse health effects. Chronic excessive intake of iodine, known as iodine toxicity, can lead to thyroid dysfunction, autoimmune thyroid disease, and other health problems. Therefore, it is important to consume iodine in moderation and avoid excessive intake from supplements or iodine-rich foods.

In summary, iodine is an essential mineral that plays a critical role in thyroid function and overall health. Consuming a balanced diet that includes iodine-rich foods is important for preventing iodine deficiency and supporting optimal thyroid function. However, excessive intake of iodine should be avoided to prevent adverse health effects.

Plant-Based Foods Contain Iodine

While iodine is most commonly associated with seafood and dairy products, there are some plant-based sources available. Here are some plant-based foods that are relatively high in iodine:

1. **Seaweed (Nori, Kelp, Wakame, Dulse):**

- Seaweed is one of the richest sources of iodine, with some varieties containing exceptionally high levels. Nori, commonly used in sushi rolls, and kelp are particularly iodine-rich. Seaweed can be incorporated into soups, salads, stir-fries, or used as a seasoning in dishes.

2. **Iodized Salt:**
    - Some brands of table salt are fortified with iodine to help prevent iodine deficiency. Using iodized salt in cooking or seasoning food can contribute to your iodine intake.
3. **Potatoes (with skin):**
    - Potatoes, especially when consumed with the skin, contain moderate levels of iodine. Enjoy baked potatoes, mashed potatoes, or roasted potatoes as part of your meals to add a source of iodine.
4. **Cranberries:**
    - Cranberries are a good source of iodine and can be enjoyed fresh, dried, or in juice form. They can be added to salads, smoothies, oatmeal, or used to make sauces and jams.
5. **Strawberries:**
    - Strawberries contain small amounts of iodine and can be enjoyed fresh as a snack or added to salads, yogurt, smoothies, or desserts.
6. **Organic Soy Products:**
    - Some organic soy products, such as tofu and soy milk, may contain higher levels of iodine compared to conventional varieties. Incorporating organic soy products into your diet can provide a source of iodine.
7. **Lima Beans:**
    - Lima beans are a legume rich in various nutrients, including iodine. Enjoy lima beans cooked and added to soups, stews, salads, or served as a side dish.
8. **Prunes:**
    - Prunes, also known as dried plums, contain small amounts of iodine and can be enjoyed as a snack or added to baked goods, salads, or oatmeal.

While these plant-based foods can contribute to iodine intake, it's essential to consume them as part of a balanced diet to ensure adequate nutrition. If you have specific concerns about iodine intake, consult with a healthcare professional or registered dietitian for personalized advice.

Manganese

What is Manganese?

Manganese is an essential trace mineral that plays a vital role in numerous physiological processes within the human body. It is required for the functioning of various enzymes and is involved in processes such as metabolism, bone formation, wound healing, and the synthesis of connective tissues. Manganese also acts as an antioxidant, helping to protect cells from oxidative stress and damage caused by free radicals.

One of the primary functions of manganese is its role as a cofactor for several enzymes involved in carbohydrate, amino acid, and lipid metabolism. These enzymes help convert food into energy and support the proper functioning of various metabolic pathways in the body.

Manganese is also important for bone health, as it is involved in the formation and maintenance of healthy bones and cartilage. It helps stimulate the production of osteoblasts, the cells responsible for building new bone tissue, and plays a role in the synthesis of collagen, a protein that provides structural support to bones and other connective tissues.

In addition, manganese is essential for the synthesis of glycosaminoglycans (GAGs), a type of carbohydrate molecule found in connective tissues such as cartilage, tendons, and ligaments. GAGs help maintain the structure and function of these tissues and are important for joint health and mobility.

Manganese also acts as an antioxidant, helping to neutralize harmful free radicals and protect cells from oxidative damage. It works in concert with other antioxidants, such as vitamin C, vitamin E, and selenium, to maintain cellular health and reduce the risk of chronic diseases associated with oxidative stress, such as cardiovascular disease, cancer, and neurodegenerative disorders.

While manganese deficiency is relatively rare, it can occur in individuals with certain medical conditions, such as malabsorption disorders or liver disease, or in those with poor dietary intake. Symptoms of manganese deficiency may include impaired growth and development, skeletal abnormalities, reproductive issues, and neurological symptoms.

On the other hand, excessive intake of manganese can lead to toxicity, known as manganism, which can cause symptoms such as tremors, muscle stiffness, cognitive impairment, and psychiatric disturbances. Chronic manganese toxicity is rare and is more commonly associated with occupational exposure, such as in industries involving mining or welding.

Good dietary sources of manganese include nuts, seeds, whole grains, legumes, leafy green vegetables, tea, and pineapple. Consuming a balanced diet that includes manganese-rich foods is important for ensuring adequate manganese intake and supporting overall health and well-being.

Plant-Based Foods High in Manganese

Manganese is an essential mineral that is naturally present in many foods and is also found in the environment, including soil, water, and air. It is considered a trace mineral because the body requires it in small amounts, but it plays a crucial role in various physiological processes, including metabolism, bone health, and antioxidant defense. Here are some plant-based foods that are high in manganese:

1. **Nuts and Seeds:**
    - Pumpkin seeds
    - Sesame seeds
    - Sunflower seeds
    - Pine nuts
    - Almonds
    - Pecans
    - Walnuts
2. **Whole Grains:**
    - Brown rice
    - Quinoa
    - Oats
    - Barley
    - Buckwheat
    - Spelt
    - Amaranth
3. **Legumes:**
    - Soybeans
    - Lentils
    - Chickpeas (garbanzo beans)
    - Black beans
    - Lima beans
    - Navy beans

- Pinto beans

4. **Leafy Green Vegetables:**
    - Spinach
    - Kale
    - Swiss chard
    - Collard greens
    - Beet greens
    - Mustard greens
    - Turnip greens
5. **Other Vegetables:**
    - Sweet potatoes
    - Peas
    - Brussels sprouts
    - Broccoli
    - Cauliflower
    - Green beans
    - Asparagus
6. **Fruits:**
    - Pineapple
    - Raspberries
    - Strawberries
    - Blueberries
    - Avocado
    - Bananas
    - Kiwi

Incorporating these plant-based foods into your diet can help ensure an adequate intake of manganese, supporting overall health and wellbeing. Remember to consume a varied and balanced diet to obtain a wide range of essential nutrients.

Fluoride

What is Fluoride?

Fluoride is a naturally occurring mineral found in water, soil, rocks, and various foods. It is also commonly added to drinking water, toothpaste, and dental products for its dental health benefits. Fluoride plays a crucial role in dental health by helping to prevent tooth decay and cavities.

When fluoride is consumed, it becomes incorporated into the structure of tooth enamel, the outer layer of the teeth. Fluoride helps strengthen tooth enamel and makes it more resistant to acid erosion caused by bacteria and sugars in the mouth. This protective effect helps prevent the formation of cavities and slows down the progression of existing dental decay.

In addition to its topical benefits when applied directly to the teeth, fluoride also has systemic effects when ingested. Drinking fluoridated water or consuming foods and beverages containing fluoride can help provide systemic protection against tooth decay by increasing the fluoride concentration in saliva and dental plaque.

Fluoride is particularly beneficial during childhood when teeth are developing and becoming more susceptible to decay. The Centers for Disease Control and Prevention (CDC) and the American Dental Association (ADA) recommend community water fluoridation as one of the most effective and cost-effective public health measures for preventing dental caries.

While fluoride is generally considered safe and effective for preventing tooth decay when used appropriately, excessive fluoride intake can lead to potential side effects and adverse health effects. Some of the side effects of fluoride include:

1. Dental fluorosis: Dental fluorosis is a condition characterized by changes in the appearance of tooth enamel, such as white or brown discoloration, mottling, or pitting. Dental fluorosis typically occurs during tooth development in childhood and is more common when children consume excessive amounts of fluoride from multiple sources, such as fluoridated water, toothpaste, and supplements.
2. Skeletal fluorosis: Skeletal fluorosis is a bone disorder that occurs due to excessive accumulation of fluoride in the bones. In mild cases, skeletal fluorosis may cause stiffness and joint pain, while severe cases can lead to skeletal deformities, decreased bone density, and an increased risk of fractures. Skeletal fluorosis is more commonly associated with long-term exposure to high levels of fluoride, particularly from drinking water with naturally high fluoride levels.
3. Thyroid dysfunction: Some research suggests that excessive fluoride intake may interfere with thyroid function and contribute to thyroid dysfunction, including hypothyroidism (underactive thyroid) or hyperthyroidism (overactive thyroid). However, more studies are needed to fully understand the relationship between fluoride exposure and thyroid health.

4. Neurological effects: Some studies have suggested a potential link between fluoride exposure and adverse effects on neurological development and cognitive function, particularly in children. However, the evidence is limited and conflicting, and further research is needed to determine the potential neurological effects of fluoride exposure.
5. Allergic reactions: In rare cases, individuals may experience allergic reactions or skin irritation in response to fluoride-containing dental products, such as toothpaste or mouthwash. Symptoms may include rash, itching, swelling, or difficulty breathing. If you experience any allergic reactions to fluoride products, discontinue use and consult with a healthcare professional.

It's important to note that the risk of experiencing adverse effects from fluoride is generally low when fluoride-containing products are used appropriately and as directed. Additionally, the benefits of fluoride in preventing tooth decay and promoting dental health typically outweigh the potential risks, especially when fluoride exposure is carefully monitored.

In addition to its dental health benefits, fluoride has also been shown to have positive effects on bone health. Fluoride helps increase bone density and reduce the risk of osteoporosis and fractures, particularly in older adults.

Overall, fluoride is an important mineral for maintaining dental health and preventing tooth decay. It can be obtained from fluoridated water, fluoride-containing dental products, and certain foods and beverages. However, it's important to use fluoride-containing products as directed and to consult with a dentist or healthcare provider about appropriate fluoride intake, especially for young children.

Plant-Based Foods Contain Fluoride

Fluoride is a mineral that occurs naturally in various foods and water sources, although the levels can vary significantly depending on factors such as soil composition and water fluoridation practices. While fluoride is most commonly associated with dental health, it also plays a role in bone health and preventing tooth decay. Here are some plant-based foods that contain fluoride:

1. **Tea:**
    - Tea leaves naturally accumulate fluoride from the soil, particularly green and black tea. Drinking tea, whether hot or cold, can contribute to fluoride intake.
2. **Spinach:**
    - Spinach is a leafy green vegetable that contains some fluoride, albeit in lower amounts compared to tea. Including spinach in salads, soups, stir-fries, or smoothies can provide a modest amount of fluoride.

3. **Kale:**
    - Kale, another leafy green vegetable, contains small amounts of fluoride. Enjoy kale raw in salads, sautéed as a side dish, or blended into smoothies.
4. **Cabbage:**
    - Cabbage, including green cabbage and red cabbage, contains trace amounts of fluoride. Incorporating cabbage into coleslaw, stir-fries, salads, or soups can contribute to fluoride intake.
5. **Parsley:**
    - Parsley, an herb commonly used as a garnish or flavoring agent, contains fluoride. Adding fresh parsley to salads, soups, sauces, or dips can provide a source of fluoride.
6. **Cilantro (Coriander):**
    - Cilantro, another herb used in various cuisines, contains small amounts of fluoride. Including fresh cilantro in salads, salsas, marinades, or as a garnish can add flavor and a touch of fluoride.
7. **Almonds:**
    - Almonds are a nut rich in various nutrients, including fluoride. Snacking on almonds, adding them to salads, oatmeal, or trail mixes can contribute to fluoride intake.
8. **Potatoes:**
    - Potatoes, especially when consumed with the skin, contain small amounts of fluoride. Enjoy baked potatoes, mashed potatoes, or roasted potatoes as part of your meals to add a source of fluoride.

It's important to note that the fluoride content of plant-based foods can vary depending on factors such as growing conditions, soil composition, and processing methods. Additionally, fluoride intake from plant-based foods is typically lower compared to other sources such as fluoridated water or dental products. If you have specific concerns about fluoride intake, consult with a healthcare professional or dentist for personalized advice.

Chromium

What is Chromium?

Chromium is an essential trace mineral that plays a crucial role in various physiological processes within the human body. It is required in small amounts for normal carbohydrate, fat, and protein metabolism, as well as for maintaining proper glucose metabolism and insulin sensitivity.

One of the primary functions of chromium is its role in enhancing the action of insulin, a hormone produced by the pancreas that helps regulate blood sugar levels. Chromium helps insulin transport glucose from the bloodstream into cells, where it can be used for energy production. This process is particularly important for individuals with insulin resistance or type 2 diabetes, as chromium supplementation may help improve insulin sensitivity and glucose control.

In addition to its role in glucose metabolism, chromium is also involved in lipid metabolism, where it helps regulate the synthesis, storage, and breakdown of fats in the body. Chromium may help lower levels of LDL ("bad") cholesterol and triglycerides while increasing levels of HDL ("good") cholesterol, which can reduce the risk of cardiovascular disease.

Chromium is also believed to play a role in maintaining proper weight management and body composition. Some studies suggest that chromium supplementation may help reduce food cravings, suppress appetite, and promote fat loss while preserving lean body mass. However, more research is needed to fully understand the effects of chromium on weight loss and body composition.

While chromium deficiency is rare, certain factors such as poor diet, aging, pregnancy, and certain medical conditions may increase the risk of deficiency. Symptoms of chromium deficiency may include impaired glucose tolerance, insulin resistance, elevated blood sugar levels, fatigue, and weight changes.

Good dietary sources of chromium include meats, poultry, fish, whole grains, nuts, seeds, fruits, and vegetables. However, the chromium content of foods can vary depending on factors such as soil quality and processing methods.

In summary, chromium is an essential trace mineral that plays important roles in glucose metabolism, insulin sensitivity, lipid metabolism, and weight management. Consuming a balanced diet that includes chromium-rich foods is important for ensuring adequate intake of this vital nutrient and supporting overall health and well-being. Additionally, chromium supplementation may be beneficial for individuals with insulin resistance, type 2 diabetes, or certain other health conditions, under the guidance of a healthcare professional.

Plant-Based Foods Contain Chromium

Chromium is a trace mineral that plays a role in glucose metabolism and insulin sensitivity. While chromium is primarily found in animal-based foods, there are also some plant-based sources available. Here are some plant-based foods that contain chromium:

1. **Broccoli:**
    - Broccoli is a cruciferous vegetable that contains small amounts of chromium. Enjoy broccoli steamed, roasted, or stir-fried as a side dish or incorporated into salads, soups, and casseroles.
2. **Green Beans:**
    - Green beans, also known as string beans or snap beans, contain trace amounts of chromium. Incorporate green beans into stir-fries, salads, or as a side dish for added nutrition.
3. **Whole Grains (especially Whole Wheat and Barley):**
    - Whole grains such as whole wheat and barley contain small amounts of chromium. Enjoy whole wheat bread, barley salads, or barley porridge as part of your meals to add a source of chromium.
4. **Oats:**
    - Oats are a nutritious whole grain that contains some chromium. Start your day with a bowl of oatmeal topped with fresh fruit and nuts for a wholesome breakfast rich in chromium.
5. **Potatoes (with skin):**
    - Potatoes, especially when consumed with the skin, contain trace amounts of chromium. Enjoy baked potatoes, mashed potatoes, or roasted potatoes as part of your meals to add a source of chromium.
6. **Green Leafy Vegetables (such as Spinach and Kale):**
    - Green leafy vegetables like spinach and kale contain small amounts of chromium. Incorporate these nutrient-rich greens into salads, smoothies, soups, or stir-fries for added health benefits.
7. **Tomatoes:**
    - Tomatoes contain trace amounts of chromium and can be enjoyed fresh in salads, sandwiches, or as a base for sauces and soups.

8. **Romaine Lettuce:**

    - Romaine lettuce is a variety of lettuce that contains some chromium. Use romaine lettuce as a base for salads, wraps, or sandwiches for a refreshing and nutritious meal.

While these plant-based foods can contribute to chromium intake, it's essential to consume them as part of a balanced diet to ensure adequate nutrition. If you have specific concerns about chromium intake, consult with a healthcare professional or registered dietitian for personalized advice.

Molybdenum

What is Molybdenum?

Molybdenum is a trace mineral that is essential for human health. It is found naturally in many foods and is also available as a dietary supplement. Molybdenum plays a crucial role in various physiological processes within the body, including metabolism, detoxification, and the functioning of certain enzymes.

One of the primary functions of molybdenum is its role as a cofactor for several enzymes involved in the metabolism of carbohydrates, fats, and proteins. These enzymes, known as molybdoenzymes, catalyze important chemical reactions in the body, including the conversion of sulfite to sulfate, the metabolism of sulfur-containing amino acids, and the breakdown of certain toxins and drugs.

Molybdenum is also involved in the synthesis of purines and pyrimidines, which are essential components of DNA and RNA. It plays a role in the formation of uric acid, a waste product that is excreted from the body through urine. Additionally, molybdenum is important for the proper functioning of the nervous system and may play a role in preventing neurodegenerative disorders.

Dietary sources of molybdenum include legumes (such as beans, lentils, and peas), nuts, seeds, whole grains, leafy green vegetables, and certain animal products (such as liver and kidney). The molybdenum content of plant-based foods can vary depending on factors such as soil quality and growing conditions.

Molybdenum deficiency is rare in humans, as the mineral is found in many common foods and is required in only small amounts. However, certain medical conditions or dietary factors may increase the risk of deficiency. Symptoms of molybdenum deficiency may include fatigue, weakness, loss of appetite, and neurological symptoms.

On the other hand, excessive intake of molybdenum is also rare and is more likely to occur through occupational exposure or from high-dose supplements. Chronic excessive intake of molybdenum may interfere with copper metabolism and lead to copper deficiency, which can cause anemia, neurological symptoms, and other health problems.

In summary, molybdenum is an essential trace mineral that plays important roles in metabolism, detoxification, enzyme function, and neurological health. Consuming a balanced diet that includes molybdenum-rich foods is important for ensuring adequate intake of this essential nutrient and supporting overall health and well-being. If you have concerns about molybdenum intake or deficiency, it's important to consult with a healthcare professional for personalized guidance and recommendations.

Plant-Based Foods Contain Molybdenum

Molybdenum is a trace mineral that plays a crucial role in various physiological processes, including enzyme function and metabolism. While molybdenum is found in relatively small amounts in plant-based foods compared to animal-based sources, there are still several plant-based options that contain this essential mineral. Here are some plant-based foods that are sources of molybdenum:

1. **Legumes (Beans, Lentils, Peas):**
    - Legumes are excellent sources of molybdenum. Beans (such as black beans, kidney beans, and navy beans), lentils, and peas contain significant amounts of this mineral. Enjoy them in soups, stews, salads, or as a side dish to boost your molybdenum intake.
2. **Whole Grains (Barley, Oats, Quinoa):**
    - Whole grains like barley, oats, and quinoa also contain molybdenum. Incorporate these grains into your meals as a source of complex carbohydrates, fiber, and molybdenum. Enjoy them as porridge, salads, pilafs, or in baked goods.
3. **Leafy Green Vegetables (Spinach, Kale):**
    - Leafy green vegetables like spinach and kale contain small amounts of molybdenum. Include these nutrient-rich greens in salads, smoothies, stir-fries, or soups to add molybdenum to your diet.
4. **Nuts and Seeds (Sunflower Seeds, Sesame Seeds):**
    - Certain nuts and seeds, such as sunflower seeds and sesame seeds, are good sources of molybdenum. Snack on them raw or roasted, sprinkle them over salads or oatmeal, or use them in homemade energy bars or granola for a molybdenum boost.
5. **Cruciferous Vegetables (Broccoli, Cauliflower):**
    - Cruciferous vegetables like broccoli and cauliflower contain small amounts of molybdenum. Enjoy them steamed, roasted, or stir-fried as part of your meals to reap their nutritional benefits, including molybdenum.
6. **Soy Products (Tofu, Tempeh, Edamame):**
    - Soy products, such as tofu, tempeh, and edamame, contain molybdenum. Incorporate these plant-based protein sources into stir-fries, curries, salads, or grain bowls to add molybdenum to your diet.
7. **Potatoes (with skin):**
    - Potatoes, especially when consumed with the skin, contain small amounts of molybdenum. Enjoy baked potatoes, mashed potatoes, or roasted potatoes as part of your meals to add a source of molybdenum.

Including a variety of these plant-based foods in your diet can help ensure you meet your molybdenum needs and support overall health and wellbeing. If you have specific concerns about molybdenum intake, consult with a healthcare professional or registered dietitian for personalized advice.

Choline

What is Choline?

Choline is an essential nutrient that plays several important roles in the body. It is often grouped with the B vitamins, although it's not officially classified as one. Choline is crucial for various bodily functions, including:

Cell structure: Choline is a component of phospholipids, which are essential for the structure and function of cell membranes. It helps maintain cell integrity and facilitates cell communication.

Neurotransmission: Choline is a precursor to acetylcholine, a neurotransmitter involved in muscle control, memory, and cognitive function. Sufficient choline intake is necessary for optimal brain function.

Fat metabolism: Choline is involved in the transport and metabolism of fats and cholesterol. It helps prevent the accumulation of fats in the liver and promotes the export of fats from the liver.

DNA synthesis: Choline is required for the synthesis of phosphatidylcholine, a component of DNA and a precursor to cell membranes.

Methylation reactions: Choline is involved in methylation reactions, which are essential for regulating gene expression and various metabolic processes.

Good dietary sources of choline include eggs, meat, poultry, fish, dairy products, nuts, and certain vegetables like broccoli and Brussels sprouts. In some cases, dietary intake may not be sufficient, and choline supplements may be recommended, especially for pregnant and breastfeeding women to support fetal brain development. However, it's essential to consult with a healthcare professional before starting any supplement regimen.

Plant-Based Foods High in Choline

Choline is an essential nutrient that plays a crucial role in various bodily functions, including liver health, brain development, and muscle function. While animal products are often rich sources of choline, there are plant-based foods that also provide this nutrient. Here is a list of plant-based foods high in choline:

1. **Broccoli:**
    - Broccoli is a cruciferous vegetable that contains a moderate amount of choline. It's also rich in other vitamins and minerals, making it a nutritious addition to your diet.
2. **Brussels Sprouts:**
    - Brussels sprouts are another cruciferous vegetable that contains a good amount of choline. They are also high in fiber and vitamin C.

3. **Quinoa:**
    - Quinoa is a grain that contains a decent amount of choline. It is also a complete protein, providing all nine essential amino acids.
4. **Peanuts:**
    - Peanuts and peanut butter are good sources of choline. They are also rich in healthy fats and protein.
5. **Soy Products (Tofu, Tempeh):**
    - Soy-based products such as tofu and tempeh are good sources of choline. They are versatile ingredients in vegetarian and vegan diets.
6. **Chickpeas:**
    - Chickpeas, also known as garbanzo beans, contain a moderate amount of choline. They are a great plant-based protein source.
7. **Baked Potatoes:**
    - Potatoes, especially when baked with the skin on, contain a reasonable amount of choline. Ensure you eat the skin to maximize the choline content.
8. **Spinach:**
    - Spinach and other leafy greens provide some choline. They are also rich in iron, calcium, and other essential nutrients.
9. **Almonds:**
    - Almonds are nuts that contains a moderate amount of choline. They are also a good source of healthy fats, protein, and vitamin E.
10. **Flaxseeds:**
    - Flaxseeds, including flaxseed meal, contain a moderate amount of choline. They are also rich in omega-3 fatty acids and fiber.

It's important to note that while these plant-based sources contain choline, the levels may vary. A well-balanced diet that includes a variety of these foods can contribute to meeting your choline requirements, especially for individuals following vegetarian or vegan lifestyles.

Here is a list of animal-based foods high in choline:

Animal-Based Sources:

1. **Eggs:**
    - Eggs are one of the richest sources of choline. The yolk, in particular, contains a significant amount.
2. **Beef Liver:**
    - Beef liver is exceptionally high in choline. However, it's important to consume liver in moderation due to its high vitamin A content.
3. **Chicken Liver:**
    - Like beef liver, chicken liver is a potent source of choline.
4. **Salmon:**
    - Salmon is a fatty fish that provides a good amount of choline along with omega-3 fatty acids.
5. **Chicken Breast:**
    - Chicken breast is a lean source of choline and protein.
6. **Pork:**
    - Various cuts of pork, such as pork chops or pork loin, contain choline.
7. **Shrimp:**
    - Shellfish, including shrimp, is a seafood source of choline.

Including a variety of these foods in your diet can contribute to meeting your choline requirements, supporting overall health and well-being.

Water

What is Water?

Water is a transparent, tasteless, and odorless chemical substance composed of two hydrogen atoms bonded to one oxygen atom, with the chemical formula H2O. It is the most abundant molecule on Earth and is essential for life. Water plays numerous vital roles in the human body, and its benefits include:

1. **Hydration:** Water is crucial for maintaining proper hydration levels in the body. It serves as a medium for transporting nutrients to cells, regulating body temperature through sweating and respiration, and removing waste products through urine and perspiration.
2. **Lubrication:** Water lubricates joints, tissues, and organs, helping to reduce friction and facilitate smooth movement. Adequate hydration is essential for maintaining joint health and preventing conditions like arthritis.
3. **Digestion:** Water aids in the digestion and absorption of nutrients by breaking down food particles, assisting in the production of digestive enzymes, and promoting the movement of food through the digestive tract. Drinking water before meals can also help reduce appetite and support weight management.
4. **Detoxification:** Water helps flush toxins and waste products from the body through urine, sweat, and bowel movements. Staying hydrated supports proper kidney function and prevents the buildup of waste substances that can harm health.
5. **Skin Health:** Drinking enough water helps keep the skin hydrated and moisturized, promoting elasticity, suppleness, and a healthy complexion. Proper hydration can also reduce the risk of skin problems like dryness, acne, and premature aging.
6. **Cognitive Function**: Adequate hydration is essential for maintaining optimal cognitive function, including concentration, alertness, and memory. Even mild dehydration can impair cognitive performance and mood.
7. **Energy Levels:** Water plays a crucial role in energy metabolism, as it is involved in the production of adenosine triphosphate (ATP), the body's primary energy currency. Staying hydrated can help prevent fatigue and support physical performance and endurance.
8. **Immune Function:** Drinking water helps support the immune system by maintaining proper lymphatic function, which is essential for transporting immune cells and fighting off infections and illnesses.
9. **Weight Management**: Water has zero calories and can help promote feelings of fullness when consumed before or with meals, leading to reduced calorie intake and supporting weight loss or weight maintenance efforts.

10. **Regulation of Body Temperature:** Water helps regulate body temperature by absorbing and releasing heat through perspiration and evaporation. Staying hydrated is particularly important during hot weather or physical activity to prevent dehydration and heat-related illnesses.

Overall, staying adequately hydrated by drinking water throughout the day is essential for maintaining optimal health and well-being. The exact water intake needs vary depending on factors like age, sex, body weight, activity level, climate, and overall health status, but a general recommendation is to drink about 8 glasses (64 ounces) of water per day, or more if needed.

Fiber

What is Fiber?

Fiber, also known as dietary fiber or roughage, refers to the indigestible portion of plant foods. It is found in fruits, vegetables, grains, nuts, seeds, and legumes. There are two main types of fiber:

1. **Soluble Fiber:** This type of fiber dissolves in water to form a gel-like substance. It can help lower cholesterol levels and regulate blood sugar levels by slowing down the absorption of sugar into the bloodstream. Foods rich in soluble fiber include oats, barley, beans, lentils, fruits (such as apples, oranges, and berries), and vegetables (such as carrots and broccoli).
2. **Insoluble Fiber**: This type of fiber does not dissolve in water and adds bulk to the stool, helping to promote regular bowel movements and prevent constipation. It also helps to prevent hemorrhoids and diverticulosis. Foods rich in insoluble fiber include whole grains (such as wheat bran, brown rice, and whole wheat bread), nuts, seeds, and the skins of fruits and vegetables.

The benefits of fiber include:

Improved Digestive Health:

Fiber adds bulk to the stool, softens it, and helps move it through the digestive tract more efficiently, reducing the risk of constipation, hemorrhoids, and diverticulosis.

Weight Management:

High-fiber foods are often lower in calories and can help you feel full longer, reducing overall calorie intake and aiding in weight management.

Heart Health: Soluble fiber can help lower LDL cholesterol levels (the "bad" cholesterol), thereby reducing the risk of heart disease and stroke.

Blood Sugar Control:

Soluble fiber can slow down the absorption of sugar into the bloodstream, helping to regulate blood sugar levels and reduce the risk of type 2 diabetes.

Improved Gut Health:

Fiber acts as a prebiotic, providing fuel for beneficial bacteria in the gut, which can promote a healthy gut microbiome and improve overall gut health.

Reduced Risk of Certain Diseases:

A high-fiber diet has been associated with a reduced risk of certain diseases, including colorectal cancer, breast cancer, and cardiovascular disease.

It's recommended to consume a variety of high-fiber foods as part of a balanced diet to reap the many health benefits that fiber offers. The daily recommended intake of fiber varies depending on age, gender, and other factors, but most adults should aim for at least 25-30 grams of fiber per day.

Phytonutrients

What are Phytonutrients?

Phytonutrients, also known as phytochemicals, are natural compounds found in plants that have various health-promoting properties. These compounds are responsible for the vibrant colors, flavors, and aromas of fruits, vegetables, herbs, spices, nuts, seeds, and whole grains. While they are not essential nutrients like vitamins and minerals, phytonutrients have been shown to provide numerous health benefits. Some common types of phytonutrients include:

1. **Carotenoids:** These pigments give fruits and vegetables their yellow, orange, and red colors. Examples include beta-carotene (found in carrots, sweet potatoes, and pumpkin), lycopene (found in tomatoes and watermelon), and lutein (found in leafy greens like spinach and kale). Carotenoids act as antioxidants, helping to protect cells from damage caused by free radicals, and they may also support eye health and reduce the risk of certain cancers.

2. **Flavonoids**: This large class of phytonutrients includes compounds like quercetin (found in apples, onions, and citrus fruits), catechins (found in green tea), and anthocyanins (found in berries and red cabbage). Flavonoids have antioxidant and anti-inflammatory properties, and they may help reduce the risk of heart disease, improve blood vessel function, and support brain health.

3. **Polyphenols**: Polyphenols are found in a wide variety of plant foods, including cocoa, grapes, berries, tea, and nuts. They have antioxidant and anti-inflammatory effects, and research suggests they may help reduce the risk of chronic diseases such as heart disease, cancer, and neurodegenerative disorders.

4. **Sulfur**-containing compounds: Phytonutrients like glucosinolates (found in cruciferous vegetables like broccoli, cabbage, and Brussels sprouts) and allyl sulfides (found in garlic and onions) have been shown to have anti-cancer properties and may help support detoxification pathways in the body.

5. **Phytoestrogens:** These compounds, found in soybeans, flaxseeds, and other legumes, have a structure similar to estrogen and may have hormone-balancing effects. They have been studied for their potential role in reducing the risk of hormone-related cancers and managing symptoms of menopause.

The benefits of phytonutrients include:

- **Antioxidant activity:** Phytonutrients help protect cells from oxidative damage caused by free radicals, thereby reducing the risk of chronic diseases like cancer, heart disease, and diabetes.

- **Anti-inflammatory effects:** Many phytonutrients have anti-inflammatory properties, which can help reduce inflammation in the body and lower the risk of inflammatory diseases.
- **Immune support:** Some phytonutrients have been shown to support immune function and help the body defend against infections and diseases.
- **Hormone balance:** Certain phytonutrients may have hormone-balancing effects, which can be beneficial for reproductive health and managing symptoms of hormonal imbalances.
- **Detoxification support:** Phytonutrients like glucosinolates help support the body's natural detoxification pathways, aiding in the elimination of toxins and harmful substances.

Including a variety of colorful fruits, vegetables, herbs, spices, nuts, seeds, and whole grains in your diet is an excellent way to ensure you're getting a wide range of phytonutrients and reaping their many health benefits.

Omega-3 Fatty Acids

What is Omega-3 Fatty Acids?

Omega-3 fatty acids are a group of essential polyunsaturated fatty acids that are important for maintaining overall health. They are considered essential because the body cannot produce them on its own, so they must be obtained through diet. There are three main types of omega-3 fatty acids:

1. **Alpha-linolenic acid (ALA):** This is found in plant sources such as flaxseeds, chia seeds, walnuts, and hemp seeds.
2. **Eicosapentaenoic acid (EPA): This** is found mainly in fatty fish such as salmon, mackerel, sardines, and trout.
3. **Docosahexaenoic acid (DHA):** This is also found in fatty fish and is particularly abundant in seafood.

Sources of Omega -3 Fatty acid

1. **Dietary Sources**: The primary source of omega-3 fatty acids is through the consumption of foods rich in these nutrients. Sources include:

   - ALA: Found in plant-based foods such as flaxseeds, chia seeds, hemp seeds, walnuts, and soybeans.
   - EPA and DHA: Found primarily in fatty fish such as salmon, mackerel, sardines, herring, and trout. These marine sources of omega-3 fatty acids are particularly rich in EPA and DHA.

2. **Conversion of ALA to EPA and DHA**: While ALA is the most common omega-3 fatty acid found in plant-based foods, the body can convert a portion of ALA into EPA and DHA. However, this conversion process is inefficient, and only a small amount of ALA is converted into EPA and DHA. Therefore, it's important to consume adequate sources of EPA and DHA from marine sources or supplements, especially for individuals following a vegetarian or vegan diet.

3. **Supplements**: Omega-3 fatty acid supplements, such as fish oil capsules or algae oil capsules, are available and can provide a concentrated source of EPA and DHA. These supplements can be particularly beneficial for individuals who do not consume enough fatty fish or who have specific dietary restrictions.

In summary, the body obtains omega-3 fatty acids through dietary sources, primarily from fatty fish rich in EPA and DHA, as well as from plant-based sources rich in ALA. Consuming a balanced diet that includes a variety of omega-3-rich foods is important for ensuring an adequate intake of these essential nutrients and supporting overall health and well-being.

The benefits of omega-3 fatty acids include:

Heart Health:

Omega-3 fatty acids have been shown to help reduce the risk of heart disease by lowering triglyceride levels, reducing inflammation, improving blood vessel function, and lowering blood pressure. They may also help prevent the formation of blood clots and reduce the risk of stroke.

Brain Health:

DHA, in particular, is important for brain development and function. It is a major component of the brain and plays a crucial role in cognitive function, memory, and learning. Omega-3 fatty acids may also help reduce the risk of age-related cognitive decline and Alzheimer's disease.

Eye Health:

DHA is also found in high concentrations in the retina of the eye, where it helps support healthy vision and may reduce the risk of age-related macular degeneration.

Joint Health:

Omega-3 fatty acids have anti-inflammatory properties that can help reduce joint pain and stiffness in conditions like rheumatoid arthritis and osteoarthritis.

Mental Health:

Some research suggests that omega-3 fatty acids may help improve mood and reduce symptoms of depression and anxiety. They may also have a protective effect against other mental health disorders such as schizophrenia and bipolar disorder.

Pregnancy and Infant Development:

Omega-3 fatty acids are important for fetal brain and eye development during pregnancy. They may also help reduce the risk of preterm birth and may be beneficial for infant development and cognitive function.

Skin Health: Omega-3 fatty acids may help maintain healthy skin by reducing inflammation and supporting skin barrier function. They may also help improve symptoms of certain skin conditions like eczema and psoriasis.

Including omega-3-rich foods in your diet, such as fatty fish, flaxseeds, chia seeds, walnuts, and hemp seeds, or taking omega-3 supplements if needed, can help ensure you get an adequate intake of these essential fatty acids and reap their many health benefits. However, it's important to consult with a healthcare professional before starting any supplementation regimen, especially if you have any underlying health conditions or are taking medications.

Antioxidant -Essential Compounds

What are Antioxidants?

Antioxidants are compounds that help protect the body against damage caused by free radicals. Free radicals are unstable molecules that can cause oxidative stress, a process linked to various chronic diseases and aging. Antioxidants neutralize free radicals by donating electrons, thereby preventing them from causing damage to cells, proteins, and DNA.

There are several types of antioxidants, including vitamins (such as vitamin C, vitamin E, and vitamin A), minerals (such as selenium and zinc), phytochemicals (found in plant-based foods), and enzymes (such as catalase and superoxide dismutase) produced by the body.

1. **Vitamin C (Ascorbic Acid):**
   - **Benefits:** Vitamin C is a powerful water-soluble antioxidant that helps protect cells from oxidative damage, supports immune function, promotes collagen synthesis for healthy skin, aids in wound healing, enhances iron absorption, and may reduce the risk of chronic diseases such as heart disease and certain cancers.
2. **Vitamin E (Tocopherols and Tocotrienols):**
   - **Benefits:** Vitamin E is a fat-soluble antioxidant that protects cell membranes from oxidative damage, acts as a free radical scavenger in lipid-rich areas of the body, supports immune function, promotes skin health, and may reduce the risk of age-related cognitive decline and cardiovascular disease.
3. **Beta-Carotene:**
   - **Benefits:** Beta-carotene is a provitamin A carotenoid antioxidant found in orange and yellow fruits and vegetables. It functions as a precursor to vitamin A, supports immune function, promotes healthy vision, helps maintain skin health, and may reduce the risk of certain cancers and cardiovascular disease.
4. **Selenium:**
   - **Benefits:** Selenium is a trace mineral that acts as a cofactor for antioxidant enzymes such as glutathione peroxidase. It helps protect cells from oxidative damage, supports thyroid function, boosts immune response, promotes reproductive health, and may reduce the risk of certain cancers and cardiovascular disease.
5. **Flavonoids:**
   - **Benefits:** Flavonoids are a group of polyphenolic compounds found in various plant-based foods, including fruits, vegetables, tea, and red wine. They possess antioxidant, anti-inflammatory, and anti-cancer properties, support cardiovascular

health, promote cognitive function, and may reduce the risk of chronic diseases such as diabetes and neurodegenerative disorders.

6. **Lycopene:**
    - **Benefits:** Lycopene is a carotenoid antioxidant found in red-colored fruits and vegetables, such as tomatoes, watermelon, and pink grapefruit. It exhibits potent antioxidant properties, helps protect against oxidative damage to cells and tissues, supports heart health, and may reduce the risk of certain cancers, particularly prostate cancer.
7. **Polyphenols:**
    - **Benefits:** Polyphenols are a diverse group of antioxidants found abundantly in plant-based foods, including fruits, vegetables, tea, coffee, cocoa, and red wine. They possess antioxidant, anti-inflammatory, anti-microbial, and anti-cancer properties, support cardiovascular health, promote cognitive function, and may contribute to longevity and overall well-being.
8. **Coenzyme Q10 (CoQ10):**
    - **Benefits:** CoQ10 is a fat-soluble antioxidant and a crucial component of the electron transport chain involved in cellular energy production. It helps protect cells from oxidative damage, supports heart health, enhances exercise performance, promotes skin health, and may reduce the risk of neurodegenerative diseases and migraine headaches.

Incorporating a variety of antioxidant-rich foods into your diet can help maintain optimal health, protect against oxidative stress, and reduce the risk of chronic diseases associated with free radical damage.

Free Radicals

What are Free radicals?

Free radicals are highly reactive molecules that contain one or more unpaired electrons in their outer shell. These unpaired electrons make free radicals highly unstable and reactive, as they seek to pair with electrons from other molecules in order to achieve stability. In the process of seeking to stabilize themselves, free radicals can cause damage to surrounding molecules by stealing electrons from them. This process, known as oxidative stress, can lead to cellular damage and contribute to the development of various diseases and aging processes.

Free radicals are generated as natural byproducts of cellular metabolism, particularly during processes such as respiration and energy production. Additionally, external factors such as exposure to environmental pollutants, radiation, cigarette smoke, and certain medications can also increase the production of free radicals in the body.

While some level of free radical production is normal and necessary for cellular function, excessive levels of free radicals can overwhelm the body's antioxidant defenses and lead to oxidative damage. Antioxidants are molecules that can neutralize free radicals by donating electrons without becoming destabilized themselves. Antioxidants can be obtained from dietary sources, such as fruits, vegetables, nuts, seeds, and certain spices, as well as produced by the body itself.

When free radicals are not properly neutralized by antioxidants, they can cause damage to cellular structures such as proteins, lipids, and DNA. This damage can disrupt cellular function and contribute to the development of various health conditions, including cardiovascular disease, cancer, neurodegenerative disorders, and aging-related conditions.

In summary, free radicals are highly reactive molecules that can cause damage to cells and tissues through oxidative stress. While some free radical production is normal and necessary for cellular function, excessive levels of free radicals can lead to oxidative damage and contribute to the development of various diseases and aging processes. Consuming a diet rich in antioxidants and minimizing exposure to factors that increase free radical production can help protect against oxidative damage and support overall health and well-being.

Plant-Based Foods Beneficial for Diabetes

What is Diabetes?

Diabetes is a chronic medical condition that occurs when the body either does not produce enough insulin or cannot effectively use the insulin it produces, leading to high blood sugar levels. Insulin is a hormone that regulates glucose in the bloodstream and allows it to enter cells for energy. There are three main types of diabetes: Type 1, an autoimmune condition where the body attacks insulin-producing cells; Type 2, which develops due to insulin resistance and is often linked to lifestyle factors; and gestational diabetes, which occurs during pregnancy. If left unmanaged, diabetes can lead to serious complications such as heart disease, kidney failure, nerve damage, and vision problems. Proper management includes a healthy diet, regular exercise, medication, and monitoring blood sugar levels.

Some Plant-based foods that are beneficial for managing diabetes, as they are low in glycemic index, high in fiber, and rich in nutrients that support blood sugar control:

1. **Leafy Greens** (Spinach, Kale, Swiss Chard) – Low in carbs and high in fiber and antioxidants.
2. **Berries** (Blueberries, Strawberries, Raspberries) – Low glycemic fruits with antioxidants and fiber.
3. **Chia Seeds** – High in fiber and omega-3 fatty acids, which support blood sugar stability.
4. **Flaxseeds** – Rich in fiber, healthy fats, and can help regulate blood sugar.
5. **Quinoa** – A high-protein, fiber-rich grain alternative with a low glycemic index.
6. **Avocado** – Provides healthy fats and fiber, which help slow digestion and regulate blood sugar.
7. **Broccoli** – Contains fiber and a compound called sulforaphane, which may help improve insulin sensitivity.
8. **Beans** (Black, Chickpeas, Kidney) – High in protein, fiber, and complex carbs for stable energy.
9. **Lentils** – Packed with protein, fiber, and slow-digesting carbohydrates.
10. **Sweet Potatoes** – A low glycemic alternative to regular potatoes, rich in fiber and beta-carotene.
11. **Nuts** (Almonds, Walnuts, Pecans) – High in fiber, protein, and healthy fats, promoting satiety and stable blood sugar.

12. **Oats** – A whole grain with soluble fiber that can help control blood sugar levels.

13. **Zucchini** – Low in calories and carbs, making it a good choice for blood sugar control.

14. **Tomatoes** – Low-carb and rich in antioxidants, especially lycopene.

15. **Bell Peppers** – Low in carbs and high in vitamins A and C, adding color and nutrients without spiking blood sugar.

16. **Carrots** – Despite their sweetness, they are low in glycemic impact and packed with fiber and beta-carotene.

17. **Eggplant** – Low-carb, fiber-rich, and versatile for a range of dishes.

18. **Cauliflower** – Low in carbs, can replace grains, and is rich in fiber and vitamins.

19. **Mushrooms** – Low in carbs and calories, they are good for satiety without impacting blood sugar.

20. **Apples** – Low glycemic fruit that contains fiber and antioxidants, particularly in the skin.

Incorporating these foods can help maintain steady blood sugar levels while providing essential nutrients for overall health.

Oxidative Stress

What is oxidative Stress?

Oxidative stress is a physiological imbalance between the production of reactive oxygen species (ROS) or free radicals and the body's ability to neutralize them with antioxidants. Reactive oxygen species include molecules such as superoxide radicals, hydroxyl radicals, and hydrogen peroxide, which are generated as natural byproducts of cellular metabolism, particularly during processes such as respiration and energy production.

Under normal conditions, the body's antioxidant defenses, including enzymes such as superoxide dismutase (SOD), catalase, and glutathione peroxidase, as well as non-enzymatic antioxidants such as vitamin C, vitamin E, and glutathione, help neutralize reactive oxygen species and protect cells from oxidative damage. However, when the production of reactive oxygen species exceeds the body's antioxidant capacity, oxidative stress occurs.

Oxidative stress can lead to damage to cellular structures such as proteins, lipids, and DNA. This damage can disrupt cellular function and contribute to the development of various health conditions, including cardiovascular disease, cancer, neurodegenerative disorders, inflammatory conditions, diabetes, and aging-related conditions.

Several factors can contribute to oxidative stress, including:

1. **Environmental factors:** Exposure to environmental pollutants, radiation, cigarette smoke, and certain chemicals can increase the production of reactive oxygen species and contribute to oxidative stress.
2. **Lifestyle factors:** Poor diet, lack of exercise, excessive alcohol consumption, smoking, and chronic stress can all increase oxidative stress levels in the body.
3. **Disease conditions:** Certain diseases and health conditions, such as diabetes, obesity, autoimmune disorders, and neurodegenerative diseases, can also increase oxidative stress due to inflammation and impaired antioxidant defenses.
4. **Aging:** The aging process is associated with an increase in oxidative stress and a decline in antioxidant defenses, which may contribute to age-related diseases and the aging process itself.
5. **Dietary factors:** Consumption of a diet high in processed foods, refined sugars, unhealthy fats, and low in antioxidants can increase oxidative stress levels in the body.

In summary, oxidative stress is a physiological imbalance between the production of reactive oxygen species and the body's antioxidant defenses. It can lead to damage to cellular structures and contribute to the development of various diseases and aging processes. Minimizing exposure to factors that increase oxidative stress and consuming a diet rich in antioxidants can help protect against oxidative damage and support overall health and well-being.

Cardiovascular Disease (CVD)

What is cardiovascular disease?

Cardiovascular disease (CVD) refers to a group of conditions that affect the heart and blood vessels, often leading to complications such as heart attack, stroke, or peripheral artery disease. It is one of the leading causes of death globally, accounting for millions of deaths each year.

There are several types of cardiovascular diseases, including:

1. **Coronary artery disease (CAD):** CAD occurs when the blood vessels that supply oxygen-rich blood to the heart muscle become narrowed or blocked due to the buildup of plaque (a combination of cholesterol, fat, and other substances). This can restrict blood flow to the heart and lead to chest pain (angina), heart attack (myocardial infarction), or other complications.
2. **Stroke:** A stroke occurs when the blood supply to part of the brain is interrupted or reduced, depriving brain tissue of oxygen and nutrients. This can result in brain damage, disability, or death. There are two main types of stroke: ischemic stroke, which occurs when a blood clot blocks a blood vessel in the brain, and hemorrhagic stroke, which occurs when a blood vessel in the brain ruptures and causes bleeding.
3. **Peripheral artery disease (PAD):** PAD occurs when the blood vessels outside of the heart, usually in the legs, become narrowed or blocked due to atherosclerosis (the buildup of plaque). This can result in reduced blood flow to the limbs, leading to symptoms such as leg pain, numbness, or weakness, and increasing the risk of complications such as infection or tissue damage.
4. **Heart failure:** Heart failure occurs when the heart is unable to pump enough blood to meet the body's needs. This can result from conditions such as CAD, high blood pressure, or damage to the heart muscle (e.g., from a heart attack). Symptoms of heart failure may include shortness of breath, fatigue, swelling in the legs or abdomen, and difficulty exercising.
5. **Arrhythmias:** Arrhythmias are abnormal heart rhythms that can occur when the electrical impulses that regulate the heartbeat are disrupted. This can cause the heart to beat too fast (tachycardia), too slow (bradycardia), or irregularly. While some arrhythmias may be harmless, others can be life-threatening and require medical treatment.

Risk factors for cardiovascular disease include:

- High blood pressure (hypertension)
- High cholesterol levels
- Smoking
- Diabetes

- Obesity
- Physical inactivity
- Unhealthy diet
- Family history of CVD
- Age (risk increases with age)
- Gender (men are at higher risk than premenopausal women, though the risk equalizes after menopause)
- Socioeconomic factors (such as low income or education level)

Prevention and management of cardiovascular disease involve lifestyle modifications (such as regular exercise, healthy diet, smoking cessation, and weight management), medication (such as blood pressure or cholesterol-lowering medications), and, in some cases, medical procedures or surgery (such as angioplasty, stenting, or bypass surgery). Early detection and treatment of risk factors and underlying conditions are crucial for reducing the risk of cardiovascular disease and its complications. Regular check-ups with a healthcare provider can help assess and manage individual cardiovascular risk.

Here are some plant-based foods that are rich in key nutrients known to help manage certain cardiovascular disease such as:

High Blood Pressure

Managing high blood pressure through diet is a crucial aspect of overall health. Incorporating plant-based foods rich in essential nutrients can be beneficial for maintaining healthy blood pressure levels. Here are some plant-based foods that are rich in key nutrients known to help manage high blood pressure:

Leafy greens:

- Spinach, kale, Swiss chard, collard greens, and other leafy greens are excellent sources of potassium, magnesium, and dietary nitrates, which can help relax blood vessels and lower blood pressure.

Bananas:

- Bananas are rich in potassium, an essential mineral that helps regulate blood pressure by balancing sodium levels and promoting healthy blood vessel function.
-

Berries:

- Blueberries, strawberries, raspberries, and other berries are packed with antioxidants, including flavonoids and anthocyanins, which have been associated with lower blood pressure levels.

Beets:

- Beets are high in dietary nitrates, which the body converts into nitric oxide, a compound that helps relax blood vessels and improve blood flow, thereby lowering blood pressure.

Avocados:

- Avocados are rich in potassium, magnesium, and heart-healthy monounsaturated fats, which can help lower blood pressure and improve overall cardiovascular health.

Legumes:

- Beans, lentils, chickpeas, and other legumes are excellent sources of potassium, magnesium, fiber, and protein, all of which contribute to lower blood pressure levels and improved heart health.

Sweet potatoes:

- Sweet potatoes are rich in potassium and magnesium, as well as fiber and antioxidants, making them a nutritious choice for managing blood pressure and promoting overall health.

Oats:

- Oats are high in soluble fiber, which can help lower cholesterol levels and reduce blood pressure. They also contain magnesium and potassium, which further contribute to heart health.

Nuts and seeds:

- Almonds, walnuts, flaxseeds, chia seeds, and pumpkin seeds are rich in heart-healthy fats, magnesium, potassium, and fiber, all of which support lower blood pressure levels.

Garlic:

- Garlic contains compounds that may help relax blood vessels, improve blood flow, and lower blood pressure. Incorporating fresh or cooked garlic into meals can be beneficial for cardiovascular health.

Incorporating a variety of these plant-based foods into your diet, along with reducing sodium intake, maintaining a healthy weight, regular physical activity, and managing stress, can help support healthy blood pressure levels and overall cardiovascular health. It's also important to consult with a healthcare professional or registered dietitian for personalized dietary recommendations and guidance.

High Cholesterol

Managing high cholesterol levels through diet is an important aspect of cardiovascular health. Incorporating plant-based foods rich in essential nutrients can help lower LDL ("bad") cholesterol levels and improve overall lipid profiles. Here are some plant-based foods that are particularly beneficial for managing high cholesterol:

Oats and oatmeal:

- Oats are rich in soluble fiber, specifically beta-glucan, which helps reduce LDL cholesterol levels by inhibiting its absorption in the intestines. Consuming oats or oatmeal regularly can help lower cholesterol levels and improve heart health.

Legumes:

- Beans, lentils, chickpeas, and other legumes are excellent sources of soluble fiber, protein, and plant sterols, all of which help lower LDL cholesterol levels and improve overall lipid profiles.

Nuts and seeds:

- Almonds, walnuts, flaxseeds, chia seeds, and pumpkin seeds are rich in heart-healthy fats, fiber, and plant sterols, which help lower LDL cholesterol levels and reduce the risk of heart disease.

Avocados:

- Avocados are high in monounsaturated fats, which have been shown to help raise HDL ("good") cholesterol levels and lower LDL cholesterol levels. They are also rich in fiber and antioxidants, making them a heart-healthy addition to the diet.

Fatty fish:

- Fatty fish such as salmon, mackerel, sardines, and trout are rich in omega-3 fatty acids, which help lower triglyceride levels and reduce inflammation. Consuming fatty fish regularly can help improve lipid profiles and reduce the risk of heart disease.

Berries:

- Blueberries, strawberries, raspberries, and other berries are rich in antioxidants, including anthocyanins and flavonoids, which have been shown to help lower LDL cholesterol levels and reduce the risk of heart disease.

Whole grains:

- Whole grains such as brown rice, quinoa, barley, and whole wheat are rich in soluble fiber, which helps lower LDL cholesterol levels and improve heart health. Consuming whole grains regularly can help reduce the risk of heart disease.

Leafy greens:

- Spinach, kale, Swiss chard, and other leafy greens are rich in fiber, antioxidants, and plant compounds that help lower cholesterol levels and reduce the risk of heart disease.

Soy products:

- Soybeans, tofu, tempeh, and other soy products are rich in plant proteins, fiber, and phytoestrogens called isoflavones, which help lower LDL cholesterol levels and improve heart health.

Garlic:

- Garlic contains compounds that have been shown to help lower LDL cholesterol levels and reduce the risk of heart disease. Incorporating fresh or cooked garlic into meals can be beneficial for managing cholesterol levels.

Incorporating a variety of these plant-based foods into your diet, along with reducing saturated and trans fats, limiting dietary cholesterol, maintaining a healthy weight, regular physical activity, and managing stress, can help improve lipid profiles and reduce the risk of heart disease. It's also important to consult with a healthcare professional or registered dietitian for personalized dietary recommendations and guidance.

Diabetes

Managing diabetes through diet is crucial for controlling blood sugar levels and preventing complications. Plant-based foods can be particularly beneficial for individuals with diabetes as they are typically low in saturated fats, rich in fiber, and provide essential nutrients. Here are some plant-based foods with essential nutrients that can help manage diabetes:

Leafy greens:

- Spinach, kale, Swiss chard, collard greens, and other leafy greens are low in calories and carbohydrates while being rich in fiber, vitamins, and minerals. They are excellent choices for managing blood sugar levels and supporting overall health.

Non-starchy vegetables:

- Vegetables such as broccoli, cauliflower, bell peppers, carrots, zucchini, and tomatoes are low in carbohydrates and calories but high in fiber, vitamins, and antioxidants. They can be included in meals to add flavor, texture, and nutrients without significantly affecting blood sugar levels.

Whole grains:

- Whole grains such as quinoa, brown rice, barley, oats, and whole wheat are rich in fiber, which helps slow down the absorption of glucose into the bloodstream and stabilize blood sugar levels. They also provide essential vitamins, minerals, and antioxidants.

Legumes:

- Beans, lentils, chickpeas, and other legumes are high in fiber, protein, and complex carbohydrates, making them excellent choices for managing blood sugar levels. They have a low glycemic index, which means they cause a gradual rise in blood sugar levels after consumption.

Berries:

- Berries such as strawberries, blueberries, raspberries, and blackberries are low in calories and carbohydrates but high in fiber, vitamins, and antioxidants. They can satisfy sweet cravings without causing significant spikes in blood sugar levels.

Nuts and seeds:

- Almonds, walnuts, flaxseeds, chia seeds, and pumpkin seeds are rich in healthy fats, protein, fiber, and essential nutrients. They can help stabilize blood sugar levels, reduce inflammation, and improve heart health when consumed in moderation.

Avocados:

- Avocados are rich in monounsaturated fats, fiber, and essential nutrients such as potassium and magnesium. They can help improve insulin sensitivity, reduce cholesterol levels, and promote heart health.

Sweet potatoes:

- Sweet potatoes are a nutritious source of carbohydrates, fiber, vitamins (such as vitamin A and vitamin C), and minerals. They have a lower glycemic index compared to white potatoes, meaning they cause a slower increase in blood sugar levels.

Cinnamon:

- Cinnamon is a spice that has been shown to help improve insulin sensitivity and reduce blood sugar levels. Adding cinnamon to foods and beverages can provide flavor and potential health benefits for individuals with diabetes.

Garlic and onions:

- Garlic and onions contain compounds that may help improve insulin sensitivity and reduce blood sugar levels. Incorporating them into meals can add flavor and potential health benefits for managing diabetes.

Incorporating a variety of these plant-based foods into your diet, along with portion control, regular physical activity, and blood sugar monitoring, can help manage diabetes and promote overall health and well-being. It's also important to consult with a healthcare professional or registered dietitian for personalized dietary recommendations and guidance.

Obesity

Managing obesity through diet involves choosing nutrient-dense foods that are low in calories but high in essential nutrients. Plant-based foods can be particularly beneficial for managing obesity as they are typically high in fiber, vitamins, minerals, and antioxidants while being lower in calories and saturated fats compared to animal products. Here are some plant-based foods with essential nutrients that can help manage obesity:

Leafy greens:

- Spinach, kale, Swiss chard, collard greens, and other leafy greens are low in calories and carbohydrates but high in fiber, vitamins, and minerals. They can help promote satiety and fullness while providing essential nutrients.

Non-starchy vegetables:

- Vegetables such as broccoli, cauliflower, bell peppers, carrots, zucchini, and tomatoes are low in calories and carbohydrates but high in fiber, vitamins, and antioxidants. They can be included in meals to add volume, flavor, and nutrients without significantly increasing calorie intake.

Whole grains:

- Whole grains such as quinoa, brown rice, barley, oats, and whole wheat are rich in fiber, which helps promote satiety and regulate appetite. They provide essential nutrients and can help stabilize blood sugar levels, reducing the risk of overeating.

Legumes:

- Beans, lentils, chickpeas, and other legumes are rich in fiber, protein, and complex carbohydrates, making them excellent choices for managing obesity. They help promote satiety, regulate blood sugar levels, and support weight management.

Berries:

- Berries such as strawberries, blueberries, raspberries, and blackberries are low in calories and carbohydrates but high in fiber, vitamins, and antioxidants. They can satisfy sweet cravings and provide essential nutrients without significantly increasing calorie intake.

Nuts and seeds:

- Almonds, walnuts, flaxseeds, chia seeds, and pumpkin seeds are rich in healthy fats, protein, fiber, and essential nutrients. They can help promote satiety, reduce cravings, and support weight management when consumed in moderation.

Avocados:

- Avocados are rich in monounsaturated fats, fiber, and essential nutrients such as potassium and magnesium. They can help promote satiety, reduce hunger, and support weight loss when included in a balanced diet.

Sweet potatoes:

- Sweet potatoes are a nutritious source of carbohydrates, fiber, vitamins (such as vitamin A and vitamin C), and minerals. They have a lower glycemic index compared to white potatoes and can help regulate blood sugar levels and promote satiety.

Non-dairy milk alternatives:

- Plant-based milk alternatives such as almond milk, soy milk, and oat milk are lower in calories and saturated fats compared to cow's milk. They can be used as substitutes in recipes or consumed as beverages to reduce calorie intake.

Herbs and spices:

- Herbs and spices such as cinnamon, ginger, turmeric, cayenne pepper, and black pepper can add flavor to meals without adding extra calories. They may also have metabolism-boosting or appetite-suppressing properties, supporting weight management efforts.

Incorporating a variety of these plant-based foods into your diet, along with portion control, regular physical activity, adequate sleep, and stress management, can help manage obesity and promote overall health and well-being. It's also important to consult with a healthcare professional or registered dietitian for personalized dietary recommendations and guidance.

Unhealthy Diet

Managing an unhealthy diet involves making healthier food choices rich in essential nutrients while limiting processed foods, refined sugars, unhealthy fats, and excessive salt intake. Plant-based foods can play a key role in improving dietary habits as they are typically high in fiber, vitamins, minerals, and antioxidants while being lower in calories and saturated fats compared to many animal products and processed foods. Here are some plant-based foods with essential nutrients that can help manage an unhealthy diet:

Leafy greens:

- Spinach, kale, Swiss chard, collard greens, and other leafy greens are rich in vitamins (such as vitamin A, vitamin C, and vitamin K), minerals (such as iron and calcium), and antioxidants. They can help improve overall nutrition and support a healthy diet.

Non-starchy vegetables:

- Vegetables such as broccoli, cauliflower, bell peppers, carrots, zucchini, and tomatoes are low in calories but high in fiber, vitamins, and antioxidants. They can add flavor, texture, and nutrients to meals while promoting satiety and fullness.

Whole grains:

- Whole grains such as quinoa, brown rice, barley, oats, and whole wheat are rich in fiber, vitamins, minerals, and complex carbohydrates. They provide sustained energy, promote satiety, and support digestive health.

Legumes:

- Beans, lentils, chickpeas, and other legumes are excellent sources of protein, fiber, vitamins, and minerals. They can help regulate blood sugar levels, reduce cholesterol levels, and support weight management.

Berries:

- Berries such as strawberries, blueberries, raspberries, and blackberries are low in calories but high in fiber, vitamins, and antioxidants. They can satisfy sweet cravings and provide essential nutrients without contributing to excessive calorie intake.

Nuts and seeds:

- Almonds, walnuts, flaxseeds, chia seeds, and pumpkin seeds are rich in healthy fats, protein, fiber, vitamins, and minerals. They can help reduce inflammation, support heart health, and promote satiety when consumed in moderation.

Avocados:

- Avocados are rich in monounsaturated fats, fiber, vitamins, and minerals. They can help improve cholesterol levels, reduce inflammation, and support overall health when included in a balanced diet.

Sweet potatoes:

- Sweet potatoes are nutritious root vegetables that are rich in fiber, vitamins (such as vitamin A and vitamin C), and minerals. They have a lower glycemic index compared to white potatoes and can help regulate blood sugar levels and promote satiety.

Herbs and spices:

- Herbs and spices such as garlic, ginger, turmeric, cinnamon, and black pepper can add flavor to meals without adding extra calories. They may also have anti-inflammatory, antioxidant, and metabolism-boosting properties.

Plant-based protein sources:

- Tofu, tempeh, seitan, edamame, and plant-based protein powders (such as pea protein or soy protein) are nutritious alternatives to animal protein sources. They are rich in protein, vitamins, minerals, and antioxidants and can be incorporated into a variety of dishes to improve overall nutrition.

Incorporating a variety of these plant-based foods into your diet, along with reducing processed foods, refined sugars, and unhealthy fats, can help manage an unhealthy diet and promote overall health and well-being. It's also important to practice mindful eating, portion control, and regular physical activity for optimal health outcomes. Consulting with a healthcare professional or registered dietitian can provide personalized dietary recommendations and guidance based on individual needs and preferences.

Plant-Based Foods Beneficial for Cancer Prevention and Support

Some plant-based foods beneficial for cancer prevention and support. They are rich in antioxidants, anti-inflammatory compounds, fiber, and essential nutrients that help protect cells, reduce oxidative stress, and inhibit cancer growth:

1. **Broccoli** – Contains sulforaphane, a compound that may inhibit cancer cell growth, especially in breast, prostate, and colon cancers.
2. **Berries (Blueberries, Strawberries, Raspberries)** – High in antioxidants like anthocyanins that help prevent cell damage and reduce inflammation.
3. **Leafy Greens (Spinach, Kale, Swiss Chard)** – Rich in folate, carotenoids, and antioxidants that may lower the risk of certain cancers, including colon cancer.
4. **Garlic** – Contains allicin, which may help protect against stomach and colon cancers by enhancing detoxification processes.
5. **Turmeric** – Contains curcumin, known for its powerful anti-inflammatory and antioxidant properties that may help inhibit cancer growth.
6. **Tomatoes** – High in lycopene, an antioxidant that has been linked to reduced risk of prostate cancer and other cancers.
7. **Flaxseeds** – Rich in omega-3 fatty acids and lignans, which may slow the growth of hormone-related cancers, like breast and prostate.
8. **Walnuts** – Contain omega-3s, antioxidants, and polyphenols that may help reduce the risk of certain cancers.
9. **Ginger** – Known for its anti-inflammatory properties, which may help reduce tumor growth and protect cells from damage.
10. **Pomegranate** – Contains polyphenols with antioxidant properties, which may help slow cancer cell growth.
11. **Beans (Black, Kidney, Lentils)** – High in fiber and antioxidants that support detoxification and may reduce the risk of colorectal cancer.
12. **Green Tea** – Contains catechins and polyphenols, which may inhibit cancer cell growth and reduce oxidative stress.
13. **Apples** – High in fiber and antioxidants like quercetin, which may protect cells and reduce cancer risk.
14. **Citrus Fruits (Oranges, Lemons, Grapefruit)** – Rich in vitamin C and flavonoids, which help boost immune function and reduce inflammation.
15. **Carrots** – Packed with beta-carotene, which has been shown to reduce the risk of several cancers, including lung and prostate.

16. **Whole Grains (Oats, Brown Rice, Quinoa)** – Contain fiber and lignans, which support gut health and may reduce colorectal cancer risk.

17. **Cruciferous Vegetables (Cauliflower, Brussels Sprouts)** – High in glucosinolates, which activate enzymes that detoxify carcinogens.

18. **Beets** – Contain betalains, antioxidants that support detoxification and protect cells from oxidative damage.

19. **Chia Seeds** – Provide omega-3s, fiber, and antioxidants that may reduce inflammation and support cell health.

20. **Soursop** – Contains high levels of antioxidants, anti-inflammatory properties, and acetogenins—compounds that may inhibit cancer cell growth and support the immune system in targeting abnormal cells.

21. **Mushrooms (Shiitake, Maitake, Reishi)** – Rich in beta-glucans and selenium, which help modulate the immune system and may reduce cancer risk.

Including these plant-based foods as part of a balanced diet can support cellular health, boost immunity, and potentially lower the risk of cancer.

Plant-Based Foods Beneficial for Chronic Obstructive Pulmonary Disease (COPD)

Some plant-based foods beneficial for managing Chronic Obstructive Pulmonary Disease (COPD), primarily due to their anti-inflammatory, antioxidant, and nutrient-dense properties that support lung health.

1. **Leafy Greens (Spinach, Kale, Swiss Chard)** – High in vitamins A, C, and E, which support lung tissue repair and reduce inflammation.
2. **Berries (Blueberries, Strawberries, Raspberries)** – Packed with antioxidants like anthocyanins, which protect lung cells from oxidative damage.
3. **Broccoli** – Contains sulforaphane, an antioxidant that may help reduce lung inflammation and improve overall respiratory health.
4. **Beets** – High in nitrates that improve oxygen flow and support lung function, which may help with breathing.
5. **Turmeric** – Contains curcumin, a powerful anti-inflammatory compound that may reduce lung inflammation in COPD patients.
6. **Ginger** – Known for its anti-inflammatory properties, ginger can help ease respiratory symptoms and reduce airway inflammation.
7. **Apples** – Rich in quercetin, an antioxidant that may help improve lung function and reduce the risk of COPD.
8. **Garlic** – Contains allicin, which has antioxidant and anti-inflammatory effects that support lung health and immune function.
9. **Olive Oil** – High in anti-inflammatory compounds and healthy fats, which help reduce inflammation in the lungs.
10. **Tomatoes** – A source of lycopene, which can help reduce inflammation and improve lung function.
11. **Chia Seeds** – High in omega-3 fatty acids and fiber, which can reduce inflammation and improve oxygen flow.
12. **Walnuts** – Another good source of plant-based omega-3s that can help reduce inflammation and support lung health.
13. **Pineapple** – Contains bromelain, an enzyme with anti-inflammatory properties that may help reduce lung inflammation and improve breathing.
14. **Carrots** – High in beta-carotene and vitamin A, which support lung tissue health and repair.

15. **Bananas** – High in potassium, which can improve lung function by aiding in muscle contraction and relaxation for better airflow.
16. **Citrus Fruits (Oranges, Lemons)** – Rich in vitamin C and antioxidants that boost immune function and may improve lung health.
17. **Pumpkin** – High in beta-carotene, which can protect lung tissue and reduce the risk of respiratory complications.
18. **Lentils** – A good source of fiber, magnesium, and folate, which help reduce inflammation and support respiratory health.
19. **Pomegranate** – Contains antioxidants that may improve lung function and protect against damage from pollutants.
20. **Green Tea** – Contains antioxidants and anti-inflammatory compounds like catechins, which can improve respiratory health and support lung function.

These foods offer nutrients that support lung tissue, reduce inflammation, and improve oxygen flow, which can be beneficial for people managing COPD.

Plant-Based Foods Beneficial for Cold and Flu

Some plant-based foods that are beneficial for combating the common Cold and Flu. These foods are rich in vitamins, antioxidants, and immune-boosting compounds that help the body fight infections, reduce inflammation, and speed up recovery:

1. **Citrus Fruits (Oranges, Lemons, Limes, Grapefruit)** – High in vitamin C, which boosts immune function and helps reduce cold duration.
2. **Ginger** – Contains anti-inflammatory compounds and antioxidants that soothe sore throats and help reduce inflammation.
3. **Garlic** – Rich in allicin, which has antiviral and antibacterial properties that may help fight off infections.
4. **Turmeric** – Contains curcumin, a powerful anti-inflammatory and antioxidant that supports immune health.
5. **Broccoli** – High in vitamin C, vitamin E, and antioxidants, which strengthen the immune system and aid in recovery.
6. **Spinach** – Packed with vitamin C, beta-carotene, and antioxidants, which help increase immune function and reduce infection risk.
7. **Berries (Blueberries, Strawberries, Blackberries)** – High in antioxidants, particularly vitamin C, which supports immune health and reduces inflammation.
8. **Almonds** – A good source of vitamin E, an antioxidant that helps boost the immune system, especially when combined with vitamin C.
9. **Red Bell Peppers** – High in vitamin C, which supports immune response and helps the body fight infections.
10. **Mushrooms (Shiitake, Maitake, Reishi)** – Contains beta-glucans, compounds that may help boost immune function and fight off infections.
11. **Green Tea** – Rich in catechins, antioxidants that have antiviral properties and help improve immune function.
12. **Carrots** – High in beta-carotene, which the body converts into vitamin A, supporting immune health and mucus membranes.
13. **Pumpkin** – Contains beta-carotene and vitamin C, which help strengthen immunity and fight off viruses.
14. **Pomegranate** – Contains polyphenols with antiviral properties, which may help reduce symptoms and speed up recovery.
15. **Watermelon** – Hydrating and high in vitamin C, which supports immune function and keeps mucus membranes moist.

16. **Papaya** – High in vitamin C, antioxidants, and digestive enzymes that support immune health and reduce inflammation.

17. **Kiwi** – Rich in vitamins C, K, and E, which help boost immune function and reduce cold symptoms.

18. **Apples** – Contain quercetin, an antioxidant with immune-boosting and antiviral properties that may help prevent infections.

19. **Oats** – High in beta-glucans, which have immune-enhancing effects and help the body respond to infections.

20. **Coconut Water** – Hydrating and contains electrolytes, which help maintain hydration and support the immune system during illness.

These foods provide essential vitamins, minerals, and antioxidants that support immune function, helping the body resist and recover from colds and flu faster. Incorporating these foods into your diet can help strengthen your immune system and potentially reduce the severity and duration of cold and flu symptoms.

Plant-Based Foods Beneficial for Diabetes

Some Plant-based foods that are beneficial for managing diabetes, as they are low in glycemic index, high in fiber, and rich in nutrients that support blood sugar control:

1. **Leafy Greens (Spinach, Kale, Swiss Chard)** – Low in carbs and high in fiber and antioxidants.
2. **Berries (Blueberries, Strawberries, Raspberries)** – Low glycemic fruits with antioxidants and fiber.
3. **Chia Seeds** – High in fiber and omega-3 fatty acids, which support blood sugar stability.
4. **Flaxseeds** – Rich in fiber, healthy fats, and can help regulate blood sugar.
5. **Quinoa** – A high-protein, fiber-rich grain alternative with a low glycemic index.
6. **Avocado** – Provides healthy fats and fiber, which help slow digestion and regulate blood sugar.
7. **Broccoli** – Contains fiber and a compound called sulforaphane, which may help improve insulin sensitivity.
8. **Beans (Black, Chickpeas, Kidney)** – High in protein, fiber, and complex carbs for stable energy.
9. **Lentils** – Packed with protein, fiber, and slow-digesting carbohydrates.
10. **Sweet Potatoes** – A low glycemic alternative to regular potatoes, rich in fiber and beta-carotene.
11. **Nuts (Almonds, Walnuts, Pecans)** – High in fiber, protein, and healthy fats, promoting satiety and stable blood sugar.
12. **Oats** – A whole grain with soluble fiber that can help control blood sugar levels.
13. **Zucchini** – Low in calories and carbs, making it a good choice for blood sugar control.
14. **Tomatoes** – Low-carb and rich in antioxidants, especially lycopene.
15. **Bell Peppers** – Low in carbs and high in vitamins A and C, adding color and nutrients without spiking blood sugar.
16. **Carrots** – Despite their sweetness, they are low in glycemic impact and packed with fiber and beta-carotene.
17. **Eggplant** – Low-carb, fiber-rich, and versatile for a range of dishes.
18. **Cauliflower** – Low in carbs, can replace grains, and is rich in fiber and vitamins.
19. **Mushrooms** – Low in carbs and calories, they are good for satiety without impacting blood sugar.

20. **Apples** – Low glycemic fruit that contains fiber and antioxidants, particularly in the skin.

Incorporating these foods can help maintain steady blood sugar levels while providing essential nutrients for overall health.

Plant-Based Foods Beneficial for Heart Disease

Some plant-based foods that are beneficial for managing heart disease, along with reasons for their effectiveness:

1. **Leafy Greens (Spinach, Kale, Swiss Chard)** – High in nitrates, potassium, and antioxidants, which help lower blood pressure and improve artery function.
2. **Berries (Blueberries, Strawberries, Raspberries)** – Contain polyphenols and anthocyanins, which reduce oxidative stress and inflammation linked to heart disease.
3. **Avocado** – Rich in heart-healthy monounsaturated fats, potassium, and fiber, which help reduce cholesterol and blood pressure.
4. **Nuts (Walnuts, Almonds)** – Provide omega-3 fatty acids, fiber, and healthy fats, which lower LDL cholesterol and inflammation.
5. **Olive Oil** – Contains monounsaturated fats and antioxidants, such as oleic acid, that reduce LDL cholesterol and inflammation.
6. **Flaxseeds** – High in omega-3 fatty acids, fiber, and lignans, which help reduce blood pressure and cholesterol.
7. **Chia Seeds** – Contain omega-3s, fiber, and antioxidants, which support cholesterol and blood pressure management.
8. **Oats** – Rich in beta-glucan, a soluble fiber that can help lower cholesterol and improve blood vessel health.
9. **Tomatoes** – Provide lycopene, an antioxidant that lowers LDL cholesterol and reduces the risk of heart disease.
10. **Beans (Black, Kidney, Chickpeas)** – High in fiber, protein, and folate, which help lower cholesterol and support heart health.
11. **Whole Grains (Brown Rice, Quinoa)** – High in fiber and nutrients like magnesium that reduce cholesterol and blood pressure.
12. **Garlic** – Contains allicin, a compound that can reduce blood pressure and cholesterol levels.
13. **Citrus Fruits (Oranges, Lemons)** – High in vitamin C, fiber, and flavonoids, which help lower blood pressure and improve heart health.
14. **Carrots** – High in fiber and antioxidants, which help reduce blood pressure and cholesterol.
15. **Green Tea** – Contains catechins and flavonoids that improve blood flow, reduce cholesterol, and lower blood pressure.

16. **Broccoli** – Packed with fiber, potassium, and antioxidants that support healthy blood pressure and cholesterol levels.

17. **Sweet Potatoes** – Rich in potassium, fiber, and antioxidants, which help lower blood pressure and reduce heart disease risk.

18. **Beets** – Contain nitrates that help dilate blood vessels, improve circulation, and reduce blood pressure.

19. **Pumpkin Seeds** – High in magnesium, fiber, and antioxidants, which support heart health by lowering blood pressure and inflammation.

20. **Pomegranate** – Rich in polyphenols and antioxidants that help reduce cholesterol buildup and improve blood vessel health.

These plant-based foods contribute essential nutrients, healthy fats, fiber, and antioxidants that help support cardiovascular health, manage blood pressure, and reduce inflammation, which are key factors in preventing and managing heart disease.

Plant-Based Foods Beneficial for Hypertension (High Blood Pressure)

Some plant-based foods beneficial for managing high blood pressure, along with reasons for their effectiveness:

1. **Leafy Greens (Spinach, Kale, Swiss Chard)** – High in potassium and magnesium, which help regulate blood pressure by balancing sodium levels.
2. **Berries (Blueberries, Strawberries, Raspberries)** – Rich in antioxidants, especially anthocyanins, which improve blood vessel function and reduce blood pressure.
3. **Beets** – Contains nitrates that help relax blood vessels, improving blood flow and lowering blood pressure.
4. **Bananas** – A potassium-rich fruit that helps counteract the effects of sodium and reduces tension in blood vessel walls.
5. **Oats** – High in fiber, especially beta-glucan, which has been shown to reduce blood pressure by improving cholesterol and blood sugar levels.
6. **Garlic** – Contains allicin, which may help relax blood vessels and improve circulation, reducing blood pressure.
7. **Flaxseeds** – High in fiber and omega-3 fatty acids, which support heart health and lower blood pressure.
8. **Tomatoes** – Rich in lycopene and potassium, both beneficial for lowering blood pressure and supporting heart health.
9. **Nuts (Almonds, Walnuts)** – Contain magnesium and healthy fats that improve circulation and reduce blood pressure.
10. **Avocado** – High in potassium, healthy fats, and antioxidants that can help regulate blood pressure levels.
11. **Citrus Fruits (Oranges, Lemons)** – High in vitamin C and flavonoids, which improve blood vessel function and reduce blood pressure.
12. **Carrots** – Contain potassium and antioxidants, which support heart health and can help lower blood pressure.
13. **Celery** – Contains phthalides, compounds that may help relax blood vessel walls, improving blood flow and reducing pressure.
14. **Whole Grains (Brown Rice, Barley, Quinoa)** – High in fiber and magnesium, which helps reduce arterial stiffness and maintain healthy blood pressure.
15. **Pomegranate** – Contains antioxidants that improve blood vessel health and may reduce blood pressure.

16. **Legumes (Beans, Lentils, Chickpeas)** – High in fiber, protein, and potassium, all of which support healthy blood pressure levels.
17. **Chia Seeds** – Packed with fiber, omega-3 fatty acids, and minerals like magnesium and potassium that aid in blood pressure control.
18. **Apples** – Contain fiber and polyphenols that help improve blood vessel function and reduce blood pressure.
19. **Sweet Potatoes** – High in potassium and fiber, both of which support lower blood pressure by reducing sodium levels and promoting healthy digestion.

20.Broccoli – Rich in fiber, potassium, and antioxidants like flavonoids, which help improve blood vessel function and regulate blood pressure.

Incorporating these nutrient-dense, plant-based foods into your diet can support healthy blood pressure levels, benefiting overall cardiovascular health.

Plant-Based Foods Beneficial for Kidney Disease

Some plant-based foods that are beneficial for kidney health, particularly for individuals managing kidney disease. These foods are rich in essential nutrients like antioxidants, fiber, and anti-inflammatory compounds that support kidney function and help reduce the burden on the kidneys:

1. **Leafy Greens (Spinach, Kale, Swiss Chard)** – Rich in vitamins, minerals, and antioxidants, although individuals with kidney disease should monitor potassium intake from some leafy greens.
2. **Cauliflower** – A low-potassium vegetable packed with vitamin C and fiber, which supports kidney function.
3. **Berries (Blueberries, Strawberries, Raspberries)** – High in antioxidants, especially anthocyanins, which help reduce inflammation and protect kidney cells.
4. **Red Bell Peppers** – Low in potassium and rich in vitamin C, which supports kidney health and helps reduce inflammation.
5. **Garlic** – Contains sulfur compounds that have anti-inflammatory properties and may help reduce the buildup of waste products in the kidneys.
6. **Cabbage** – High in antioxidants, fiber, and vitamin K, which help reduce inflammation and support kidney function.
7. **Olive Oil** – Rich in healthy fats and antioxidants that may help protect kidney cells from damage.
8. **Apples** – Contain pectin, a type of fiber that helps lower cholesterol and support kidney health by promoting detoxification.
9. **Cucumbers** – Low in potassium and a good source of hydration, supporting kidney function by keeping the body hydrated.
10. **Carrots** – High in beta-carotene and vitamin A, which promote healthy kidney tissue and function.
11. **Pumpkin** – Packed with vitamins, antioxidants, and fiber, which support kidney function and help reduce inflammation.
12. **Cherries** – Rich in antioxidants, particularly anthocyanins, which may help reduce inflammation and protect kidney function.
13. **Beans (Black, Kidney, Lentils)** – Provide plant-based protein and fiber, though they should be consumed cautiously in advanced kidney disease due to their potassium and phosphorus content.
14. **Zucchini** – A low-potassium vegetable that is high in water content, promoting hydration and kidney health.

15. **Quinoa** – A complete plant-based protein that provides essential amino acids, while being lower in phosphorus compared to animal-based protein.

16. **Sweet Potatoes** – High in vitamin A, beta-carotene, and fiber; moderate potassium content requires monitoring for those with advanced kidney disease.

17. **Turmeric** – Contains curcumin, a powerful anti-inflammatory compound that may help reduce kidney inflammation and protect against kidney damage.

18. **Pears** – Low in potassium and high in fiber, pears support kidney health and help maintain proper fluid balance.

19. **Mangoes** – Rich in vitamins A and C, antioxidants, and fiber, which support kidney health and help manage oxidative stress.

20. **Watermelon** – High in water content and low in potassium, providing hydration and helping to flush out toxins from the kidneys.

These plant-based foods support kidney health by offering nutrients that help manage fluid balance, reduce inflammation, and protect against oxidative damage, which is essential for those managing kidney disease. Always consult with a healthcare provider or dietitian for personalized dietary recommendations, particularly if you have advanced kidney disease.

Plant-Based Foods Beneficial for Mental Health

Some plant-based foods that can support mental health, especially for managing depression and anxiety. These foods contain nutrients like antioxidants, B vitamins, magnesium, and omega-3s that play a role in brain function, mood regulation, and reducing inflammation:

1. **Leafy Greens (Spinach, Kale, Swiss Chard)** – Rich in folate and magnesium, which help produce mood-regulating neurotransmitters.
2. **Berries (Blueberries, Strawberries, Blackberries)** – High in antioxidants, which reduce oxidative stress linked to depression.
3. **Avocados** – Provide healthy fats, B vitamins, and potassium, supporting brain function and mood stability.
4. **Chia Seeds** – Contain omega-3 fatty acids, which reduce inflammation and promote brain health.
5. **Walnuts** – High in omega-3s and antioxidants, which can help improve mood and cognitive function.
6. **Bananas** – Rich in vitamin B6, which helps produce serotonin, the "feel-good" neurotransmitter.
7. **Oats** – Complex carbs that provide steady energy and help keep blood sugar levels stable, reducing mood swings.
8. **Oranges** – High in vitamin C, which reduces cortisol (a stress hormone) and helps boost the immune system.
9. **Turmeric** – Contains curcumin, an anti-inflammatory compound that may improve mood and reduce symptoms of depression.
10. **Dark Chocolate (70% cacao or higher)** – Contains polyphenols and flavonoids that improve mood and cognitive function.
11. **Quinoa** – A complex carb high in protein and fiber, which supports stable blood sugar and energy levels, promoting better mood.
12. **Pumpkin Seeds** – High in magnesium and zinc, which help regulate the nervous system and reduce stress.
13. **Sweet Potatoes** – Contain fiber and complex carbs for steady energy, plus vitamin B6 for serotonin production.
14. **Green Tea** – Contains L-theanine, an amino acid that promotes relaxation and reduces anxiety.
15. **Broccoli** – High in folate and vitamin C, supporting brain function and reducing oxidative stress.

16. **Beans (Black, Kidney, Lentils)** – Provide folate, magnesium, and fiber, supporting brain health and mood regulation.
17. **Citrus Fruits (Grapefruit, Lemons, Limes)** – High in vitamin C and antioxidants, which help reduce stress.
18. **Tomatoes** – Contain lycopene and folate, which support brain health and may help reduce depressive symptoms.
19. **Asparagus** – High in folate and tryptophan, which are important for serotonin production and mood stability.
20. **Beets** – Contain betaine and folate, which support serotonin production and reduce inflammation.

These plant-based foods support mental health by offering essential nutrients that help regulate mood, reduce inflammation, and maintain steady energy levels.

Plant-Based Foods Beneficial for Osteoarthritis

Here are some plant-based foods that are beneficial for managing osteoarthritis, primarily due to their anti-inflammatory properties, high antioxidant content, and joint-supporting nutrients:

1. **Turmeric** – Contains curcumin, a powerful anti-inflammatory compound that may help reduce joint pain and stiffness.
2. **Ginger** – Known for its anti-inflammatory properties, which can relieve osteoarthritis symptoms when used regularly.
3. **Berries (Blueberries, Strawberries, Raspberries)** – High in antioxidants and anthocyanins, which help reduce inflammation.
4. **Broccoli** – Contains sulforaphane, an antioxidant that may slow cartilage damage in osteoarthritis.
5. **Spinach** – Rich in vitamins K and C, as well as antioxidants that protect joint tissues from damage.
6. **Cherries** – Especially tart cherries, which contain anthocyanins that have anti-inflammatory effects.
7. **Walnuts** – High in omega-3 fatty acids and antioxidants, both of which help reduce inflammation in joints.
8. **Flaxseeds** – A plant-based source of omega-3 fatty acids that helps reduce inflammation and joint pain.
9. **Olive Oil** – Contains oleocanthal, a compound with anti-inflammatory effects similar to ibuprofen.
10. **Garlic** – Contains diallyl disulfide, an anti-inflammatory compound that may reduce the progression of osteoarthritis.
11. **Carrots** – High in beta-carotene, an antioxidant that helps protect joint tissues from damage.
12. **Sweet Potatoes** – Rich in beta-carotene and vitamin C, which help reduce inflammation and support cartilage health.
13. **Pineapple** – Contains bromelain, an enzyme with anti-inflammatory properties that may relieve joint pain.
14. **Oranges** – High in vitamin C, which helps support collagen production for healthy cartilage.
15. **Green Tea** – Contains polyphenols and antioxidants that reduce inflammation and protect joint cells.

16. **Brussels Sprouts** – Rich in vitamin K, which supports bone health and may help reduce cartilage damage.
17. **Avocado** – High in healthy fats and antioxidants that help reduce inflammation around joints.
18. **Citrus Fruits (Lemons, Limes)** – High in vitamin C, essential for joint health and reducing inflammation.
19. **Beets** – Contains betalains, which have antioxidant and anti-inflammatory effects that may help protect joints.
20. **Tomatoes** – Rich in lycopene and other antioxidants that help reduce inflammation in the body.

Including these foods in a balanced diet can help manage inflammation and support joint health, potentially alleviating some osteoarthritis symptoms.

Plant-Based Foods Beneficial for Osteoporosis

Some plant-based foods that are beneficial for managing osteoporosis. These foods are rich in calcium, magnesium, vitamin K, vitamin D, and other nutrients essential for maintaining strong bones:

1. **Kale** – High in calcium, magnesium, and vitamin K, which are essential for bone strength.
2. **Collard Greens** – Packed with calcium and vitamin K, helping to support bone density.
3. **Broccoli** – Contains calcium, magnesium, and vitamin C, which help with collagen formation for bone health.
4. **Spinach** – A good source of calcium, magnesium, and vitamin K, all essential for bone health.
5. **Bok Choy** – High in calcium, magnesium, and vitamin K, helping to strengthen bones.
6. **Almonds** – Contain calcium, magnesium, and healthy fats that support bone health.
7. **Tahini (Sesame Seed Paste)** – High in calcium, magnesium, and phosphorus, which support bone density.
8. **Chia Seeds** – Provide calcium, phosphorus, and omega-3 fatty acids, all beneficial for bone strength.
9. **Flaxseeds** – Rich in omega-3 fatty acids and magnesium, which help reduce bone breakdown and support bone structure.
10. **Tofu** – A great source of plant-based calcium, often fortified, and contains magnesium and protein, which support bone health.
11. **Fortified Plant Milks (Almond, Soy, Oat)** – Often fortified with calcium and vitamin D, essential for bone density.
12. **Sweet Potatoes** – Contain magnesium and potassium, which are essential for bone health and strength.
13. **Prunes** – Studies suggest prunes may help prevent bone loss and improve bone density.
14. **Oranges** – Provide vitamin C, which helps with collagen production, an important component of bone structure.
15. **Figs** – Rich in calcium, potassium, and magnesium, which support bone density.
16. **Pumpkin Seeds** – Contain magnesium, which is essential for calcium metabolism and bone health.
17. **Quinoa** – Provides magnesium and phosphorus, both essential for bone strength and density.

18. **Lentils** – High in protein, magnesium, and phosphorus, which are beneficial for bone health.

19. **Avocado** – Contains vitamin K, magnesium, and healthy fats that aid in calcium absorption.

20. **Bananas** – High in potassium and magnesium, which help prevent calcium loss and maintain bone health.

Incorporating these plant-based foods can help support bone density and strength, offering essential nutrients to help manage osteoporosis.

Plant-Based Foods Beneficial for Respiratory Infectious Disease

Some plant-based foods that can help support the respiratory system and overall immune health, making them beneficial for managing and potentially alleviating symptoms of respiratory infections like COVID-19, the common cold, flu, and other respiratory illnesses:

1. **Lime** - Rich in vitamin C, antioxidants, and natural acids that boost immune function, reduce mucus buildup, and help fight off respiratory infections.
2. **Ginger** – Contains gingerol, an anti-inflammatory compound that helps reduce throat soreness, improve respiratory health, and relieve congestion.
3. **Garlic** – Rich in allicin, which has antiviral and antibacterial properties that support the immune system and help fight respiratory infections.
4. **Turmeric** – Contains curcumin, an anti-inflammatory and antioxidant that can help reduce lung inflammation and support immune function.
5. **Broccoli** – High in vitamins C and K, as well as antioxidants that support lung health and reduce oxidative stress in respiratory tissues.
6. **Spinach** – Packed with vitamins A, C, and E, and antioxidants that strengthen the immune system and help clear respiratory passages.
7. **Red Bell Peppers** – High in vitamin C, which is essential for immune function and may reduce inflammation in the respiratory system.
8. **Mushrooms (Shiitake, Maitake, Reishi)** – Contain beta-glucans and other immune-boosting compounds that may help fight respiratory infections.
9. **Oranges and Citrus Fruits** – Rich in vitamin C and antioxidants that support immune response and may alleviate cold and respiratory symptoms.
10. **Pineapple** – Contains bromelain, an enzyme with anti-inflammatory properties that may help reduce mucus and ease breathing.
11. **Berries (Blueberries, Strawberries, Raspberries)** – High in antioxidants that support immune health and help reduce inflammation in respiratory tissues.
12. **Apples** – Contain quercetin, a flavonoid with antioxidant and anti-inflammatory properties that supports lung function and immune health.
13. **Carrots** – Rich in beta-carotene, which converts to vitamin A and helps protect and maintain healthy respiratory tissues.
14. **Green Tea** – Contains catechins, which are antioxidants with anti-inflammatory and antiviral properties that may help reduce respiratory symptoms.
15. **Cabbage** – High in antioxidants and vitamin C, supporting immune function and helping to clear out mucus.

16. **Oats** – High in beta-glucans, which have immune-enhancing properties that help the body fight off infections.
17. **Peppermint** – Contains menthol, which acts as a natural decongestant and helps open up airways, making breathing easier.
18. **Beets** – Contain nitrates that support blood flow and oxygenation, helping to improve lung function and breathing.
19. **Thyme** – Contains compounds with antimicrobial properties that may help clear respiratory infections and reduce congestion.
20. **Kiwi** – Packed with vitamins C, E, and K, which support immune function and protect the respiratory system.
21. **Watercress** – A nutrient-dense leafy green that helps reduce inflammation, clears mucus, and supports respiratory health.

These plant-based foods provide nutrients that support the immune system, reduce inflammation, and aid respiratory function, making them beneficial for preventing and managing respiratory infections. Incorporating these foods into your diet can help support your body's natural defenses against respiratory illnesses.

Nutrients Daily Recommendations

Here's a comprehensive list of essential nutrients for optimal health along with their recommended daily intake:

Macronutrients:

- **Carbohydrates:** Provide energy for the body.
    - Recommended intake: **45-65% of total daily calories.**
- **Proteins:** Essential for building and repairing tissues.
    - Recommended intake: **0.8 grams per kilogram of body weight.**
- **Fats:** Important for cell structure, hormone production, and insulation.
    - Recommended intake: **20-35% of total daily calories.**

Vitamins:

- **Vitamin A:** Supports vision, immune function, and skin health.
    - Recommended intake: **700-900 micrograms for adults.**
- **Vitamin C:** Acts as an antioxidant, supports immune function, and aids in collagen synthesis.
    - Recommended intake: **75-90 milligrams for adults.**
- **Vitamin D:** Facilitates calcium absorption, important for bone health and immune function.
    - Recommended intake: **600-800 IU for adults.**
- **Vitamin E:** Acts as an antioxidant, supports immune function, and protects cell membranes.
    - Recommended intake: **15 milligrams for adults.**
- **Vitamin K:** Essential for blood clotting and bone metabolism.
    - Recommended intake: **90-120 micrograms for adults.**
- **Vitamin B-complex (B1, B2, B3, B5, B6, B7, B9, B12):** Essential for energy metabolism, nervous system function, and red blood cell production.
    - Recommended intake varies for each B-vitamin, typically ranging from a few micrograms to several milligrams.

Minerals:

- **Calcium:** Vital for bone and teeth health, muscle function, and nerve transmission.
    - Recommended intake: **1000-1200 milligrams for adults.**
- **Iron:** Essential for hemoglobin production and oxygen transport in the blood.
    - Recommended intake: **8-18 milligrams for adults.**
- **Magnesium:** Involved in over 300 biochemical reactions in the body, including energy metabolism and muscle function.
    - Recommended intake: **310-420 milligrams for adult males, 320-400 milligrams for adult females.**
- **Potassium:** Important for fluid balance, nerve transmission, and muscle contractions.
    - Recommended intake: **3400-4700 milligrams for adults.**
- **Sodium:** Essential for fluid balance, nerve function, and muscle contractions.
    - Recommended intake: **Less than 2300 milligrams per** day (lower for certain individuals such as those with hypertension).
- **Zinc:** Supports immune function, wound healing, and DNA synthesis.
    - Recommended intake: **8-11 milligrams for adult males, 8-9 milligrams for adult females.**

Other Essential Nutrients:

- **Water:** Essential for hydration, temperature regulation, and nutrient transport.
    - Recommended intake: **Approximately 3.7 liters (for adult males) to 2.7 liters (for adult females)** from all beverages and foods combined.

These recommended daily intakes are general guidelines and may vary depending on factors such as age, gender, activity level, and individual health status. It's essential to maintain a balanced diet that includes a variety of nutrient-rich foods to meet your body's needs for optimal health and well-being. If you have specific dietary concerns or health conditions, consult with a healthcare professional or registered dietitian for personalized recommendations.

Nutrient-Rich Foods that Grows in less than 100 Days

Here are some nutrient-rich foods along with a brief overview of their growth process and approximate time to maturity:

Dill

Dill (Anethum graveolens) is a relatively fast-growing herb that can be cultivated from seed to harvest in a relatively short period. Here's a detailed overview of the growth stages and timeline for dill:

Germination (7-14 days):

- Dill seeds typically germinate within 7 to 14 days when planted in moist, well-draining soil with temperatures ranging between 60°F to 70°F (15°C to 21°C). Providing consistent moisture during this stage is crucial for successful germination.

Seedling Stage (2-4 weeks):

- After germination, dill seedlings emerge from the soil. During this stage, they develop their first true leaves and establish their root system. Dill seedlings are delicate and may require protection from harsh weather conditions, pests, and diseases.

Vegetative Growth (4-6 weeks):

- As the dill seedlings mature, they enter a phase of vegetative growth, focusing on developing foliage and stems. With adequate sunlight, water, and nutrients, dill plants grow rapidly during this stage, reaching heights of 18 to 24 inches (45 to 60 centimeters).

Flowering (6-8 weeks):

- Dill plants typically begin to flower about 6 to 8 weeks after planting. The flowers are small, yellow, and arranged in umbrella-like clusters called umbels. Flowering signals that the dill plant is nearing maturity and transitioning from vegetative growth to seed production.

Seed Formation (2-3 weeks):

- After flowering, dill plants focus on producing seeds. The seeds develop within the umbels and gradually change from green to brown as they mature. It's essential to allow some of the seeds to fully mature on the plant if you want to collect them for future planting.

Harvesting (8-10 weeks):

- Dill leaves can be harvested as soon as the plants reach a suitable size, typically about 8 to 10 weeks after planting. Snip off individual leaves as needed or cut the entire plant down to about 2 inches (5 centimeters) above the soil level to encourage regrowth.
- If you're harvesting dill seeds, wait until the seeds are fully mature and turning brown on the plant. Cut the seed heads from the plant and hang them upside down in a well-ventilated area to dry. Once dry, shake the seed heads to release the seeds, and store them in an airtight container for future use.

By following this timeline and providing proper care and maintenance, you can enjoy a bountiful harvest of fresh dill leaves or seeds within a relatively short timeframe.

Edamame

Edamame, which are immature soybeans harvested at the peak of their flavor, generally take about 80 to 100 days to grow from planting to harvest. Here's a breakdown of the typical timeline for growing edamame:

1. **Preparation and Planting (Day 1-10):**
    - Prepare the soil by tilling it well and adding compost or organic matter if needed.
    - Plant the seeds directly in the soil after the danger of frost has passed and the soil temperature reaches at least 60°F (15°C). This is usually around late spring to early summer.
    - Plant the seeds about 1 to 1.5 inches deep and space them 2 to 4 inches apart in rows that are about 2 feet apart.
2. **Germination and Seedling Stage (Day 10-21):**
    - The seeds will germinate within 7 to 14 days under optimal conditions.
    - Once germinated, the seedlings will begin to emerge from the soil.
    - During this stage, it's important to keep the soil consistently moist but not waterlogged to support healthy growth.
3. **Vegetative Growth (Day 21-60):**
    - As the seedlings mature, they will develop into full-grown plants with multiple leaves.
    - Continue to water regularly, ensuring the soil remains consistently moist.

- It's also essential to provide adequate sunlight or partial shade, as soybeans require full sun for optimal growth.

4. **Flowering Stage (Day 40-60):**
    - Around 4 to 6 weeks after planting, the plants will begin to produce flowers.
    - These flowers are necessary for pollination and the subsequent development of pods.
5. **Pod Formation (Day 60-80):**
    - After successful pollination, small pods will start to develop where the flowers were located.
    - These pods will gradually enlarge and fill with developing edamame beans.
6. **Maturation and Harvest (Day 80-100):**
    - Depending on the variety and growing conditions, the pods will reach maturity in about 80 to 100 days after planting.
    - Edamame pods are ready for harvest when they are plump and firm, typically about 2 to 3 inches long.
    - Harvesting should be done carefully to avoid damaging the plants. Simply pick the pods by hand when they are ready.
7. **Post-Harvest (Day 100+):**
    - After harvesting, the plants can be composted or tilled back into the soil to enrich it for future crops.
    - If you're planning to save seeds for the next growing season, allow some pods to fully mature and dry on the plant before harvesting the seeds.

By following these steps, you can expect to harvest fresh and delicious edamame from your garden in about 80 to 100 days after planting.

Endive

The time it takes for endive to grow depends on several factors, including the variety of endive, growing conditions, and desired harvest size. Here's a detailed timeline of the typical growth stages of endive:

1. Seed Germination (7-14 days):

- Endive is typically grown from seeds, which are sown directly into the soil or started indoors and transplanted later.
- Germination usually occurs within 7 to 14 days under optimal conditions, including adequate moisture, warmth, and light.

2. Seedling Stage (2-4 weeks):

- After germination, endive seedlings emerge from the soil and begin to develop their first true leaves.
- During this stage, seedlings require consistent moisture and moderate temperatures to establish healthy root systems and foliage.

3. Vegetative Growth (4-6 weeks):

- As the seedlings mature, they enter a phase of vegetative growth, during which they develop additional leaves and establish a strong root system.
- Endive plants require regular watering and sufficient sunlight or artificial light to support healthy growth.

4. Head Formation (6-8 weeks):

- Endive leaves continue to grow and form a compact head or rosette at the center of the plant.
- The duration of this stage can vary depending on the specific variety of endive and growing conditions.

5. Harvesting (8-12 weeks):

- Endive can be harvested at various stages of maturity, depending on the desired size and flavor preferences.
- Baby endive leaves can be harvested as soon as they reach a usable size, typically within 8 to 10 weeks after planting.
- Full-sized endive heads are usually ready for harvest within 10 to 12 weeks after planting, once they have reached their mature size and developed a crisp texture.

Factors Affecting Growth Time:

- Temperature: Endive grows best in cool temperatures between 60°F and 70°F (15°C to 21°C). Warmer temperatures may accelerate growth, while extreme heat can cause bolting (premature flowering).
- Soil Conditions: Endive prefers well-draining, fertile soil with a pH between 6.0 and 7.0. Amending the soil with compost or organic matter can promote healthy growth.
- Watering: Consistent moisture is essential for endive growth, but overwatering can lead to root rot. Water the plants deeply and evenly, allowing the soil to dry slightly between waterings.
- Light: Endive requires ample sunlight or artificial light to photosynthesize and produce healthy foliage. Providing 6 to 8 hours of sunlight per day is ideal for optimal growth.

By following these guidelines and providing proper care, you can expect to harvest flavorful and nutritious endive within 8 to 12 weeks of planting, depending on the specific growing conditions and variety chosen.

Eggplant

The time it takes for eggplants to grow from planting to harvest varies depending on several factors, including the variety of eggplant, growing conditions, and climate. However, on average, it takes about 70 to 85 days for most eggplant varieties to reach maturity and become ready for harvest. Here's a detailed overview of the stages involved in the growth of eggplants:

1. **Seed Germination (7-10 days)**:
    - The first stage in the growth of eggplants is seed germination. Eggplant seeds typically germinate within 7 to 10 days when planted in warm and moist soil conditions. During this stage, the seeds absorb water and begin to sprout, sending out roots and shoots.
2. **Seedling Stage (2-4 weeks)**:
    - After germination, the eggplant seeds develop into seedlings. During this stage, the seedlings require adequate sunlight, water, and nutrients to grow strong and healthy. They develop their first true leaves and start to establish their root system.
3. **Transplanting (6-8 weeks)**:
    - Once the seedlings have grown to a suitable size and have developed a few sets of true leaves, they are ready to be transplanted into the garden or larger containers. This typically occurs 6 to 8 weeks after germination, once the danger of frost has passed and the weather has warmed up.

4. **Vegetative Growth (4-6 weeks)**:
    - After transplanting, the eggplant plants enter a period of vegetative growth, where they focus on developing foliage and establishing a strong root system. During this stage, the plants require regular watering, fertilization, and protection from pests and diseases.
5. **Flowering (6-8 weeks)**:
    - Eggplant plants typically begin to flower about 6 to 8 weeks after transplanting. The flowers are usually small and star-shaped, and they may be purple, white, or lavender in color. Each flower has the potential to develop into a fruit (eggplant) if pollinated.
6. **Fruit Development (4-6 weeks)**:
    - After pollination, the flowers develop into small, green fruits, which gradually grow larger and mature over the next 4 to 6 weeks. During this stage, it's essential to provide the plants with adequate water and nutrients to support fruit development.
7. **Harvesting (70-85 days)**:
    - Eggplants are typically ready for harvest about 70 to 85 days after transplanting, depending on the variety. The fruits should be firm, glossy, and fully colored, with a slight give when pressed gently. Use a sharp knife or pruning shears to cut the eggplants from the plant, leaving a short stem attached.

By following proper growing practices and providing optimal growing conditions, you can help ensure a successful eggplant harvest within the expected timeframe.

Fava Beans / Broad Beans

Broad beans, also known as fava beans, have a relatively longer growing season compared to some other vegetables. The time it takes for broad beans to grow from planting to harvest can vary depending on factors such as the variety of broad bean, weather conditions, and growing practices. Here's a detailed breakdown of the growth stages of broad beans:

1. **Preparation and Planting (Day 1-10):**
    - Prepare the soil by loosening it and incorporating organic matter to improve drainage and fertility.
    - Plant broad bean seeds directly in the garden soil in early spring, once the soil has warmed up and the danger of frost has passed.
    - Sow the seeds about 1 to 2 inches deep and space them 4 to 6 inches apart in rows that are 18 to 24 inches apart.

2. **Germination and Seedling Stage (Day 10-21):**
    - Broad bean seeds typically germinate within 10 to 21 days, depending on soil temperature and moisture levels.
    - Keep the soil consistently moist but not waterlogged to support seedling emergence and early growth.
3. **Vegetative Growth (Week 3-8):**
    - Once germinated, the broad bean plants enter the vegetative growth stage, during which they develop leaves, stems, and roots.
    - Provide adequate water and sunlight to promote healthy growth, and monitor for signs of pests or diseases.
4. **Flowering Stage (Week 8-12):**
    - Broad bean plants typically begin flowering about 8 to 12 weeks after planting, depending on growing conditions.
    - The flowers are usually white or pale pink and are pollinated by insects, including bees.
5. **Pod Development (Week 12-16):**
    - After successful pollination, the broad bean plants start producing pods, which contain the developing beans.
    - The pods gradually enlarge and fill out as the beans inside mature.
6. **Maturation and Harvest (Week 16-20):**
    - Broad beans are typically ready for harvest about 16 to 20 weeks after planting, depending on the variety and growing conditions.
    - Harvest the pods when they are still green and firm but have reached their full size, usually about 4 to 6 inches long.
    - To harvest, simply grasp the pod and gently pull it away from the plant.
7. **Post-Harvest Care:**
    - After harvesting, shell the beans from the pods and enjoy them fresh or store them in the refrigerator for up to a week.
    - Broad beans can also be blanched and frozen for longer-term storage.

By following these general timelines and care practices, you can successfully grow broad beans and enjoy a bountiful harvest of delicious, nutritious legumes.

Fennel

The time it takes for fennel to grow from seed to harvest can vary depending on various factors such as climate, soil conditions, and the specific variety of fennel being grown. However, on average, fennel takes approximately 80 to 100 days to reach maturity. Here's a detailed breakdown of the growth stages of fennel:

1. **Seed Germination (7-14 days):**
    - Fennel seeds typically germinate within 7 to 14 days under optimal conditions. During this stage, the seeds absorb water and sprout, forming seedlings.
2. **Seedling Stage (2-4 weeks):**
    - After germination, fennel enters the seedling stage, where the young plants develop their first true leaves and establish a root system. During this period, it's essential to ensure adequate moisture and sunlight for healthy growth.
3. **Vegetative Growth (4-6 weeks):**
    - As the seedlings mature, they continue to grow and develop more leaves, stems, and roots. Fennel plants require consistent watering and well-drained soil to thrive during this stage.
4. **Bulb Formation (6-10 weeks):**
    - Depending on the variety, some types of fennel produce a bulbous, edible base. Bulb formation typically occurs around 6 to 10 weeks after planting. During this period, the plants may require additional nutrients, such as nitrogen, to support bulb development.
5. **Maturation (10-14 weeks):**
    - Fennel reaches maturity approximately 10 to 14 weeks after planting. At this stage, the bulbs are fully developed and ready for harvest. The foliage may also become dense and lush.
6. **Harvesting:**
    - Fennel can be harvested once the bulbs have reached the desired size, typically about 3 to 4 inches in diameter for most varieties. Harvesting can be done by cutting the bulbs at ground level using a sharp knife or shears. It's essential to harvest fennel promptly to ensure optimal flavor and texture.
7. **Post-Harvest Care:**
    - After harvesting, remove any remaining foliage and roots from the plants. Fennel bulbs can be stored in the refrigerator for several weeks or used fresh in various culinary dishes. The seeds of fennel can also be harvested once the plant has matured and dried, typically around 100 to 120 days after planting.

By following these general timelines and care practices, you can successfully grow fennel and enjoy its flavorful bulbs, fronds, and seeds in your garden or culinary creations.

Flaxseed

The growth timeline of flaxseed, from planting to harvest, varies depending on several factors such as climate, soil conditions, and the specific variety of flax being cultivated. However, here's a general breakdown of the growth stages of flaxseed:

1. **Preparation and Planting (Day 1-10):**
    - Prepare the soil by tilling it well and removing any weeds or debris.
    - Flaxseed is typically sown directly into the ground in early spring, after the danger of frost has passed.
    - The seeds are planted at a depth of about 0.5 to 1 inch (1.3 to 2.5 cm) and spaced approximately 1 to 2 inches (2.5 to 5 cm) apart in rows that are 6 to 12 inches (15 to 30 cm) apart.
2. **Germination and Seedling Stage (Day 10-21):**
    - Flaxseed germinates relatively quickly, typically within 7 to 14 days under favorable conditions.
    - Once germinated, the seeds develop into seedlings with two cotyledon leaves.
3. **Vegetative Growth (Week 3-6):**
    - During the vegetative growth stage, flax plants develop additional leaves and establish a strong root system.
    - The plants require regular watering to support growth, especially during dry periods.
4. **Flowering Stage (Week 6-10):**
    - Flax plants typically begin flowering about 6 to 10 weeks after planting, depending on the variety and growing conditions.
    - The flowers are small and usually blue, although some varieties may have white or pink flowers.
5. **Seed Formation (Week 10-14):**
    - After pollination, the flowers give way to seed capsules, which contain the developing flaxseeds.
    - The seed capsules gradually mature and turn brown as the seeds inside ripen.

6. **Maturation and Harvest (Week 14-18):**
   - Flaxseed is typically ready for harvest about 14 to 18 weeks after planting, although the exact timing can vary depending on factors such as weather and growing conditions.
   - Harvesting is typically done when the majority of seed capsules have turned brown and begin to crack open, revealing the mature seeds inside.
   - Flaxseed is harvested using specialized equipment such as a combine harvester, which separates the seeds from the rest of the plant material.
7. **Post-Harvest Processing:**
   - After harvesting, flaxseed may undergo additional processing steps to remove any remaining plant material and debris.
   - The cleaned seeds are then dried to reduce moisture content and ensure long-term storage stability.

By following these general timelines and care practices, you can successfully grow flaxseed and harvest a bountiful crop of nutritious seeds for consumption or further processing.

Kale:

For those with green thumbs, cultivating Kale is a rewarding endeavor. Discover the ideal growing conditions, planting techniques, and harvesting tips to ensure a bountiful yield. Be mindful of common pests and diseases that may affect Kale plants.

Garden Cultivation:

The time it takes for kale to grow from seed to harvest varies depending on several factors, including the variety of kale, environmental conditions, and cultivation practices. However, here's a detailed breakdown of the typical growth timeline for kale:

1. **Seed Germination (5-10 days):**
   - Kale seeds are planted in well-draining soil, either directly in the garden or started indoors in seed trays. Germination typically occurs within 5 to 10 days, although it can vary depending on factors such as soil temperature and moisture levels.
2. **Seedling Stage (2-4 weeks):**
   - After germination, kale seedlings emerge from the soil. During this stage, they develop their first true leaves and establish a strong root system. Seedlings require consistent moisture, adequate sunlight, and proper spacing to support healthy growth. This stage usually lasts 2 to 4 weeks.

3. **Vegetative Growth (4-6 weeks):**
   - As kale plants mature, they enter a phase of vigorous vegetative growth. During this stage, the plants continue to develop additional leaves and increase in size. Adequate spacing between plants is essential to allow for proper air circulation and minimize competition for nutrients. Vegetative growth typically lasts 4 to 6 weeks, depending on the variety and growing conditions.
4. **Maturity and Harvest (8-12 weeks):**
   - Kale is typically ready for harvest when the leaves reach a suitable size and texture for consumption. The exact time to harvest depends on the desired maturity level and whether you prefer baby kale or mature leaves. Baby kale can be harvested as early as 4 to 6 weeks after planting, while mature kale may take 8 to 12 weeks or longer. Harvesting individual leaves from the outer portions of the plant encourages continued growth and prolongs the harvest period.
5. **Bolting and Flowering (varies):**
   - In some cases, kale plants may bolt, or send up flower stalks, especially in response to heat stress or long daylight hours. Bolting can negatively impact leaf quality and taste, so it's generally best to harvest kale before this occurs. However, some varieties are more resistant to bolting than others.

Overall, the entire growth cycle of kale, from seed to harvest, typically takes approximately 8 to 12 weeks under optimal growing conditions. Proper care and maintenance throughout each stage of growth, including adequate watering, fertilization, and pest control, are essential for successful kale cultivation. Additionally, harvesting kale regularly encourages continued production and ensures a steady supply of fresh, nutritious leaves.

Container Gardening:

Kale is well-suited for container gardening, making it accessible for individuals with limited space. Choose a large container with good drainage, fill it with nutrient-rich potting soil, and sow kale seeds or transplant seedlings. Place the container in a sunny location and water regularly to keep the soil consistently moist. Container gardening allows for flexibility in moving the kale to optimal sunlight conditions and provides easy access for harvesting. Regularly trim outer leaves to encourage continuous growth.

Mustard Greens

Mustard greens are fast-growing leafy vegetables that can be harvested relatively quickly compared to many other crops. Here's a detailed overview of the growth stages and timeline for mustard greens:

1. **Germination (5-10 days)**:
    - Mustard greens seeds typically germinate within 5 to 10 days when planted in well-draining soil with temperatures between 45°F to 85°F (7°C to 29°C). Providing consistent moisture and warmth during this stage is crucial for successful germination.
2. **Seedling Stage (1-2 weeks)**:
    - After germination, mustard green seedlings emerge from the soil. During this stage, they develop their first true leaves and establish their root system. Seedlings should be thinned to allow adequate space for growth, typically leaving about 4 to 6 inches (10 to 15 centimeters) between plants.
3. **Vegetative Growth (3-4 weeks)**:
    - As the mustard green plants mature, they enter a phase of vegetative growth, focusing on developing foliage and stems. With adequate sunlight, water, and nutrients, mustard greens grow rapidly during this stage, reaching heights of 12 to 18 inches (30 to 45 centimeters).
4. **Maturity and Harvesting (6-8 weeks)**:
    - Mustard greens are typically ready for harvest about 6 to 8 weeks after planting. However, you can begin harvesting individual leaves as soon as they reach a suitable size, typically about 4 to 6 inches (10 to 15 centimeters) in length.
    - To harvest mustard greens, use scissors or garden shears to cut the outer leaves from the plant, leaving the inner leaves to continue growing. Harvesting in this manner allows the plants to continue producing new leaves for an extended harvest period.
5. **Bolting and Flowering (8-10 weeks)**:
    - If left to grow for an extended period without harvesting, mustard greens may begin to bolt, or produce flower stalks. Bolting typically occurs 8 to 10 weeks after planting, especially in warm weather.
    - Once mustard greens bolt and flower, the leaves become bitter and less palatable. To prevent bolting and prolong the harvest period, harvest the leaves regularly and plant mustard greens in cooler weather if possible.

By following this timeline and providing proper care and maintenance, you can enjoy a bountiful harvest of fresh mustard greens within a relatively short timeframe. Additionally, succession planting can help ensure a continuous supply of greens throughout the growing season.

Lettuce:

Lettuce (*Lactuca sativa*) is a fast-growing, cool-season leafy vegetable that thrives in well-drained soil and consistent moisture. It can be grown in garden beds, containers, or raised beds.

Varieties

- **Loose-leaf** (e.g. Green Leaf, Red Leaf) – ~30–40 days
- **Romaine (Cos)** – ~60–75 days
- **Butterhead** (e.g. Bibb, Boston) – ~55–75 days
- **Crisphead (Iceberg)** – ~70–90 days (slower, needs more care)

Step-by-Step Growing Process

1. Choose Your Location

- Lettuce prefers full sun but will tolerate partial shade, especially in warmer climates.

a). Germination (Days 1–7)

- **When**: Early spring or fall (cool temps between 45–75°F / 7–24°C)
- **How**: Sow seeds 1/4 inch deep in moist, loose soil.
- **Germination Time**: 2–7 days (faster in warmer soil)

b). Prepare the Soil

- Soil should be well-drained, moist, and rich in organic matter.
- Ideal pH: 6.0 to 6.8
- Avoid direct sun if temps are hot—shade or mulch may help.
- Mix compost or aged manure into the top 6–8 inches of soil to improve fertility and drainage.

c). Sowing Seeds

- Direct sow in the ground or start indoors in seed trays.
- Plant seeds 1/8 to 1/4 inch deep.
- Space rows 12–18 inches apart. For loose-leaf varieties, thin plants to 4 inches apart; for head varieties, thin to 10–12 inches apart.

d). Watering

- Keep soil consistently moist, especially during germination.
- Water deeply but avoid waterlogging.
- Mulch around plants to retain moisture and reduce weeds.

2. Seedling Stage (Days 7–21)

- **What Happens**: Cotyledons (first leaves) appear, followed by true leaves.
- **Care**:
    - Thin seedlings to 4–6 inches apart for leaf lettuce, 10–12 inches for head varieties.
    - Keep soil evenly moist—not soggy.
    - Provide partial shade if very sunny or hot.

Thinning Seedlings

- When seedlings are 1–2 inches tall, thin them to avoid overcrowding.
- Use the thinned plants as baby greens in salads.

3. Vegetative Growth (Days 21–50)

- **What Happens**: Leaves grow rapidly, rosettes form (for leaf types), or heads begin forming (for romaine and crisphead).
- **Tips**:
    - Water regularly (about 1 inch per week).
    - Watch for pests: aphids, slugs, snails—use neem oil or natural deterrents.

3a). Fertilizing

- Lettuce is a light feeder, but a balanced liquid fertilizer (e.g., 10-10-10) every few weeks helps maintain steady growth.
- Avoid over-fertilizing; too much nitrogen can cause bitterness.

4. Head Formation (for Head Types) (Days 45–75)

- **What Happens**: Romaine, Butterhead, and Iceberg varieties begin forming compact heads.
- **Care**:
    - Maintain consistent watering.
    - Avoid disturbing roots or soil.

4a). Pest and Disease Control

- Common pests: aphids, slugs, snails, cutworms
- Natural remedies: Neem oil spray, insecticidal soap, crushed eggshells or diatomaceous earth for slugs
- Watch for mildew or rot in humid conditions. Water at the base of plants early in the day to avoid wet leaves overnight.

5. Harvest (Days 30–90 depending on variety)

- **Loose-Leaf Lettuce**: ~30–45 days – Harvest leaves individually from the outside as soon as they are large enough to eat.
- **Romaine & Butterhead**: ~60–75 days – Cut whole head at base when firm and mature.
- **Crisphead (Iceberg)**: ~70–90 days – Best to harvest in the morning when leaves are crisp and cool once head is firm.

Bolting Warning

- Avoid waiting too long —lettuce may bolt (flower and become bitter) in hot weather (above 80°F/27°C).
- To prevent:
    - Choose bolt-resistant varieties.
    - Provide afternoon shade.
    - Harvest before plants elongate.

Aftercare & Storage

- Wash thoroughly to remove soil and insects.
- Store in a plastic bag in the refrigerator; fresh lettuce lasts up to 1 week.
- For continuous harvest, sow seeds every 2–3 weeks (succession planting).

Lettuce Growth Timeline Summary

Stage	Days	What Happens
Germination	2–7 days	Seeds sprout
Seedling	7–21 days	True leaves emerge
Vegetative Growth	21–50 days	Leaves grow, heads start forming
Head Formation	45–75 days	(for romaine & iceberg)
Harvest	30–90 days	Depending on type

Conclusion

As we reach the culmination of our journey through "The Book of Life – Natural Healing," we reflect upon the profound insights and transformative wisdom that have illuminated our path towards optimal health and vitality. Through the exploration of natural ways to a healthy lifestyle, rooted in the abundance of plant-based foods, we have uncovered the keys to nourishing body, mind, and soul.

In these pages, we have delved into the myriad benefits of embracing a diet rich in fruits, vegetables, whole grains, nuts, seeds, and legumes – nature's pharmacy of essential nutrients. From the vibrant colors of antioxidant-rich berries to the nourishing power of leafy greens, each plant-derived food offers a symphony of flavors, textures, and nutrients that support our journey towards radiant health.

By incorporating essential nutrients such as vitamins, minerals, phytonutrients, and omega-3 fatty acids into our daily diet, we have embraced a holistic approach to wellness that nurtures every aspect of our being. We have learned that true health is not merely the absence of disease, but a state of vibrant vitality and well-being that emanates from within.

As we bid farewell to these pages, let us carry forth the wisdom of God gleaned from "The Book of Life – Natural healing" into our daily lives. Let us honor the earth and its bountiful offerings, savoring the flavors of wholesome, plant-based foods with gratitude and reverence. Let us cultivate mindfulness in our eating habits, sowing the seeds of health and vitality with each nourishing bite.

May "The Book of Life – Natural healing" serve as a beacon of inspiration and empowerment on your journey towards optimal health and wellness. May its empowering information guide you towards a life of balance, harmony, and abundance – a life nourished by the wisdom of nature and the transformative power of plant-based nutrition.

In closing, I extend my deepest gratitude first to God and to you, dear reader, for joining me on this journey of discovery and growth. May your path be illuminated by the radiant light of health, vitality, and joy.

With warmest wishes,

Niddia Alexander

Psalm 23

"The Lord is my shepherd; I shall not want.

He maketh me to lie down in green pastures:

He leadeth me beside the still waters. He restoreth my soul:

He leadeth me in the paths of righteousness for his name's sake.

Yea, though I walk through the valley of the shadow of death,

I will fear no evil: for thou art with me; thy rod and thy staff they comfort me.

Thou preparest a table before me in the presence of mine enemies: thou anointest my head with oil; my cup runneth over.

Surely goodness and mercy shall follow me all the days of my life: and I will dwell in the house of the Lord forever."

AMEN

End

www.ingramcontent.com/pod-product-compliance
Lightning Source LLC
LaVergne TN
LVHW070844210926
848482LV00016B/867
9798999730671